# The Nursing Process

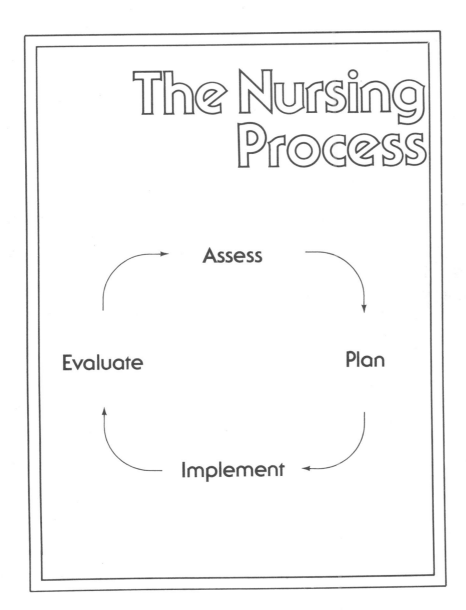

Assess

Plan

Implement

Evaluate

# Fundamentals of Nursing Care

Ellen McNulty Feeley, R.N., Ed.D.
Georgetown University

Moira Shannon Shine, R.N., Ed.D.
George Mason University

Sharon Bernier Sloboda, R.N., M.S.N.
Howard University

D. Van Nostrand Co.
New York   Cincinnati   Toronto   London   Melbourne

To our families and friends,
who supported us in writing this book.

D. Van Nostrand Company Regional Offices:
New York   Cincinnati

D. Van Nostrand Company International Offices:
London   Toronto   Melbourne

Published by D. Van Nostrand Company
135 West 50th Street, New York, N.Y. 10020

10   9   8   7   6   5   4   3   2   1

# Preface

The goal of this textbook is to introduce concepts, principles and procedures fundamental to nursing care. While team-teaching the fundamentals course in an undergraduate baccalaureate program, the authors felt a need for a comprehensive text that presented skills, issues, and concepts essential to nursing.

*Fundamentals of Nursing Care* is intended for students entering or reentering nursing education programs. Prevention is seen as a major focus. Health is seen as a dynamic, changing point on a continuum from high-level wellness to illness and death. The biophysical, psychosocial, spiritual, and cultural aspects of the individual client are considered as well as the interrelationships of the client with the family and the larger community.

The nursing process, which includes the four steps of assessing, planning, implementing, and evaluating, is described in detail. Since assessment is an integral part of the nursing process, the book deals with beginning skills in physical and psychosocial assessment. The authors recognize that many quality audiovisual materials and supplementary guides may be used to supplement this learning. Assessment has been integrated into appropriate chapters throughout this textbook.

Part 1 describes the common human experiences of growth and development, sexuality, and grief. Chapter 1 describes caring as an essential part of nursing. Chapter 2 focuses on human growth and development and their implications for nursing care through the life cycle. Chapter 3 is devoted to human sexuality, emphasizing basic biophysical and psychosocial processes. Chapter 4 deals with loss, grief and dying, underlining the importance of self-awareness for the nurse confronted with these significant universal events.

Part 2 develops the interrelationships between the individual and the family and the larger community. Cultural and environmental considerations are discussed. This part of the textbook presents a unique approach to the important role of the nurse within the larger social system.

Part 3 emphasizes the nursing process and the importance of communication in establishing and maintaining the nurse-client relationship. These chapters contain an introduction to basic physical and psychological assessment techniques that are further developed in Part 4.

Part 4 describes nursing interventions basic to the care of individuals with existing or potential health problems. Each of these chapters contains boxed inserts called "Performance Checklists" to guide students step-by-step through nursing procedures.

Part 5 includes chapters on nursing trends past and present and current health care concerns. Chapter 23 follows the historical development of nursing education, practice, and research including a discussion of professional and legal responsibilities. Chapter 24 discusses the overall health care delivery system.

The textbook includes a number of features to facilitate learning. Each chapter begins with an outline of its contents and a set of behavioral objectives and key terms for mastery. All key terms are defined in the glossary at the back of the textbook. Each chapter ends with a summary, a list of learning activities, and references and suggested readings. Numerous illustrations have been included in the book. A table of significant nursing symbols and abbreviations is printed on the back endpapers. An Instructor's Manual available separately includes the following elements: chapter objectives, outline of chapter contents, teaching/learning activities, including suggested simulation activities, evaluation methods, including sample test questions, and additional resources and references.

To facilitate the use of pronouns, the person of the nurse is referred to as "she." This represents the majority but not the exclusive composition of the profession. The pronoun "he" is used to refer to the client, solely as an arbitrary contrast to the "she" used for the nurse.

The word "client" has been chosen by the authors to denote the recipient of nursing care. This term reflects the authors' view that a person is expected to assume appropriate responsibility for his or her self-care, as contrasted with the dependent connotation of "patient."

The authors gratefully acknowledge the contributions of the following persons to this text: Gertrude M. Stanchfield; Charlet Grooms; Frank R. Engler, Jr., Acting Director, Medical and Dental Communications, Georgetown University Medical Center; and publisher Judith Joseph of D. Van Nostrand Company.

We are grateful for the comments and suggestions of the critical reviewers: Barbara A. Backer, Herbert H. Lehman College; Laurel Eisenhauer, Boston College; Anne Kibrick, Boston State College; Leda McKenry, University of Miami; Virginia Smith, University of Connecticut; Helen Vandenburg, Bergen Community College; Sandra Wardell, Rutgers University.

# Contents

## Part 4: Basic Procedures in Nursing Care

# Fundamentals of Nursing Care

# 1

# Nursing Care Throughout the Life Span

# The Concept of Caring
# Nursing and the Developmental Process
# Human Sexuality
# Loss, Grief, and Dying

Part 1 introduces the essence of nursing—the caring relationship. Nursing care is focused on the whole person and considers the stages of biophysical and psychosexual development from birth to death. To assist the nurse in preparing to offer comprehensive nursing care to clients, a conceptual introduction to foundational theory in the areas of growth and development, sexuality and reproduction, and grief and dying is presented in Part 1.

# 1

# The Concept of Caring

## Behavioral Objectives

Upon completion of this chapter, the student will be able to:

1. Define the concept of caring.
2. Describe the meaning of self-care.
3. Identify the major ingredients of caring.
4. Describe the elements of a caring relationship.

## Key Terms

| | | |
|---|---|---|
| adaptive | inquisitiveness | self-care |
| caring | maladaptive | sympathy |
| empathy | mentor | tactile |

## Introduction

Nursing is caring. Nursing literature is replete with phrases that include the word *CARE*, including nursing care, nursing care plan, caring relationship. To say that caring is nursing is not enough, however.

This chapter will look at the relationship of caring to nursing and attempt to focus on caring as one of the most important foundations of nursing. Caring involves helping others and thus will necessitate looking at self-care and the role of the caring relationship in nursing.

Historically, the concept of nursing goes beyond the time of Florence Nightingale (1820–1910). Nursing as we know it today, however, defines itself from the time of Nightingale's important work, and one of the things that Miss Nightingale continually professed was the importance of considering the wholeness of the individual.

## CARING

Considering the individual in this holistic manner may be seen as the essence of caring in nursing. Mayeroff (1971) has defined caring as the process of helping another person to grow and actualize himself. The student may recognize an important ingredient in this definition: self-help.

### Self-Care

Self-care has been defined by Orem (1971) as the practice of activities that individuals personally initiate and perform on their own behalf to maintain life, health, and well-being. This can occur at any level of wellness. For example, a person who has a colostomy and incorporates this into a normal productive life by practicing good nutrition and elimination habits is maintaining his personal optimal level of wellness by practicing self-care.

Nursing, in its caring role, strives to help the individual grow and become responsible for himself. Caring is not always a reciprocal process, but through caring for someone else, the nurse lives the meaning of her own life.

### Major Ingredients of Caring

Mayeroff (1971) has identified eight important ingredients in the caring process:

1. **Knowing.** In order to care for another person it is necessary to know his needs. The nurse, therefore, must know what the person's powers and limitations are and how to respond to them. She must also recognize her own powers and limitations in any caring situation.

2. **Alternating rhythms.** One cannot care the same way everytime. It is necessary to be flexible and able to adjust caring to the individual who is identified as needing assistance.

3. **Patience.** This may be the most important ingredient in the caring process. Patience means allowing the other person to grow in his own time and in his own way. It implies a nonjudgmental acceptance of the other person. Patience reflects respect for the other person and tolerance for mistakes in the growth process. An example of patience in caring can be seen in the parent who assists the toddler in toilet training in a positive, tolerant manner (see Chapter 2).

4. **Honesty.** This ingredient implies an ability for the caring person as well as the recipient of the care to accept criticism and to be open to change. An honest relationship implies genuineness and self-honesty.

5. **Trust.** The caring person must trust her own capacity to care. Trust encompasses elements of knowing, patience, and honesty in that there must be a belief that the other person will grow in time and that mistakes will be growth-producing. There is an element of risk in trust. The nontrusting

person will dominate or force the other person into a set of behaviors. This would not be caring.

6. Humility. The caring process means reciprocal learning. The caring person must be able to learn from the other.

7. Hope. This essential ingredient in caring expresses the fact that through caring the other person will grow. Since growth in this sense is difficult to measure, hope means sticking with or standing by the other person no matter how difficult it may seem at times.

8. Courage. This ingredient is the essence of the caring process and possibly the essence of nursing. For it is courage that allows the nurse to be able to go into the unknown of human behavior, her own and her client's.

## THE CARING RELATIONSHIP

Caring has been defined in the first section of this chapter as helping another person to grow. In any relationship there is an implicit understanding that at least two persons are interacting in some manner. This section will look at the nurse-client caring relationship.

### The Nurse

How does one recognize caring behaviors?

An essential task is to become knowledgeable about oneself in relation to others. Some guidelines for achieving this are:

1. Inquisitiveness. This is the process of seeking as much knowledge and information as possible about human behavior and human relations.

2. Observation. The student needs to always look closely and carefully at herself and at others. The use of the communication skills of listening and observing of nonverbal behavior are important here (see Chapter 4).

3. Recognition of personal feelings and beliefs. All persons have certain ideas, philosophies, and thoughts regarding the customs and rituals of others. The student needs to try consciously to be aware of her responses to various problems and situations which may arise. This is especially true in the United States where there is great cultural, religious, and economic diversity.

4. Seek a mentor. A mentor is generally defined as a wise and trusted counselor. For the student nurse a mentor may be an instructor or a more experienced nurse. It is with this person that the student will be able to exchange ideas, experiences, and observations. The relationship allows the student to experience being cared for in a growing way herself.

### The Relationship

Certain elements or tasks are important in establishing a relationship. These tasks are similar in many ways to the necessary ingredients for caring.

Tasks in the relationship:

1.  Establishing trust
2.  Supporting adaptive behaviors, assistance with maladaptive behaviors
3.  Facilitating growth
4.  Achieving optimal self-help

The student can see that from step 1 through step 4 the goal of the relationship is optimum self-care for the individual.

The care-giving aspects of nursing can be viewed as the "independent" functions that contribute to nursing's uniqueness (Moidel, Giblin, and Wagner, 1976).

Within the limits of the caring relationship, there are many nursing functions of a one-to-one nature. The nurse functions in a preventive and rehabilitative role when she is involved in providing physical care, manipulating the environment for optimal comfort, and using technical skills to insure safety and security. Therapeutically the nurse uses herself as a comforter, teacher, listener, and administrator. The therapeutic atmosphere is created through words (skilled communication), touch, and empathy. (Communication skills are discussed in greater depth in Chapter 4.)

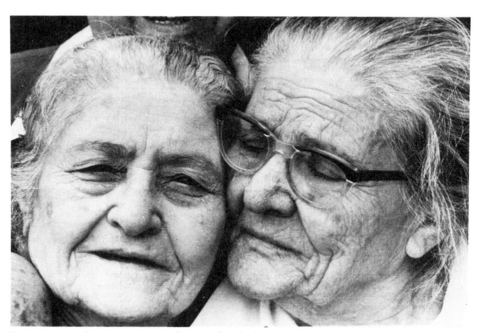

**Figure 1-1.**   *Caring encompasses all ages and can be demonstrated by touch, word, or glance.   (United Press International photo)*

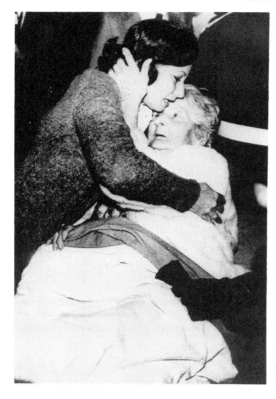

Figure 1-2.  *This mother and daughter exemplify the power of touch.  (United Press International photo)*

## Empathy

Empathy can best be defined as the ability to put oneself inside the other person and experience what he is experiencing while not losing sight of objectivity. It could be expressed as "walking in another's shoes." The nurse who is empathic is able to have a caring relationship. Sympathy is closely related to empathy in emotional content. In sympathy, however, the person loses objectivity and becomes involved in the other's problem to a point where caring is hindered, and helping another to grow does not occur.

## Touch

Touch has been described by Simon (1976) as the most basic nonverbal human communication. Touch delivers the most assuring message two persons can exchange, "I am here, you are here, and we care" (Simon, 1976).

Touch often becomes one of the most important ingredients in the caring relationship. All persons enter this world with a need to be touched and this need persists until death. Considering the developmental stages there appear to be dramatic changes in socially sanctioned touching depending on one's age, situation in life, and cultural influence. Our society wholeheartedly supports touching and cuddling of babies and small children. Grandparents can caress, hug, and pet their grandchildren openly. However, warm, caring, soothing touches between the grandparents would be less enthusiastically accepted. We have difficulty in separating a sexual touch from one of caring, especially in certain age groups. Touching in most families decreases as children grow older, until by late adolescence the only touching within the family may be in rough-housing, contact sports, or a routine good-night kiss.

In the caring relationship respectful, aware, and tender touching can be one of the most healing and therapeutic experiences a person can have. The elderly and the very sick are often touched only during physical care and nursing procedures. This kind of touching is not usually considered emotional and tactile nourishment for the client. As nurses we need to be aware of how much a warm, caring touch means to another person. Often just taking an extra moment to touch a client's hand gently while telling him what procedure is to be done will help to lessen fears and thus make care more effective.

## The Lifespan

Nursing considerations across the lifespan are discussed in detail in Chapter 2. It is appropriate here, however, to briefly look at the responses a nurse may have in a caring relationship depending on the age of the client.

In most instances nurses, like the general population, are warm and caring without effort when dealing with children. The exception to this might be seen when a child has a fatal illness and is near death or if the child is physically distorted by birth defects or a chronic disease.

It is more difficult to continue in a caring way when the client is physically unattractive (in the sense of showing us what disease can do) or if death is near. These types of conditions remind us too clearly of our own humanness. This is where the ingredients of hope and courage are so important to the caring relationship.

By the time a person reaches adolescence, the interaction of growing and seeking self-identity and the routines of hospitals or health care units often cause misunderstandings between the adolescent and the caring person. The nurse who is aware of this and who can remember her own adolescence will be able to establish trust and caring with the client.

Young adults who enter the health care system are in a stage of development where choosing a vocation and establishing a lifestyle are important tasks. Illness, accidents, and chronic disease cause serious disruptions in these tasks.

The middle-aged adult entering the health care system is generally concerned about health, stamina, aging, and death (see Chapter 4). The implications for the need to educate both of these age groups are many. Listening and assistance with problem-solving are very important nursing measures. The nurse, for example, can be aware of the fact that women and men are seeking to redefine their lives: children have become independent, and elderly parents are becoming more dependent upon them.

The elderly person faces loss of independence, loss of friends and spouse, and loss of health. The caring relationship becomes one of the most cherished for many elderly people.

In the care of all clients, the nurse's awareness of the need to extend the caring relationship to the family or significant other persons in the client's life, will make the process of building the caring relationship more effective. This is true in any caring situation whether it be in health, illness, or death. It is through this caring that persons are able to work through their losses and subsequent grieving (see Chapter 4).

## SUMMARY

Caring is a foundational concept in nursing. Within the concept, self-care has been considered an important ingredient of caring. Eight specific ingredients have been discussed. The relationship of the caring ingredients to the caring relationship has been identified. Finally there has been a brief discussion of the relationship of caring to life cycle experiences.

This introduction hopefully prepares the student for more detailed discussions of caring as it relates to growth and development, family and culture, and nursing procedures as they affect the individual.

## LEARNING ACTIVITIES

1.  Identify at least one caring relationship you have had. Were the eight ingredients identifiable? If not, which ones were not? Why?

2.  Seek out an adult friend or parent and talk with him or her about mentors. Has he or she ever had a mentor? What were the important elements in the relationship?

3.  In a clinical experience attempt to establish caring relationships with two persons of differing age, e.g., child and elderly, adult and adolescent. What differences did you notice in yourself in response to the two clients? Can you explain this in terms of age?

4.  Identify elements of self-care you might expect to encounter in client care.

## REFERENCES AND SUGGESTED READINGS

Benjamin, A., 1969.  *The helping interview.*  Boston: Houghton Mifflin.

Bower, F. L. and Bevis, E. D., 1979.  *Fundamentals of nursing practice.*  St. Louis: C. V. Mosby.

Hall, J. E. and Weaver, B. R., 1977.  *Distributive nursing practice: a systems approach to community health.*  Philadelphia: J. B. Lippincott.

Mayeroff, N., 1971.   *On caring.*   New York: Harper and Row.

Mitchell, P. H., 1977.   *Concepts basic to nursing.* 2nd ed.   New York: McGraw-Hill.

Moidel, H. C.; Giblin, E. C.; and Wagner, B. M., 1976.   *Nursing care of the patient with medical–surgical disorders.* 2nd ed.   New York: McGraw-Hill.

Orem, D. E., 1971.   *Nursing: concepts of practice.*   New York: McGraw-Hill.

Palmer, I. S., 1976.   Florence Nightingale, founder of modern nursing. Nursing Archive, Division of Special Collections, Boston U. Libraries.

Roy, Sr. C., 1976.   *Introduction to nursing: an adaptation model.*   Englewood Cliffs, N. J.: Prentice-Hall.

Schorr, T. M.   Editorial: The lost art of mentorship. *American Journal of Nursing,* November, 1978, p. 1873.

————.   Editorial: Mentor remembered. *American Journal of Nursing*, January, 1979, p. 65.

Simon, S. B., 1976.   *Caring, feeling, touching.*   Niles, Illinois: Argus Communications.

# 2

# Nursing and the Developmental Process

### Behavioral Objectives

Upon completion of this chapter, the student will be able to:

1. Describe the factors affecting growth and development.
2. Describe the basic concepts of the theories of psychosexual, psychosocial, cognitive, and moral development.
3. Compare the four major stage theories of growth and development.
4. Describe the expected developmental behaviors of a client based on age.
5. Plan nursing care based on a client's developmental needs at any age.

### Key Terms

| | | |
|---|---|---|
| accommodation | development | maturation |
| assimilation | egocentrism | moral development |
| autonomy | epigenetic principle | psychosexual development |
| biological imperative | equilibration | psychosocial development |
| cognitive development | growth | puberty |
| critical periods | maternal deprivation | separation anxiety |

## Introduction

There is a certain orderly scheme to all human growth and development. Exceptions and deviations occur along the normal continuum, but there has been a predictable pattern of growth and development over time. Theories have been developed based on this predictability. Most theories have dealt with some pattern of development based on social, psychological, environmental, cognitive, or moral premises.

This chapter focuses on tasks for stages of development based on the theories of Freud (psychosexual), Erikson (psychosocial), Piaget (cognitive), and Kohlberg (moral reasoning). From these it will be possible for the student to form a picture of how the whole person develops. The chapter should also serve as a building block, based on previous learning, for the nursing student who has already studied general psychology and growth and development. It will also assist the student in recognizing the similarities and differences in theories. Where there are complementary ideas at play, the student will be able to understand the relationship of these to the developmental process and to the concept of major life tasks. Finally, it is hoped that the student will be able to apply this information in her plan of care for clients of any age or stage of life.

## OVERVIEW OF GROWTH AND DEVELOPMENT

Establishing a foundation of principles of growth and development is basic to understanding theoretical concepts. The terms *growth* and *development* are generally used together: growth may be defined as the increase in size, differentiation of structure, and alteration of form of the living organism beginning at the cellular level; development may be defined as the orderly and irreversible stages that every organism must go through from conception to death. The pattern of growth and development is predictable and orderly, but the pace may differ with each individual. This explains the range of differences one sees in the development of motor skills in children, such as walking, bike riding, and throwing a ball.

Several factors may affect growth and development.

### Emotional Factors

The early experiences of the infant in learning to trust and be trusted may affect his way of relating in later stages of development. For example, children who are severely intimidated by adults and not allowed to speak freely may suffer from speech retardation. Maternal deprivation as seen in the studies of children who are institutionalized for long periods of time is another well-known example of the relationship of emotional factors to development. These children exhibit lethargy, apathy, and may even die (Spitz and Wolf, 1946).

### Nutritional Factors

Nutrition is believed to be directly related to the rate and speed of growth as well as to one's final adult stature. Studies have revealed that the first year of life is the most critical in determining intelligence, and that good nutrition is basic to normal brain growth.

## Physical Health

From conception the health of the fetus may affect growth and development by restricting the "normative sequence" of growth. This sequence is the obvious orderly process of development from conception. If an infant suffers from a debilitating illness or prematurity, for example, there will be limited motor activity resulting in slower muscle development and slower gross and fine motor ability. It has been clearly shown that children with congenital anomalies grow neither as fast nor as well as "normal" children (Sutterly and Donnelly, 1973).

## Environmental Factors

Crowding, uncleanliness, lack of sanitation and other factors may affect growth and development. With crowding, a condition so often seen in inner-city ghettos and poor rural areas, whole families may live in one or two rooms and children may sleep several to a bed. Sleep deprivation and sleep disturbance are common in these situations. Problems related to cleanliness and sanitation often lead to chronic illnesses such as upper respiratory infections, streptoccal infections, and the like.

If these four major factors are considered across a lifespan, it is possible to see how they all could be crucial to persons regardless of their developmental stage. For example, the elderly are often isolated, poorly nourished, and living in an environment not conducive to good mental and physical health.

## STAGE THEORIES OF GROWTH AND DEVELOPMENT

The theories to be discussed in this chapter all have orderly stages a person must pass through in the course of "normal" development. Since there is no skipping or reordering of stages, they are referred to as invariant. With the theory of psychosocial development (Erikson), for example, the person has passed through all eight stages once he reaches old age and faces the prospect of death. The relative success of the passage through the stages is dependent on many factors. Some people will be unable to go through all prescribed stages because of an interruption by illness or death. The important points for the student to remember are:

1.  The transition from one stage to another is gradual and occurs over time, and is not spontaneous.
2.  Each individual travels at his own rate through the stages.
3.  There are expected age limits within which a person must have transcended a particular stage.
4.  The successful mastery of the stages of development is influenced by factors affecting growth and development: emotional, nutritional, physical, and environmental.

## Psychosexual Development

Sigmund Freud's theory is based on stages of maturational development. The libido is the basic element and is seen as changing its site of emphasis in the body depending upon the developmental stage. For example, during the oral stage the libido is focused around the mouth and the sensations therein. The libido, in Freud's theory, is seen as the basic motive force or drive in the individual. It is the sum total of all desires and strivings the person has, with the primary force ultimately manifested in the sexual drives or instincts. The effects of each stage on the person's psychosexual functioning are believed to be most influenced by individual life experiences (Lerner, 1976). Table 2-1 outlines the stages of psychosexual development.

### Table 2-1 Freud's Stages of Psychosexual Development

| | |
|---|---|
| **Oral (first year)** | 1. Mouth source of pleasure, libido centered here, gratification through sucking and biting. |
| | 2. Feelings of dependency develop due to close relationship with mothering person. |
| | 3. Pleasure principle—need for immediate gratification. |
| | 4. Prototypes of later character traits develop: |
| |    a. oral incorporation—smoking, guilibility, excessive eating, seeking wealth or power. |
| |    b. oral aggressive—sarcastic, argumentative. |
| **Anal (1 to 3 years)** | 1. Anal region center of gratification (libido). |
| | 2. Reality principle—begins to learn to delay gratification in form of postponing relief of anal tension, can hold on and let go at will. |
| | 3. First experience with external regulation of instinctual (id) impulses. |
| | 4. Ego begins to emerge. |
| | 5. Prototype of later character traits develop: |
| |    a. anal retentive personality—too demanding toilet training, bowels considered dirty and needing strict control. Results in obstinate and stingy personality. |
| |    b. anal expulsive personality—too severe or too punitive toilet training results in cruelty, temper tantrums, sloppiness. |
| |    c. toilet training of positive, praising nature results in a creative and productive personality. |
| **Phallic (3 to 5 years)** | 1. Major conflict is Oedipus complex. |
| |    a. boy wants to possess mother and remove father; girl wants to possess father and displace mother. |
| |    b. castration anxiety results, boy fears jealous father will castrate him so decides to identify with father. |

Table    2-1    Freud's Stages of Psychosexual Development Continued

|  | c. penis envy results when girl realizes she and mother have no penis, identifies with mother in this loss. |
|  | 2. Superego develops through identification process with same sex parent. Child begins to see parent as "ideal" and incorporates morals and values of the parent. Results in formation of conscience. |
| **Latency (6 to 12 years)** | 1. Repression of Oedipal conflict. |
|  | 2. Regression of sexual development. |
|  | 3. Meant to refer to *genital* latency only. |
|  | 4. A period generally ignored by Freudians because of lack of overt evidence of instinctual processes. |
| **Genital (13 years)** | 1. Emergence of genital sexual instincts—adolescent lust. |
|  | 2. Necessary to separate from parents and find another love object: |
|  |   a. son reconciled with father—releases sexual desires of mother. |
|  |   b. daughter releases sexual desires of father. |
|  | 3. Oral, anal, and phallic stages become fused and synthesized with genital impulses. |
|  | 4. Biological function of reproduction matures. |
|  | 5. Final organization of personality is represented by contributions of all four stages. |

## Psychosocial Development

Erik Erikson's theory of development has as its foundation ego development, function, and accommodation. He is a student of the Freudian school and sees his theory as complementary to psychosexual development.

Erikson's theory (1963) is concerned with a person's development throughout the lifespan. The major premise is based upon the interrelation of the ego and ever-present, ever-changing societal forces. The ego must continually adjust to society's demands. Thus, with each stage of development there are new demands placed on the ego and new emotional crises emerge. Erikson labeled these crises "critical periods," meaning that there is only a specified amount of time in which to master each stage-specific capability. If it is not mastered, the capability for mastery of that stage is lost forever.

In his epigenetic principle, Erikson states that the ego does not have all of the capabilities necessary for becoming fully developed at birth. Therefore, each part of the ego has a specific time for development, a time when all energy is focused on this part and the only time for developing this part. So if a basic feeling of trust is not developed in the first year of life, the individual will move on to the next stage and the capability to fully develop trust will be lost forever. Table 2-2 outlines Erikson's stages of psychosocial development.

Table   2-2      Erikson's Stages of Psychosocial Development

### Trust vs. Mistrust (First Year)

Trust—            experiences are positive, warm, pleasant, and reinforcing; world is safe and supporting.

Mistrust—         frustration of needs, hostility, hurt, and sometimes pain.

### Autonomy vs. Shame and Doubt (1-3 Years)

Autonomy—         gains control over all muscles, begins to see self as separate from mother, individuality develops, bowel and bladder control of holding on and letting go.

Shame and Doubt—  failure to develop control and independence, doubts own ability, shamed by disapproval of significant others such as parents.

### Initiative vs. Guilt (3-5 Years)

Initiative—       play age, purposeful activity, roleplaying, experimentation and reality testing; imitation important, begins to see self as a person, sex identification, self-confidence, has expectations of others; major accomplishment is language development.

Guilt—            if unsuccessful in moving out and becoming more independent feels guilt over not living up to society's expectations.

### Industry vs. Inferiority (6-11 Years)

Industry—         school age, social skills learned, academic cooperation, competence, duty, and responsibility; more freedom, success in competition may build self-esteem.

Inferiority—      failure in social and academic skills may lead to inferiority, sees self in comparison to peers as failure.

### Identity vs. Role Confusion (12-16 Years)

Identity—         independence-dependence conflict, development of intellectual reasoning i.e., problem solving; physiological and psychological crises with development of primary and secondary sex characteristics, identity crisis: "Who am I?," "What is my role?"; harsh superego, commitment, loyalty, ideals.

Role Confusion—   failure to resolve identity crisis leads to diffuse feeling of lack of direction and belonging.

### Intimacy vs. Isolation (16 Years to Adulthood)

Intimacy—         period where self-identity must be achieved, experiences of love, heterosexuality, and belonging, must be able to give and share with another.

Isolation—        inability to share and be shared totally, socially isolated.

Table   2-2      Erikson's Stages of Psychosocial Development Continued

### Generativity vs. Stagnation (Adult to Late Adulthood)

| | |
|---|---|
| Generativity— | concern with establishing and guiding the next generation, caring, other-directed, community involvement, productive and creative. |
| Stagnation— | egocentric, nonproductive, self-absorbed, narcissistic. |

### Integrity vs. Despair and Disgust (Late Adulthood)

| | |
|---|---|
| Integrity— | sense of continuity, order and meaningfulness in life, wisdom, altruistic love; an acceptance of the life cycle, and a trust in the integrity of the future generation. |
| Despair and Disgust— | unable to accept limitations, feeling of being cheated in life, angry with future prospects. |

Erikson views all of the bipolar attributes (trust vs. mistrust) as being on a continuum where neither pole is considered ideal. For example, to be totally trusting is as maladaptive as being totally mistrusting. The ideal for healthy ego development is somewhere beyond midpoint toward the positive pole (see Figure 2-1).

## Cognitive Development

Jean Piaget's theory of cognition is concerned with the study of the mental processes involved in the acquisition and utilization of knowledge. Piaget views cognition or intelligence as a biological system much like the respiratory or gastrointestinal systems. Like all biological systems, there are two basic aspects always present and functioning: organization and adaptation. This means that cognition always functions with an organization and it is always an adaptive system. The process of adaptation is then divided into two complementary components:

1. **Assimilation.**   This is the taking-in process whereby the person incorporates things, people, ideas, customs, and tastes into the self. For example, when children listen to those around them, they take in such things

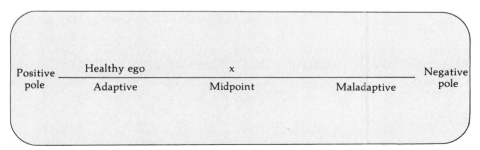

**Figure   2-1.** *Model of continuum for Erikson's bipolar attributes.*

as the language and expressions they hear and make these a part of their repertory.

2. **Accommodation.** This is the balancer of assimilation, the outgoing, adjusting process of adapting one's own internal experience to the external environmental imperatives. The child who at first speaks in unclear words or short forms of words—for example, "bankie" for blanket or "dada" for daddy—will learn from the adults in his social surroundings that these words have a proper pronunciation. The child will accommodate by learning the accepted way of speaking.

The theory of cognitive development is also dependent on stages that are time-bound to some extent, and that correspond roughly to the previous two psychological theories. Table 2-3 outlines these stages.

**Table   2-3   Piaget's Stages of Cognitive Development***

### Sensory-Motor Period (First Two Years)

| | |
|---|---|
| Stage 1 (0–1 Month). | Neonatal reflexes and gross, uncoordinated body movements. Stage of complete egocentrism with no distinction between self and outer reality; no awareness of self as such. |
| Stage 2 (1–4 Months). | New response patterns formed by chance from combinations of primitive reflexes. The baby's fist accidentally finds its way into his mouth through a coordination of arm moving and sucking. |
| Stage 3 (4–8 Months). | New response patterns are coordinated and repeated intentionally in order to maintain interesting changes in the environment. |
| Stage 4 (8–12 Months). | More complex coordinations of previous behavior patterns, both motor and perceptual. Baby pushes aside obstacles or uses parent's hand as a means to a desired end. Emergence of anticipatory and intentional behavior; beginning of search for vanished objects. |
| Stage 5 (12–18 Months). | Familiar behavior patterns. Emergence of directed groping toward a goal, and new means-end for manipulation of desired objects. |
| Stage 6 (1½–2 Years). | Internalization of sensory-motor behavior patterns and beginnings of symbolic representation. Invention of new means through internal experimentation. |

### Preoperational Period (2-7 Years)

| | |
|---|---|
| | Characterized by egocentric thinking expressed in animism, artificialism, realism, and magic omnipotence. |

Table   2-3      Piaget's Stages of Cognitive Development* Continued

| | |
|---|---|
| Preconceptual Stage (2–4 Years). | Development of perceptual constancy and of representation through drawings, language, dreams, and symbolic play. Beginnings of first overgeneralized attempts at conceptualization, in which representatives of a class are not distinguished from the class itself, e.g., all dogs are called by the name of the child's own dog. |
| Perceptual or Intuitive Stage (4–7 Years). | Prelogical reasoning appears, based on perceptual appearances untempered by reversibility, e.g., Grandma in a new hat is no longer recognized as Grandma. Trial and error may lead to an intuitive discovery of correct relationships, but the child is unable to take more than one attribute into account at one time, e.g., brown beads cannot at the same time be wooden beads. |

**Concrete Operational (7-11 Years)**

Characterized by thought that is logical and reversible. The child understands the logic of classes and relations and can coordinate series and part-whole relationships dealing with concrete things.

**Formal Operations (11 Years to Adulthood)**

Characterized by the logic of prepositions, the ability to reason from a hypothesis to all its conclusions, however theoretical. This involves second-order operations, or thinking about thoughts or theories rather than concrete realities.

*From Pulaski, M. A. *Understanding Piaget.* New York: Harper & Row 1971, pp. 207–208.

## Moral Reasoning

Lawrence Kohlberg (cited in Lerner, 1976) studied the manner in which children of different ages were able to resolve a moral dilemma by requiring them to make a choice in solving a moral problem. Children were rated not on their choice but on the reasons for their choice. From these studies of moral judgment of children, Kohlberg proposed a developmental timetable for the acquisition of moral reasoning closely related to Piaget's stages of cognitive development. It appeared that the way in which people learned to think, act, and feel morally about things was closely related to their cognitive understanding (Lerner, 1976).

Given a moral dilemma a person will decide a course of action which results in a decision. In Kohlberg's levels of moral reasoning, the stages reflect a more complex and balanced way of perceiving things as the person matures developmentally and cognitively. There is a sequential timetable, and it is not possible to skip a stage in the moral reasoning process. The six stages are

Table  2-4    Kohlberg's Levels of Moral Judgment

**Level I: Preconventional**

(4–10 Years)

Emphasis is on external control, and gratification is modified by rewards and punishments.

**Stage 1.**   Punishment and obedience orientation. The child fears punishment and so obeys the rules. There is no concept of right.

**Stage 2.**   Instrumental relativist orientation. Behavior is based on self-pleasure or reward. What will you give me (reward) if I do this (task, act) for you?

**Level II: Conventional**

(10–13 Years)

Conduct is controlled by the anticipation of social praise and blame. Decisions based on how parents or peers would behave in a similar situation. A need for acceptance, to one of the group, conformity, and stereotypical behavior.

**Stage 3.**   Good-boy, nice-girl morality. Object is to maintain good relationships and gain approval of others.

**Stage 4.**   "Law and order" orientation. Respect for authority and doing one's duty. Many persons never go beyond this stage. (I.e., "We do it because it is the law," "I was only obeying the rules," "The Bible tells us so.")

**Level III: Postconventional**

(13 Years to Adulthood)

Principled level. Often not reached by individuals. Attainment of true morality. Person regulates his behavior by an ideal which he holds, regardless of immediate social praise and blame.

**Stage 5.**   Morality of contract, of individual rights, and of democratically accepted law. Concept of human rights emerges. There is an emphasis on personal standards of social responsibility.

**Stage 6.**   Morality of individual principles of conscience. Life and personality of each individual is to be respected. Need to act in ways to satisfy one's own conscience.

divided by three levels which define a right or moral action. Table 2-4 outlines these levels.

The following are important points regarding the development of moral reasoning:

1.  Theories in moral reasoning are relatively new and therefore have not yet been studied extensively for efficacy.

2. The speed with which a person moves through the stages is closely related to cognitive development.

3. All persons do not necessarily achieve level three of moral reasoning.

4. Life experience plays an important part in the development of moral reasoning.

With this brief discussion, the student can begin to recognize the complementary qualities of the theories reviewed here. The subject of growth and development with its many interrelations is an exciting opportunity to know oneself better and to relate to others better at their level of development. From the theories flow the assigned tasks of life for the stages of development. It is important to try to keep in mind these stages as the discussion of life tasks unfolds.

## MAJOR DEVELOPMENTAL TASKS OF LIFE STAGES

The nurse is in a unique position, a position not enjoyed by most persons in the helping professions, because most nurses at one time or another come into contact with individuals in all stages of the lifespan. Nurses, therefore, can have a greater impact on the health and wellness of persons at all stages of life. Through example, educational programs, supportive modeling behaviors, and effective communication (see Chapter 10), the nurse is able to influence the health practices of the clients, friends, and communities she comes in contact with in her professional and personal life. For these reasons, it is essential that nurses have a strong foundation not only in theories of development, but also in their knowledge of expected behaviors for the various life stages.

### Infancy (Birth to 18 Months)

This is the period of life noted for the total dependence of the infant on others to care for him and to meet all of his basic needs: nutrition, shelter, love, physical and emotional stimuli. It is also, paradoxically, a period marked by major developmental strides, from a totally helpless neonate (first month of life) to an emerging personality with the ability to walk, make his needs known, and exhibit basic socializing behaviors.

One of the most important developments in the neonatal period is establishment of the maternal-infant relationship. This is accomplished through development of consistent patterns and behaviors in the care and daily routine of the infant. Feelings of safety and security are reinforced by confident loving care of the infant, and by the consistency with which his demands are met by the primary caretaker. Concurrent with this is the assimilation of the infant into the family.

The infant is taken into the family, which provides the dynamic structure and social foundation for its present and future. Parent and sibling relationships begin to be formed as they participate in the care and loving of the infant.

Identity foundations are laid by the ways in which family and friends relate to the infant. Most of these reactions are responses learned through enculturation and seem to come naturally. For example, long before the infant learns cognitively of sex-genital differences, the groundwork for masculine and feminine behaviors is laid. Studies have shown that male babies tend to be held and treated more roughly than female babies; custom still suggests blue attire for boys and pink for girls; and mothers tend to coo and cuddle female babies more than males (Stone and Church, 1973).

Table   2-5    Developmental Tasks of the Infant

**Birth**
  Sleep and wakefulness transient
  Changes position often
  Reflex behaviors
  Turns head from side to side
  Lifts head for short periods
  Head sags when not supported
**1 Month**
  Head not self-supporting
  Stares at surroundings
  Eye movements coordinated most of the time
  Listens to soft sounds
  Stops bodily activity to concentrate
**4 Months**
  Controls head
  Hands engage, unite at midline
  Contemplates objects held in hands
  Observes
  Sits with support
  Plays with hands, feet, and other objects
  Chuckles, laughs, coos
**7–8 Months**
  Sits alone for short periods
  Attempts to crawl and then does crawl—abdomen on floor, fish-like motion
  Rolls over from back to stomach
  Stands with help
  Thumb opposition
  Babbles
**10–12 Months**
  Creeps on hands and knees
  Grasps with index finger and thumb
  Stands with support
  Creeps and cruises well
  Says "mama" and "dada" with meaning

Table   2-5     Developmental Tasks of the Infant Continued

Stacks one object on top of another
Stands and walks with help
Seats self on floor
**18 Months**
Walks alone—stiff and propulsive
Seats self
Climbs stairs one at a time
Holds glass with two hands
Can throw a ball
Longer attention span
Pulls and pushes toys
Feeds self with some spilling

Nursing Implications.    The nurse has the opportunity to teach new parents from the moment of birth about the development of their baby and the impact of birth on the family. With the great emphasis placed on prenatal teaching and care, the nurse is often involved with the parents long before the baby is born. Some points to remember when working with families with infants are:

**1.**   *Sensory needs.*    The earliest learning and building of trust comes through the sense of touch. Restless babies are often soothed by mother's touch and caress. Security, contentment, and gratification are derived from touching, talking, and visual stimuli.

**2.**   *Communication.*    The baby's only means of communication for several months is crying. Since this does not always signify hunger or wetness, parents have to begin to interpret various needs of the baby. Allowing a baby to cry to exhaustion is an unnecessary agitation for parents and baby alike. Often changing the position of the baby, rocking, singing, or walking will quickly quiet crying or fussing if hunger is not the problem.

**3.**   *Assimilation.*    If there are other children at home, parents can be helped in planning ways to include them in the care of the new baby. This helps to increase family cohesiveness and to decrease sibling rivalry.

**4.**   *Safety.*    Babies as they grow are more vulnerable to accidents because they become more mobile and venture more and more into their environment. For example, as a 10-month-old learns to crawl, safety precautions in the home become a must. Often parents overlook hazards to a baby because they are not used to thinking of safety at a basic level. The nurse can talk about the possible hazards, such as house-cleaning supplies in a floor level cabinet, and help parents plan for prevention of accidents.

**5.**   *Separation.*    Beginning at about 7 months, long separations from family should be avoided. Health professionals have realized the importance of this

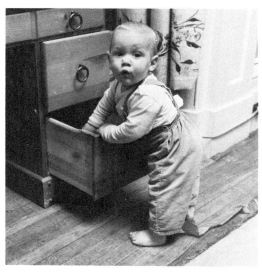

**Figure 2-2.** *The toddler exhibits independence and inquisitiveness. (Merrim/ Monkmeyer Press Photo Service)*

concept to the extent that most pediatric units have room for a parent to live in while the baby is hospitalized. "Stranger anxiety" is also evidenced by the way in which the infant clings to the parent figure. In office visits it is not uncommon for the infant to scream at the sight of the nurse or doctor at this time.

## Toddler (18 Months to 3 Years)

This age is marked by major gross musculoskeletal development, exemplified by toilet training, and also by cognitive development as seen in the acquisition of language. Although some children walk as early as 9 months, the toddler chooses the upright position and exhibits independence in his ability to move about. This self-assuredness is the mark of the toddler.

**Nursing Implications.**   Toddlers often end up in the emergency room for sutures or in the hospital due to accidental injuries. Understanding their particular emotional and physical needs is extremely important in their progression to wellness.

**1.** *Separation anxiety.*   This intense anxiety is seen when parents leave the child either to go home or even to take a short break from the child. Usually there are outbursts of screaming and a feeling of acute panic. A severely homesick child may become withdrawn and depressed. The nurse may also observe regressive behaviors, such as thumb-sucking, fetal position for sleeping, or bed-wetting. All measures possible should be employed to decrease the anxiety, most especially the continuous presence of a significant person in the child's life. There are times when the nurse must become that person and offer consistency and caring to the hospitalized child.

Table   2-6      Developmental Tasks of the Toddler

| Sensory-Motor | Personal-Social |
|---|---|
| Walks well | 3–4 word sentences |
| Kicks ball | Likes singing, rhymes |
| Runs | Solitary or parallel play |
| Jumps into air | Follows mother from room to room |
| Good hand finger coordination | Imitates and mimics |
| Builds tower of 3-5 blocks | Shows spontaneous affection |
| Feeds self with spoon | Obeys simple domestic commands |
| Undresses self, especially shoes | Shows interest in television |
| and socks | Enjoys stories and looking at pictures |
| | Makes many demands at bedtime, ritual-istic especially regarding security objects |
| | Likes rough play |
| | Temper tantrums begin |
| | Verbalizes toilet needs |

**2.** *Emotional factors.* Usually the toddler has a favorite toy or blanket which is important to his security. The nurse should be aware of this and encourage parents to have the favorite security symbol with the child during the hospital stay.

**3.** *Safety.* This is an age of great ambivalence between independence and dependence. Toddlers take risks with their safety because they lack the judgment to realize the dangers. In the hospital as well as at home discipline and supervision become important imperatives.

**4.** *Language.* Verbal skills are developing rapidly. It is through example and practice that language skills develop. Children often become quiet in the hospital because of fear, anxiety, and depression. The nurse can help to alleviate this by spending nonhurried time with the child talking, reading, or just sitting quietly with him.

**5.** *Play.* Play is an important source of intellectual and social growth for the toddler. Play, in fact, should be viewed as the work of childhood. It serves as an outlet for aggressive impulses, a way to develop creative skills, a socialization vehicle, and a time to learn to be alone with oneself (solitary play).

## Preschooler (3 Years to 5 Years)

The child in this age range is growing from the first strivings for independence to the accomplishment of leaving home for the first day of school. The major achievements of this age group are tied to this eventual leave-taking of mother and the family.

There is a move from parallel to cooperative play, and peers begin to relate to one another socially as well as verbally. This is especially evident in the nursery school experience. Children enjoy dramatic play, including imitation

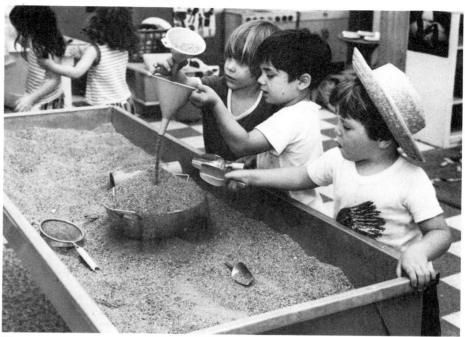

**Figure 2-3.** *These preschoolers are engaged in cooperative play.* *(Bayer/Monkmeyer Press Photo Service)*

of adult roles. Imaginary playmates are seen as fulfilling companionship needs. The 4- to 6-year-old child is easier to reason with, expresses himself more freely because of an increased vocabulary, and is able to put feelings into words.

### Table 2-7    Developmental Tasks of the Preschooler

| | Sensory-Motor | Personal-Social |
|---|---|---|
| **3 years** | Rides tricycle | Constantly asking questions |
| | Stands on one foot | Goes to bathroom independently |
| | Walks up and down stairs alternating feet | Vocabulary of about 1,000 words |
| | Buttons and unbuttons | Uses grammar correctly |
| | Tiptoes | Sex curiosity: where do babies come from? difference between sexes. |
| | Draws simple pictures | Can feel prolonged anxiety, capable of fear and jealousy. |
| | Wants to help with household chores | Interested in playing with others. |
| | Pours from a pitcher | Dreams and fantasy |
| | Feeds self well | Father becomes important |
| | Builds tower of 9 to 10 blocks | Wants to please parents |

Table  2-7    Developmental Tasks of the Preschooler Continued

| | | |
|---|---|---|
| **4 years** | Runs and jumps with ease<br>Skips and hops<br>Throws well overhand<br>Uses scissors<br>Likes to try simple motor<br>   stunts | Questioning at its peak<br>Chatters for attention<br>Can participate in long involved conversa-<br>   tions<br>Tells lengthy stories<br>Uses deception, mixes truth with fiction<br>Concept of numbers<br>Self-reliant in personal habits: dresses and<br>   undresses, knows front from back, laces<br>   shoes, brushes teeth, good at supplying<br>   alibis<br>No nap during day<br>Prone to fears: darkness, unfamiliar ani-<br>   mals or people<br>Associative play—two to three children |
| **5 years** | Balances on one foot for<br>   several minutes<br>Well-developed sense of<br>   equilibrium<br>Ready for dancing and<br>   physical exercise<br>Draws recognizable man<br>Copies square and triangle<br>Sits and stands straight<br>Solves simple geometric<br>   problems | Expresses self in clear, complete sentences<br>2,200 word vocabulary<br>Dramatic play about home and business<br>Asks the meaning of words<br>Can give name and address<br>Dependable and obedient<br>Very sociable<br>Elementary sense of shame, disgrace, and<br>   status<br>Chooses own clothing for the day<br>Likes to impress friends<br>Likes excursions, collections and<br>   masquerades |

## Nursing Implications

1. *Emotional.*    The most outstanding personality development of this stage is the resolution of the Oedipal conflict (see Table 2-1). With this resolution, there is an increased interest in the body and the way it functions. Children undergoing surgical procedures have enormous fears concerning body intactness and integrity. The nurse can offer appropriate support and understanding with this knowledge.

2. *Identity.*    There is an increased interest in the genital area and in the differences between the sexes. Children feel consoled and secure when they can fondle their genitals, especially if they are in a highly anxiety-producing situation. This often causes parents to feel distressed unless they can be given explanations for the behavior. The nurse should bring the subject up in a

casual manner in order to educate parents and to decrease the possibility of additional anxiety for parents and child.

**3.** *Play.*   Since imitative play is an important aspect of this age, it can be used to help the preschooler act out some of his fears and anxieties. Many hospitals have orientation programs for children and their parents and allow the children to play with syringes, dolls, and dressup in doctor and nurse clothes. This gives them an opportunity to verbalize and act out some of their feelings. The astute nurse will pay close attention to the verbal and nonverbal communication from the child at this time, and use it at a later time to help relieve tensions.

## Middle Childhood (6 Years to 12 Years)

Once the child enters school, his world enlarges to include peers, teachers, and other significant adults. The intensity of ties to home and family gradually begin to lessen, but the parents continue to be the major influence and of first importance in providing security, support, and guidance. Developmental tasks at this stage include:

**a.**   a beginning recognition of sexual identity.

**b.**   a mastery of social skills.

**c.**   consolidation of identification and ego functions leading to a better-defined self.

**d.**   establishment of peer relationships.

**e.**   gaining approval of important adults such as teachers, coaches, clergy, scout leaders, and older schoolmates.

**f.**   widening of one's own perception of the world.

**g.**   preparation for adult roles through, for instance, an interest in adult careers and occupations, in developing a sense of industry (Erikson, 1968), and more time spent away from home.

Nursing Implications.   Although children approaching puberty are on the brink of adulthood, they still have many emotions and feelings tied to childhood.

**1.** *Emotional.*   The middle child may act with bravado in the face of something frightening such as hospitalization, but at the same time may wish for supportive understanding from the nurse. Children at this age are quick to tears in anger, fear, or embarrassment, and they need caring and respect from the nurse. The 12-year-old who is hospitalized due to injury may "want his mommy" to stay with him, but fears the ridicule of adults if he asks for this. The nurse can anticipate this need and say, "I know this has been pretty upsetting to you, most of the kids ask their mom or dad to stay a night or two." This gives the needed sanction and is, therefore, not threatening to the newly established self-identity.

**2.** *Identity.*   Awareness of sexuality and some early embarrassing signs of maturity often cause excessive anxiety for the child. The nurse can allay some of this anxiety by respecting privacy needs and refraining from teasing the child in any way.

## Adolescence (13 Years to 20 Years)

The maturational sequence beginning with puberty (a physiological landmark) and ending with the attainment of young adulthood (an imprecise boundary) is referred to as adolescence. Because of the number of years this period spans and the great changes which occur, it is often subdivided into early adolescence, middle adolescence, and late adolescence.

Adolescent development is not a smooth, continuous process, but is fraught with fits and starts, regressions and transgressions, and many questions but few answers. One observes that the adolescent becomes more involved in peer and school activities and less involved with home and family. Emotions run high with sudden romantic attachments of short duration, on-again-off-again friendships, and angry outbursts of short duration, usually directed at family rather than friends. Developmental tasks of adolescence include:

a. establishment of a sexual identity.
b. making a commitment to work.
c. developing a personal moral and value system—the beginning of a personal philosophy of life.

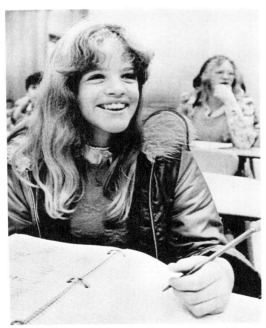

**Figure 2-4.**   *The developmental tasks of adolescence include developing a commitment to work.   (United Press International photo)*

**d.** developing the capacity for a lasting relationship.

**e.** developing the capacity for both tender and genital sexual love in heterosexual relationships.

**f.** gaining the ability to return to one's parents in a new relationship based on adult equality (Schwartz and Schwartz, 1972).

Nursing Implications

**1.** *Identity.* In the range of adolescence there is marked change in physical development and appearance. This is especially true in early adolescence with the appearance of secondary sexual characteristics, facial, body, and pubic hair; changes in body contour; voice levels; and breast appearance in girls and increased size of the male genitalia. When caring for the adolescent, therefore, the strictest attention must be paid to respect for privacy and personal integrity.

**2.** *Sexuality.* The middle years of adolescence are characterized by rebellion against parental authority, involvement and conformity with peer groups, and increased interest in sexual exploration. This often includes exploration of one's own body. During this age masturbation, the deliberate manipulation of one's sexual organs for pleasure and tension release, becomes an important part of normal sexual exploration. It is considered to be a universal practice with boys (mainly because of the obvious prominence of the genitals), and it is also a common practice with many girls. Since the subject of masturbation is fraught with anxiety, fear, embarrassment, and guilt, the nurse can help to educate both parents and adolescents regarding its practice and the role it may play in normal heterosexual development. (See Chapter 3.)

**3.** *Health.* Adolescence is usually viewed as a period of relatively good health. The most outstanding problems stem from auto and sports accidents, pregnancy, venereal disease, and drug use. The nurse becomes an important teacher regarding these possible hazards. At times the nurse takes on the role of surrogate parent in helping the adolescent to sort out difficulties relating to passage through these years. Most important to remember is that any illness or injury presents an overwhelming threat to body integrity and to the sense of self. Since independence is such an important issue, the nurse can see that the dependency nature of illness and hospitalization increases the level of anxiety to overwhelming proportions. This knowledge will help the nurse to understand behaviors such as anger, hostility, regression, and withdrawal. It will be possible to assist the adolescent in dealing with these if they are properly recognized.

## Young Adulthood (21 Years to 35 Years)

The young adult is usually healthy. Unless there is a chronic disease present such as multiple sclerosis or diabetes, or injuries occur due to accidents, the nurse will not see the young adult for illness-related problems. This age group is often health conscious, however, dieting, exercising, and seeking social activities for mental health. Prevention and health teaching are important areas for the nurse to emphasize with the young adult. Developmental tasks at this stage include:

a. establishing a career or vocation.

b. beginning to achieve a sense of intimacy with another person, usually in a heterosexual relationship.

c. solidifying a sense of self-identity.

### Nursing Implications

1. *Health.*   The nurse may find that her contacts with young adults are in relation to employment-related examinations, well-child care, pre- and postnatal care, and accident-induced injuries. The greatest need for this age group is health teaching: breast and genital self examination, pulse and blood pressure monitoring, and adequate nutrition and exercise.

2. *Sexuality.*   Young adults have premarital examinations and often seek information regarding their sexual behaviors and practices. The nurse has the opportunity to bring up subjects that otherwise might not be discussed such as planned parenthood, partner expectations, various books available on human sexuality, and can generally allow the person or couple to feel free to discuss sexual matters with her.

## Middle Adulthood (36 Years to 64 Years)

The middle adult is in a period of life where establishment of a meaningful relationship has probably occurred, there is a sense of productivity, and a sense of participating in role modeling behaviors for the future generation. Middle adults are active in community and civic organizations, socialize with established groups of friends, and seek to enhance their already established personal lifestyle through career, family life, sports activities, and social belonging. Developmental tasks of middle adulthood include:

a. establishing one's role as a member of the community.

b. beginning to accept the inevitable changes in the physiological make-up of the body: loss of muscle strength, hair loss or greying, signs of aging such as wrinkles and weight changes, and a general decline in stamina and stature.

c. beginning to recognize health needs which may not have been present in the past: heart and blood pressure concerns, ulcers, and menstrual changes in women.

d. establishing relationships with the next generation as a model, mentor, and friend.

e. reassessing the relationship with the intimate person in one's life.

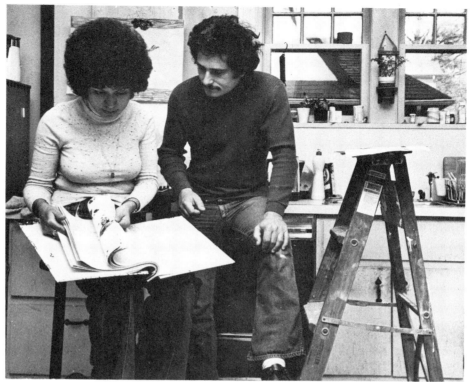

**Figure 2-5.** *Middle adulthood is a time for appreciating roles, relationships, and productivity. (Sybil Shelton/Monkmeyer Press Photo Service)*

### Nursing Implications

**1.** *Health.* The person in this age group begins to feel the physical manifestations of aging. There is an undeniable change in physical stamina, skin turgor (elasticity), and resistance to illness and infections. The nurse will see the middle adult in the hospital for surgical procedures such as hysterectomies, cholecystectomies, prostatectomies, and mastectomies, and for medical management of such conditions as ulcers, heart problems, and back ailments. Often the nurse can use the time she has with these clients to educate them regarding health practices such as regular check-ups with the doctor, and to encourage them to discuss any concerns they may have regarding their present and future life.

**2.** *Psychosocial.* It is during this stage of life that the person must begin to let go of children who have grown to young adulthood and are ready to try independence. There begins a reestablishment of relationships with children on a new adult level.

The middle adult is also often the caretaker of an elderly parent. In this sense there is an ambivalence of role, being a parent to one's own young adult children and a pseudo-parent to aging parents.

In the fast-paced society we live in there may be a phenomenon of "identity crisis" in the middle adult. Persons find themselves questioning their roles, their careers, and their feelings of self-fulfillment. It is thought that increased life expectancy has some effect on this phenomenon. When a young adult chooses a career or vocation at the age of 18 or 20 and launches into the work world, the projected time spent in this chosen career or vocation may be 40 years or more. At the same time a person marries and can anticipate living with the same person at least 40 years. The uncertainty of world affairs, the economy, and the threat to the earth's resources causes people to question their commitment to established moral and social values. Therefore, mental health becomes an issue for the middle adult as evidenced by the increased divorce rate, the epidemic proportions of depression, and the numbers of persons in their 40s seeking new careers and lifestyles.

## Late Adulthood (65 Years to Death)

The major tasks of old age are directly related to Erikson's (1963) last stage of the life cycle, ego integrity or despair. Late adulthood is marked by the approach of retirement, a decline in physical capabilities and, depending upon

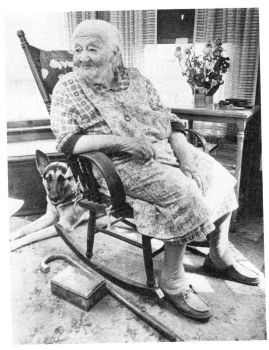

Figure 2-6. *Late adulthood may be a time of enjoyment. (United Press International photo)*

hereditary and environmental factors, possible decline in mental and cognitive capabilities.

Usually the person reaching retirement age is in relatively good health. Many persons today look forward to retirement as a time to relax and enjoy their life—families, grandchildren, and time to travel. One can plan on about 5 to 10 years of independent living barring some catastrophic event such as illness or death.

**Nursing Implications.** The person 65 to 75 years of age is seen most often in health care facilities for age-related health concerns. As the body ages normal wear and tear (stress) occurs.

**1.** *Health.* Most elderly people are in general good health. They may encounter minor problems such as limited hearing, denture discomforts, and physical difficulties: bowel and bladder dysfunctions, and respiratory and gastrointestinal upsets. Cataract surgery and injury from falls are also possible serious problems. Prevention teaching is the best treatment, especially in regard to awareness of one's own body. This includes self examinations, early detection of illness or disease by regular visits to a clinic or doctor's office, and safety measures to prevent accidents.

**2.** *Loss.* The older aged person must also be able to adjust to losses; those involving loved ones, and those involving one's physical appearance and functions. If the final stage of life is one of ego integrity, there will be the capacity for recognition of one's accomplishments and for feeling good about one's life in general. Individuals who regret some of their life stages, grieve over lost opportunities, or wish they could live their lives over tend to have feelings of depression and despair. The culmination of the developmental tasks is death. Lidz (1976) states this best:

> Death is part of the life cycle, an inevitable outcome of life that brings closure to a life story; and, because humans from early childhood are aware of their ultimate death, it influences their development and their way of life profoundly.

The person who has passed through the critical periods of life, survived stresses, and learned to adapt functionally will be prepared for this final closure to his life cycle.

## SUMMARY

The psychosexual, psychosocial, cognitive, and moral reasoning theories predict development sequentially and invariantly, one stage succeeding another with no skipping or going back. Only the psychosocial theory considers the entire lifespan of the individual, citing "critical periods" that offer a specific time in which to master the capability for that stage.

The care plan based on knowledge of growth and development introduces the dimensions of holistic nursing and caring. When utilizing the nursing process to formulate the plan of care for a client, the nurse's most valuable resource in assessment will be her knowledge of the person's developmental stage and expected behaviors for that stage. Although it is well-known and accepted that each person is unique, landmarks serve to insure the comfort of the nurse and the client.

## LEARNING ACTIVITIES

1.  Visit a school or pediatric unit and observe children of various age levels. List your observations of their behaviors and appearance for their age. Now verify with them what their age actually is and compare this with your findings.

2.  Talk with a person in the stage of late adulthood. What can you learn about this person's passage through the life stages?

3.  Look at pictures of your childhood and discuss your own development with your family. What can you learn about your own progression through the early stages?

4.  Based on developmental levels, what considerations relative to their nursing care would you expect to include for: an infant, an adolescent, a 40-year-old man with a coronary attack?

## REFERENCES AND SUGGESTED READINGS

Birthing, parenting, and nurturing. *American Journal of Nursing*, June, 1975, pp. 1679–1722.

Burnside, I., ed., 1976.   *Nursing and the aged.*   New York: McGraw-Hill.

Erikson, E. H., 1963.   *Childhood and society.*   New York: W. W. Norton.

———, 1968.   *Identity, youth and crisis.*   New York: W. W. Norton.

Kimmel, D. C., 1974.   *Adulthood and aging.*   New York: John Wiley.

Lerner, R. M., 1976.   *Concepts and theories of human development.*   Reading, Mass.: Addison-Wesley.

Lidz, T., 1976.   *The person.*   Rev. ed.; New York: Basic Books.

The middle years, a special supplement. *American Journal of Nursing*, June, 1975, pp. 993–1024.

Options for the aging. *American Journal of Nursing*, October, 1975, pp. 1799–1832.

The pangs and pains of adolescence. *American Journal of Nursing*, October, 1975, pp. 1723–1750.

Pulaski, M. A., 1971.   *Understanding Piaget: an introduction to children's cognitive development.*   New York: Harper and Row.

Schwartz, L. H. and Schwartz, J. L., 1972.    *The psychodynamics of patient care.* Englewood  Cliffs, N. J.: Prentice-Hall.

Sheehy, G., 1976.    *Passages: predictable crises of adult life.*   New York: E. P. Dutton.

Spitz, R. A. and Wolf, K.    Anaclitic depression. *Psychoanalytic Study of the Child,* 2, (1946), 313–342.

The young adult, a special feature. *American Journal of Nursing,* August, 1976, pp. 1272–1289.

# 3

# Human Sexuality

## Behavioral Objectives

Upon completion of this chapter, the student will be able to:

1. Define the concept of sexuality.
2. Describe sexual characteristics common to various stages in the life cycle.
3. Describe common male and female sexual responses.
4. Physically assess male and female sexual organs.
5. Describe the reproductive aspects of sexual functioning.
6. Describe methods of family planning.
7. Identify problems related to sexual functioning.

## Key Terms

abortion
autoeroticism
birth control pill
celibacy
climacteric
condom
contraception
diaphragm
epididymitis
family planning
fertility
heterosexual
homosexual

impotence
intrauterine device (IUD)
masturbation
menarche
menopause
menstruation
midwife
obstetrician
orgasmic dysfunction
Papanicolaou (Pap) smear
pelvic inflammatory
   disease (PID)
premature ejaculation

rape
retarded ejaculation
rhythm method of family
   planning
sexuality
sexually transmitted
   disease (STD)
speculum
sterility
tubal ligation
vaginismus
vasectomy
venereal disease (VD)

## Introduction

Sexuality has historically been recognized as one of the strongest human instincts. Its development and use is essential to the survival of the human species. Sexuality is also a treasured vehicle for sharing pleasure and a personal identification that permeates a person's lifestyle and life stages. Sexual identification begins at conception, is developed both physically and psychosocially throughout the lifespan, and ceases only with death. Sexual functioning is instinctive, but can be seriously influenced for better or for worse by sociocultural values.

Reproduction is one aspect of sexuality that affects a large percentage of the population. It is related to, and yet a separate process from sexual functioning (Figure 3-1).

The nurse needs to be familiar with basic concepts of human sexuality in relating to all clients. To assist in the self care of those persons who choose to utilize their sexual potential to create new life, the nurse needs further expertise in the areas of family nursing and obstetrics. This chapter will focus primarily on sexuality and its implications for nursing care, including a beginning understanding of health-related concerns of reproduction.

## SEXUALITY

Sexuality has been defined as a deep and pervasive aspect of the total human personality which includes feelings and behavior, not only as a sexual being,

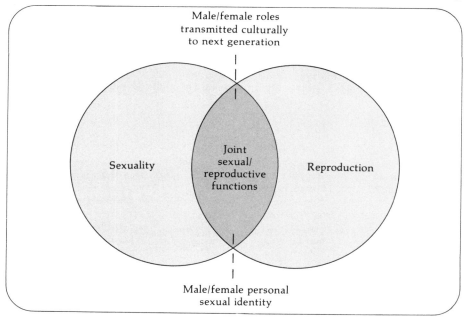

**Figure 3-1.** *Interrelationship of sexuality and reproduction.*

but also as a male or female (SEICUS, 1970). In American culture, emphasis on sexuality has shifted from evasion of the topic to considerable concentration on it in the media, entertainment, schools, and common conversations. Traditional values that placed sexuality in the context of heterosexual relationships primarily in marriage and family life, have been challenged by those who support alternative lifestyles and values. These include homosexuality, premarital and extramarital sexual activity, autoeroticism, and group sexual activities.

Some persons may take a traditional view of sexuality as a personal potential solely for the purpose of reproduction. Others may relate to sexuality purely in terms of pleasure. Between these two extreme positions is the idea that sexuality and sexual acts can be judged on an individual basis using as criteria the effect on persons involved, directly or indirectly. This so-called "new morality" prevalent in our culture today stresses individual responsibility and accountability for decision-making rather than general rules for sexual conduct. The considerations involved in a decision to choose specific sexual activity may include the responsibilities in creating and caring for new life, fidelity to a spouse if there are married persons involved, and the limiting of partners to those of the opposite sex. Traditional customs and many religious values stress that there is no compromise in such situations. Statistics on abortion, divorce, and homosexual partnerships indicate that many people make judgments that differ from traditional views and feel justified in doing so based on their individual situations.

It is the professional responsibility of the nurse to respect each client's choices in lifestyle, and no client should be burdened with the personal, possibly contrasting values of the nurse. This nonjudgmental attitude can be difficult to attain, especially if the nurse has strong sexual values that clash with those of the client. It is important that the nurse clarify and accept her own value system as distinct from that of the client. In a situation where a nurse is unable to accept a client's value system it is her professional responsibility to withdraw from the nurse-client relationship and allow another nurse to assume the responsibility for needed mutual interaction between client and nurse.

## EFFECTS OF CHANGING LIFE STAGES ON SEXUAL DEVELOPMENT

In addition to changing societal norms, the nurse must be aware of sexuality as a changing phenomenon throughout the human life cycle. Understanding of the biophysical and psychosocial characteristics of each stage assists the nurse in making a nursing assessment that is consistent with the growth and development of the client. The following sections will discuss examples of common nursing considerations at various life stages.

### Infancy

The nurse who is assisting at the birth of a child will check the external genitalia. In the male infant, it is important to note if the testicles are descended and if the foreskin is easily retractable to allow for urination and cleansing of the tip of the penis. The female infant is observed for any signs of vaginal discharge or external abnormalities in the genital area.

The biologic gender of the infant is determined prenatally by hormonal production. The psychosocial gender of the infant and the growing child is strongly influenced by the reactions of adults who are in close contact with the infant or child. From birth, parents often respond differently to girls than to boys (Woods, 1975).

The infant derives sexual and emotional pleasure primarily from the mouth. Feeding is a task crucial to psychological development as well as to nutritional status. In working with new mothers, the nurse will want to explain the importance of allowing the child to suck, and of cuddling the child often. The breast-feeding mother may need assistance and reassurance in the process of breast feeding. Interdependence between the sucking of the infant and the milk production of the mother is assumed in primitive cultures. Mothers in more "civilized" cultures, where breast feeding in public is considered socially unacceptable, may be somewhat confused by cultural norms. The La Leche Leagues are a community source of information on this topic and members are supportive to new mothers attempting to breast feed. For the mother who bottle-feeds her infant, the nurse can provide support by teaching simple techniques of bottle feeding, and stressing the importance of holding the infant close during feedings to provide the physical contact and stimulation that is essential to psychosexual nurturing.

## Childhood

The years of childhood witness many periods of physical and psychological sexual growth. The young child becomes aware of physical differences between self and members of the opposite sex. There is an awareness of pleasure in physical genital sensations. Masturbation or self-fondling occurs. In an atmosphere where self-touching may be seen as "dirty," the child is often confused between normal desires and social prohibitions. The nurse who is relating to a family with young children may be able to provide reassurance to parents and caretakers in this important area of psychosexual development. There needs to be a distinction made between socially acceptable places for behaviors and acceptance of the behavior itself. Masturbation is a normal part of sexual development and is a healthy means of self-expression that forms a foundation for subsequent sexual expression with others.

As with other healthy bodily functions, such as those of the bladder and bowel, many societies have norms which relegate these to private locations, beyond the vision of others. The nurse can support the child's normal sexual development if by her own behavior, and by parent teaching, she can affirm the healthiness of the child's awakening self-awareness of his sexuality while being realistic about prevailing social norms. The child can be taught that it is not acceptable to fondle oneself genitally in public without being taught that this is basically "bad" behavior. The nurse can suggest to parents that they allow children some privacy to explore their sexual feelings and that the expression of beginning sexual behavior in appropriate social settings, such as the privacy of the home or the bedroom, be allowed rather than punished.

In addition to becoming aware of his own sexual development, the growing child will explore the sexual characteristics of his companions. Children will often play "Doctor" or "Nurse"—games in which they undress and feel each other's private parts. It is interesting to note the childhood perception that touching and examining, particularly in the genital regions, is acceptable behavior for health professionals, but may be unacceptable for them to indulge in unless they are playing the role of doctor or nurse.

During childhood, there is an awareness of the parent of the opposite sex and an interest in this parent that differs from the feelings toward the parent of the same sex. Freud has identified this as the Oedipal complex. Further description of Freud's stages of psychosexual development through childhood are illustrated in Chapter 2, Table 2-1. Children in the pre-puberty age tend to socialize mainly with friends of the same sex.

## Adolescence

Adolescence is the growth period during which a person's sexual characteristics mature and allow for reproductive functioning. In the male, there is an increase in the size of the penis and testicles. Sperm are produced, and sometimes are discharged during nocturnal emissions or "wet dreams." Total body size increases, shoulders broaden and secondary sexual characteristics, such as deepening of the voice and growth of hair on the face, chest, axilla, and pubis develop. Boys begin to notice and be attracted to girls and may want to impress girls with their newly discovered manliness. Depending on cultural norms, various dating patterns are initiated and heterosexual experimentation may begin with affectionate cuddling and progress to various degrees of intimacy.

In the female, menarche or the beginning of menstruation occurs. Breasts enlarge and nipples protrude. Internally, the uterus is also enlarging, and the ovaries begin to produce eggs, or ova. Secondary female sexual characteristics include growth of hair in the axillary and pubic regions, and a thickening of the body through the hips and thighs. Girls are attracted to boys and within the known behaviors of any given culture, will attempt to participate in beginning heterosexual relationships. In addition to existing social and religious taboos on adolescent sexual activity, fear of pregnancy may limit female participation in heterosexual activities. The rising number of teenage pregnancies suggests that this fear is not always a deterrent. Sexually active teenage girls and boys need to be taught how to prevent an unwanted pregnancy, and how to cope with parenthood should they choose to become parents during their own adolescence.

When working with adolescents, the nurse needs to be sensitive to their embarrassment as well as their pride in their developing sexuality. The school nurse is often the person to whom the adolescent turns for guidance in

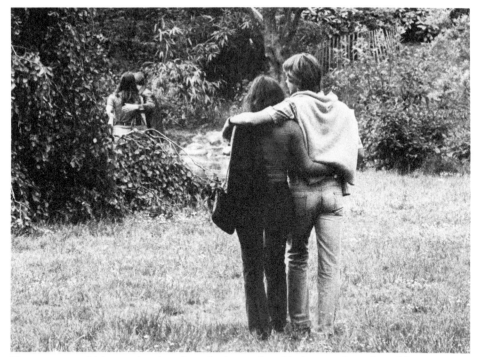

**Figure 3-2.** *Adolescence is a time of growing interest in and intimacy with members of the opposite sex. (United Press International photo)*

matters related to both the body and the emotions. Our society encourages a substantial length of time between physical readiness and social acceptability of both sexual activity and reproduction. This time lapse can be a source of great frustration to the young. The nurse can assist the adolescent in feeling good about his/her sexuality and using this as a positive life force, rather than an overwhelming desire over which the adolescent has no control.

## Adulthood

The term "adult" refers to a person who has attained full physical size and strength. Intellectual and psychological growth continue throughout the life-span but adulthood is considered here in the context of maturity of the physical aspects of the person—the so-called physical peak.

Sexual relationships are a normal and expected aspect of adulthood. Adults identify themselves as male or female, and usually engage in behaviors that are appropriate to their sex, including heterosexual interactions. Some adults choose not to express their sexuality in heterosexual behavior.

Celibacy, or abstention from sexual relations, is a sexual choice. This is a choice often made with a rationale to sublimate sexual energy into other channels perceived to be of higher value to the individual, such as a commitment to a religious vocation. A state of celibacy may also reflect an individual's choice to refrain from sexual activity in the absence of a suitable partner. This latter type of celibate choice is usually temporary and the switch to sexual activity is made when the right partner is found.

Homosexuality is another sexual choice. This choice is seen as a perversion in some societies and as an acceptable alternative to heterosexuality in others. The nurse needs to be aware of the various sexual choices that adults make, and deal with these realities in a nonjudgmental, professional manner.

Middle Age.   The midlife adult years are being increasingly examined as more people survive them and continue on in an ever-increasing life expectancy. Midlife crisis is a common word in our society today, reflecting the stresses of this period in life. As with other periods of growth and development throughout the lifespan, there are predictable and observable physical and psychosocial changes of a sexual nature.

The male climacteric or change of life may bring about a lessening in fertility, or the ability to reproduce. It does not, of itself, lessen the male's potency or sexual ability. Psychosocial considerations of this age, such as job satisfaction and security, and self esteem, may threaten a man's sense of self as a man. This insecurity is often reflected in sexual behaviors. Some men may lose interest in sex. Others may seek increased sexual activities including those with new partners. There is often a tendency to look for younger partners in an effort to regain youth which is seen as slipping away.

In the female, physical changes are more obvious. The climacteric, or menopause, is identified by cessation of menstruation. Lessening and eventual withdrawal of the estrogen hormone also causes vasomotor changes which often result in sudden, uncontrollable bouts of profuse sweating or "hot flashes." (Pedersen et al., 1978). Individual women differ in their perception of signs and symptoms of menopause (Feeley et al., 1975). Decrease in hormones can be a contributing factor to depression in midlife, although assessment of depression must include psychosocial factors of change relative to termination of parenting roles, job satisfaction, and other issues relative to self-esteem. For the woman who has remained in the home raising children for a number of years, midlife may represent the stage when her energies are no longer needed in a parent role. Increasing numbers of women in this stage are seeking a feminine identity that is separate from their families. These women may return to school, seek jobs, join feminist groups, or seek new sexual partners. Other women who have been primarily homemakers will choose to continue in that role, enjoying the lessening of family responsibilities and the increased time to pursue hobbies and leisure activities.

In working with middle-aged men and women, the nurse's awareness of possible physical, sexual, and psychosocial differences can prevent insensitive remarks. Lifestyles and values represent diverse philosophies. A further dimension that must be considered is economics. Lifestyles are usually a combination of that which is desired and that which is possible. Thus, we cannot assume that work in general or a particular job setting is chosen for its own sake by a man or woman. It may be seen by them solely as a means of support and the person may be seeking his sexual and psychosocial identity in other areas of his life.

The occupational health nurse who practices at places of employment will interact with large numbers of working adults. In addition to handling emergencies and minor complaints, the nurse in a work setting has an opportunity to plan for and implement health education programs aimed at the predominant health problems of the workers. In her counselling role, the nurse will hear of stress-producing factors that workers are experiencing, including sexual problems. Those that are beyond her level of expertise can be referred to other specially trained health professionals.

Old Age.  In many cultures, the aged are not only protected, but are revered for their assumed wisdom and life experience. Our culture has been youth-centered, and aging has been viewed as a negative process. Recent years have witnessed increased awareness of the needs of the aging in all aspects of life. Butler and Lewis (1976) have defined some of these needs in the area of sexuality. The fact that the aged population is approaching the end of the life cycle does not mean that life has ended. This occurs with death—and it is sad and usually unnecessary to witness the death of the psyche, or the social or sexual being, before the death of the body.

Sexuality is a life force—it is incompatible with death. The aged are especially in need of life forces, and yet their sexuality is often ignored or denied. Sexual functioning and response may slow down with age, but desire for sexual activity can be present and the overall need for physical contact and cuddling is as important to the very old as it is to the very young.

Physical changes in sexual characteristics occur in the elderly. Men lose their skin tone and often their hair. Enlargement of the prostate can cause urinary problems. In women, the vagina shortens and loses its elasticity. Breasts may sag, and hair often becomes coarse.

The nurse can and should assess the level of sexual functioning at any age in planning for nursing care. The elderly who are institutionalized in nursing homes are apt to be deprived of much human contact unless the members of the nursing staff realize this need and use their ability to share a sense of physical touch for the same emotional reasons they would hug and cuddle a small child. Such actions will vary with the situation and the elderly person's feelings about touch. Both the nurse and the client must be comfortable with this. But the nursing prescription for TLC (tender loving care) ought not to be limited to the child. It is a valuable and therapeutic human treatment at any age.

## SEXUAL FUNCTIONING AND RESPONSE

The Kinsey reports (1948, 1953) were the first large-scale attempt to describe sexual attitudes in American males and females. These data distin-

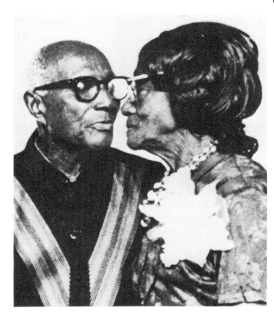

Figure 3-3. *The need for physical and emotional intimacy continues throughout the life span. (United Press International photo)*

guished patterns of human sexual response affected by social variables, such as socioeconomic class, educational level, religious involvement, and age. Physiologic aspects of human sexual response were described by Masters and Johnson (1966) following their research which monitored the sexual response cycle. This research indicated a primary physiologic response to sexual stimulation is congestion of venous blood vessels or vasocongestion. Increased muscular tension or myotonia is a secondary physiologic response to sexual stimulation. Their study described the sexual response cycle in four stages of excitement, plateau, orgasm, and resolution. Masters and Johnson dispelled the common myth that human sexual response occurred only in the genital region. They observed changes in the total body during sexual activity. Their findings also indicated that the Freudian concept of a clitoral-vaginal orgasm for women was inaccurate and that the psychosocial acceptance of sexuality is a key factor in achieving orgasm.

Bardwick (1971) defined patterns of female physiologic sexual response that differed somewhat from those of Masters and Johnson. Hite (1976) described the sexual feelings of a nationwide sample of women. Her study indicated that women's attitudes regarding sexual satisfaction differ from common sexual patterns of behavior in our culture. Cuddling and physical closeness to a partner were seen by the women interviewed as a higher value than orgasm.

The student nurse is not expected to be a sex therapist. It is important, however, that she be aware of normal sexual functioning and be comfortable in discussing it with clients should the need arise. If sexual counselling seems to be desirable, the nurse can refer the client to a reputable therapist. The American Association of Sex Educators, Counsellors and Therapists

(AASECT) is one organization that certifies health professionals who are qualified to provide these services.

## PHYSICAL EXAMINATION OF SEXUAL ORGANS

Physical assessment is an integral part of the nursing process. The examination of sexual organs should be done regularly in an effort to detect any early signs of disease. Frequently, the client can be taught to carry out his own physical examination and thus assume responsibility for preventive maintenance of his own health care.

Cancer, second only to heart disease as a cause of death in the United States, can often be detected in the reproductive organs in its early stages and be successfully treated. The importance of monthly self-examination for early detection of possible cancer is widely publicized. Nurses are often asked how this self-examination is best done.

When teaching clients how to examine their reproductive organs, the nurse needs to be aware of the fact that some persons of both sexes may have attitudes that interfere with their learning. They may never have learned to be comfortable with touching their own bodies. This reluctance must be overcome. The nurse's sensitivity in recognizing this barrier and making appropriate interventions will affect the outcome of the teaching. The nurse may want to preface her teaching with a comment such as, "Many people report they feel embarrassed when first doing a genital self-examination, but with some practice, it becomes as comfortable as bathing." By addressing the potential problems in this area, the nurse indicates to the clients that their feelings are acceptable and not unusual, and that the self-consciousness will subside. Audio-visual aids can help to clarify examining techniques.

### Testicular Self-Examination

Men can be easily taught to examine and evaluate their testicles. The testicles ordinarily lie in the scrotal sac just behind the penis. They can be palpated by using the thumb and fingers of both hands while holding the scrotum in the palms of the hands (Fig. 3-4). The testicle should feel smooth and firm and be freely movable. The presence of any lumps on the testicle should be verified by a physician. Not all lumps are malignant. They may be benign tumors or symptoms of epididymitis, an inflammation of the epididymis. This should be verified by further diagnostic tests (Murray and Wilcox, 1978). The nurse in the schools or in other clinical practice settings has an excellent opportunity to teach male clients both the value and the simplicity of regular self-examination of the testicles.

If the nurse is assisting in the assessment of a male client's genital system, some specific assessment data would be in order. Any testicular pain or swelling, discharge from the penis, or sores could be significant in assessing the possibility of illness or disease.

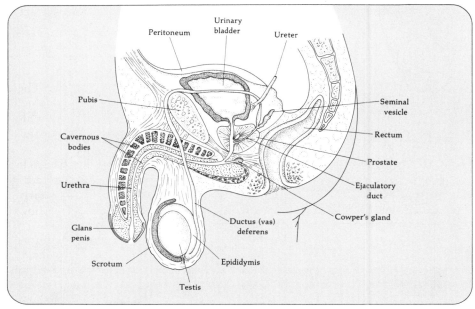

**Figure 3-4.** *Side view of the male pelvic area.* *(From* McCary's Human Sexuality, *3rd ed., by James L. McCary, D. Van Nostrand Company, 1978)*

## Breast Self-Examination

Breast self-examination is a simple yet important exercise for women in the early detection and treatment of breast cancer. It is best done about a week after the menstrual period, since the breasts may be swollen or tender premenstrually. During bath or shower is a good time for beginning self-examination, since the woman is already tending to the physical care of her body, and her fingers will move easily over wet skin. The right hand is used for the left breast, and vice versa. Fingers are moved gently over the breast to check for lumps, knots, tender areas, or any unusual change in consistency or size of the breast.

After the woman has dried herself, she should stand in front of a mirror, arms raised straight overhead, and note the symmetry of the breasts, any swelling, sunken areas, puckering of skin, pulling of the nipple, or inflammation. Next, she should observe her breasts with her hands on her hips, pressing the palms down. (Fig. 3-5).

When the breast has been thoroughly observed visually, it is time for palpation. To do this, the woman lies down on her back with a pillow under the shoulder of the side of the breast being examined, and places the hand of that side under her head. This flattens the breast and allows easier feeling of the

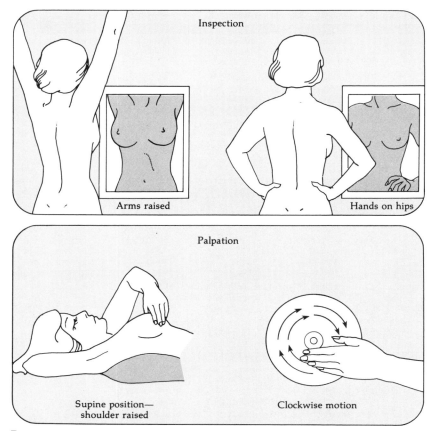

**Figure 3-5.** *Inspection and palpation of the female breasts.*

tissue. The fingers of the opposite hand are then pressed down gently, in a circular pattern, starting with the outermost circle of the breast (Fig. 3-5). After the breast itself has been examined, the nipple is gently squeezed between the thumb and index finger. The whole procedure is then repeated on the opposite side. Any lumps, discharge, or changes in the feeling of the breasts should alert the woman to consult her physician as soon as possible. Although most lumps and breast changes do not mean cancer, for the few that are early stages of cancer, it is well worth taking immediate precautions.

## Female Genital Examination

In assessing the genital system of the female, the nurse would need the individual's history including age of menarche and pattern of menstrual periods—duration, frequency, amount of flow, presence of pain, if appropriate, state of sexual activity, possible use of contraception measures if sexually active, presence of itching or vaginal discharge, bleeding unrelated to normal periods, date of last menstrual period, and frequency of Papanicolaou (Pap) smears.

Physical assessment of the female genitalia includes examination of external and internal organs that are accessible. This is done by inspection and palpation. In some clinics, women are taught to examine their own genitalia, including the vagina and cervix with a speculum. The majority of such examinations, called pelvic exams, are done by physicians or specially trained nurses and nurse midwives.

A female pelvic examination is usually done with the woman lying on her back with her knees pulled up toward her chest and her legs in stirrups attached to an examining table. This positioning allows for a clear view of the perineal region. If the woman is interested in participating in the examination, she can be assisted by propping up her shoulders and providing her with a mirror. Figure 3-6 illustrates the external female genitalia of an adult woman. Cohen, Beebe, and Duperret (1978) have described in detail the procedure for palpating both the external and internal genitalia manually.

A speculum, an instrument with two movable blades, is used to allow visual inspection of the interior vaginal walls and the cervix. Pap smears and biopsies are also obtained with the aid of a speculum. The client can be reassured that this examination is not painful and that any discomfort felt is temporary. The nurse can assist the comfort of the client by providing for maximum draping in this somewhat embarrassing position and by helping the client to relax. Running the speculum under warm water can reduce the shock of cold metal touching the sensitive vaginal area and can thereby increase client comfort.

The appearance of the perineal area will vary with a number of factors such as age, sexual activity, pregnancy, and number of deliveries, in addition to individual differences. A virgin of any age will probably have a hymen that is somewhat intact. The woman who has delivered a full-term child will usually have a larger vaginal opening then the childless woman. A pelvic examination is a sharing of an intimate part of the body which has a psychosexual as well as

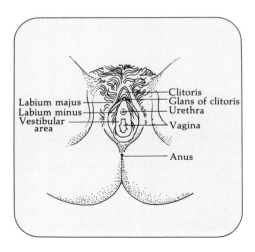

**Figure 3-6.** *Front view of the female pelvic area.*

a physical dimension. The nurse's professional yet relaxed attitude is important. As with other nursing interventions, the active participation of clients in their own care is encouraged and supported.

## REPRODUCTIVE ASPECTS OF SEXUAL FUNCTIONING

### Pregnancy

Pregnancy results when the female ova, fertilized by the male sperm, embeds itself in the lining of the woman's uterus and begins to draw its nourishment from her. Barring complications or interference, a fetus begins to develop.

The nurse will often see a pregnant woman within a few weeks after the expected date of the last menstrual period. Failure to menstruate on the usual timetable is generally considered by women to be cause to suspect pregnancy if sexual intercourse has occurred. A simple pregnancy test, which examines hormones in the urine, can be done to determine if pregnancy has occurred.

**The First Trimester.**   During the first trimester of pregnancy, the mother-to-be may experience a number of symptoms that reflect the biochemical changes that are occurring in her body. More common ones are nausea and vomiting, fatigue, and constipation. In addition to these physical changes, there are common emotional reactions to pregnancy. These include depression and feelings of vulnerability, as well as elation and a sense of creativity.

Each mother is unique in her perception of and reaction to pregnancy. The nurse must allow for this individual expression. For example, questions regarding the mother's attitude toward the pregnancy may be appropriate during a nursing assessment, but these should be open-ended such as "How do you feel about this pregnancy?" The nurse who approaches this subject with "Isn't it wonderful" or "How difficult for you" has imposed her personal value judgment on the situation and given the mother-to-be a cue regarding the expected attitude. This may form a barrier to open communication if the mother's feelings differ from those of the nurse.

Additional nutritional requirements of pregnancy should be discussed early and the mother's good diet habits encouraged. Weight control, as well as increased protein intake, is important.

**The Second Trimester.**   During the second trimester, the mother will begin to feel her child move. This is called "lightening" and is one of the absolute signs of pregnancy. Some of the earlier discomforts of the first trimester subside during the second trimester. The mother should be encouraged to keep up her general health and interests. The role of the father is also an important consideration during pregnancy. The mother is usually looking toward the father for support and encouragement in this mutual endeavor. The father is also preparing to become a parent and his attitudes will substantially affect the whole family in its adaptation to a new member. Bonding between father and child can begin prior to birth if the father is allowed and encouraged to participate in the process of pregnancy.

Classes for childbirth preparation are offered by a number of groups. Some of these classes focus on natural childbirth techniques, while others focus mainly on informing expectant parents about pregnancy, labor and delivery, and care of the newborn.

**The Last Trimester.** During the last three months of pregnancy, the impending labor and delivery become a major focus for the mother. The nurse can assist in this preparation for childbirth in a number of ways, such as informing the mother of the signs of labor, clarifying any signs and symptoms of complications which should be reported at once, encouraging the mother to be familiar with the setting in which she will deliver, and realistically describing what can be expected during labor and delivery. It is obvious that the mother who is about to deliver her first child will need much education and reassurance. It would be a mistake to assume that mothers who already have a child or children are necessarily prepared for this birth. Some questioning into previous experiences with labor and delivery will help the nurse to assess the educational needs of the mother and then to plan for any needed remedial or additional teaching.

**Birth.** The actual birth of a child is a profound human experience. It is the culmination of a sexual act between a male and female, and is the flesh and blood testimony to the human potential for generativity. Customs and rituals associated with childbirth constitute a wealth of literature and folklore (Ford, 1945).

Most births in the United States today take place in hospitals under the management of a physician. Recent years have seen many women and their partners rising in protest over the sterility in the psychological and human milieu of the hospital. In response to this, many hospitals allow helpers who have been prepared, by classes, to coach and assist the mother during labor and delivery. Rooming-in of babies with mothers is frequently an option and couples are given childbirth education courses to prepare them for active participation in the birth process.

Certified nurse midwives are allowed to manage deliveries in an increasing number of hospitals, although resistance remains on the part of some obstetricians to relinquish their supremacy in hospital delivery rooms. A practicing midwife uses the obstetrician as a back-up for complications and difficult births. Mothers who anticipate normal labor and delivery often feel they would like the option to choose between the midwife and the obstetrician for birth management. In rural areas of the country, nonnurse midwives with various levels of training and experience continue to assist in home deliveries.

Home deliveries, as an alternative to hospitalization, are sometimes chosen even in metropolitan areas. A few physicians and a larger number of midwives will assist at these, with standby arrangements at nearby hospitals in the event of unexpected complications.

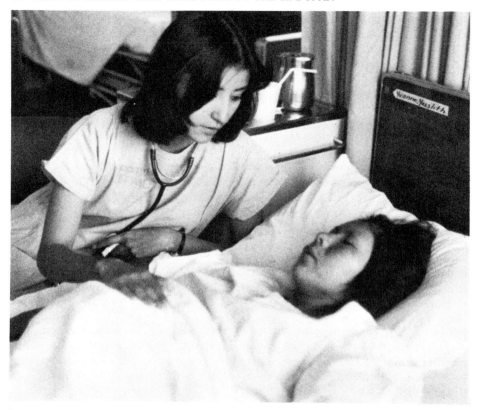

**Figure 3-7.**  *A certified nurse-midwife assists a client in labor on a Navaho reservation.  (Mimi Forsyth/Monkmeyer Press Photo Service)*

Childbearing centers are also developing popularity as a health facility offering out-of-hospital environments for labor and delivery (Lubic and Ernst, 1978; Lubic, 1979). Even the flat position necessitated by the hospital delivery table is being questioned. Studies are being done to compare the effects of upright and semiupright positions during labor (Liu, 1974). These positions are used in many "underdeveloped" countries today, and were universally accepted as "natural" before the seventeenth century and the beginnings of "modern" obstetrical medicine, including the use of instruments and anesthesia.

The development and practice of modern obstetrics is a comfort and security to women today. It is equally important that women be given a choice of the type of obstetrical management they feel is most appropriate to their individual situation. The beginning nurse can be aware of the many ways in which women choose to deliver their children, and be supportive and well-informed about these choices. Specific nursing skills for the care of the pregnant woman and her infant are developed further in more advanced nursing courses.

## FAMILY PLANNING

Before the existing knowledge of human reproduction was available, many people simply accepted the reproductive aspect of sexual behavior as a consequence beyond their control. History records many methods of attempted contraception in various cultures (Himes, 1970), some more scientific and successful than others.

Today's worldwide concerns about resources and overpopulation, combined with social and economic concerns of individuals and families, have contributed to an increasing desire for planned reproduction, or family planning. This concept remains unacceptable to some individuals for personal or religious reasons. Some religious doctrines agree with responsibility for family planning, but limit the acceptable methods of contraception to abstinence, either in total, or during anticipated times of fertility. As in other areas where values related to health are widespread and sometimes contradictory, the nurse needs a clear understanding of her personal values regarding contraception and an ability to keep these separated from those of her client.

### Contraception

There are many methods used to prevent fertilization of the ova by the sperm and the resultant beginning of the process of pregnancy. Total

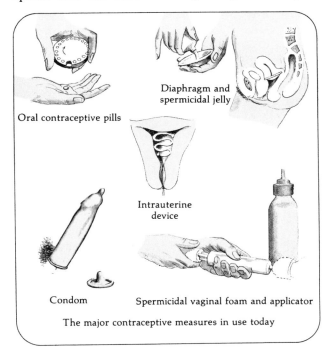

Oral contraceptive pills

Diaphragm and spermicidal jelly

Intrauterine device

Condom            Spermicidal vaginal foam and applicator

The major contraceptive measures in use today

**Figure 3-8.**   *The major contraceptive measures in use today.   (From* McCary's Human Sexuality, *3rd ed., by James L. McCary, D. Van Nostrand Company, 1978)*

abstinence from sexual intercourse with the opposite sex is the one absolutely certain way to avoid pregnancy. This method also negates the full utilization of sexual drives for purposes of human intimacy and shared pleasure. Total abstinence, or celibacy, is a chosen or at least acceptable lifestyle for some. Many others who choose to participate in sexual activity during the years when the female partner is capable of childbearing try to take responsible action to prevent the consequence of pregnancy if they are not prepared for or committed to the responsibilities of raising children.

There are a number of methods used to interfere with the potential for reproduction following sexual intercourse. These interferences may be biological, physiological, mechanical, chemical, or surgical.

The biological method of contraception utilizes the natural rhythm of the female menstrual cycle as a guide and requires abstinence during that part of the cycle when the woman is considered fertile. Methods used to determine a woman's fertility period include calendar rhythm, temperature rhythm, symptothermic rhythm, and the ovulation method. Calendar rhythm utilizes a predicted menstrual cycle with ovulation occurring midcycle. This is the most ineffective of the rhythm methods since its effectiveness requires regularity of cycles—a hard-to-predict variable.

Mechanical contraception can be achieved by inserting an intrauterine device (IUD), a diaphragm, or a condom. Correct usage of mechanical contraceptives is crucial to their success rate, so proper instruction is an important nursing responsibility. The IUD is a small device which is placed in the uterus. The presence of an IUD interferes with the implantation of a fertilized ova in the uterus and thus prevents pregnancy. An IUD is usually inserted by a physician, a nurse-midwife, or a specially trained nurse. It can be done without anesthesia and is usually done during the menstrual period.

A diaphragm is a small, rubber bowl-shaped cap that is inserted into the vaginal canal so as to cover the cervix and prevent sperm from entering the uterus. Since women vary in size and shape, a diaphragm must be individually fitted by a physician or other health professional. It is inserted prior to sexual intercourse, is usually used in combination with a spermicidal gel or foam, and is left in place for at least six hours after the last male ejaculation between the couple.

A condom is a rubber sheath which is stretched over the erect penis prior to sexual intercourse. The sperm which are ejaculated remain within the sheath which is then carefully removed. This prevents the introduction of sperm into the vagina, yet allows ejaculation to occur with the sheathed penis in the vagina. Condoms are available in a variety of textures over the counter in drug stores. They are also used to control the spread of VD by minimizing direct physical contact. Condoms may also reduce some of the sensual pleasure for the male.

Chemical interference with conception may be accomplished with spermicidal foams, jellies, and vaginal suppositories. These destroy or immobilize sperm in the vagina and cervix and thus deter their journey toward the ova. Such substances are applied just before intercourse and are often used in combination with mechanical devices.

Surgical contraception is practiced by sterilizing the male or the female. This is done in the female by severing the fallopian tubes, thus making it impossible for the ova to travel from the ovary to the uterus, or for the sperm to travel from the uterus to the ova. This procedure, called a tubal ligation, is considered a permanent method of birth control. Although there is the possibility of rejoining the sections of the fallopian tube, it is not a recommended procedure. Tubal ligation can be done by incision through the umbilicus and usually requires general anesthesia.

In the male, surgical sterility is achieved by vasectomy—severing of the vas deferens or sperm duct. This procedure is done via two small incisions on either side of the scrotum and can be done with a local anesthetic. As with the female tubal ligation, a vasectomy is considered a permanent form of contraception.

The nurse is often questioned about birth control and must be prepared to discuss available methods and the strengths and weaknesses of each. Choice of a specific method remains with the individuals involved. Acceptability of a contraceptive method is essential if the method is to be effectively used. Factors such as age, general health, religious beliefs, and personal preferences will affect the choice of a contraceptive method.

Surgical sterilization is the most effective method of contraception, except for total abstinence. Of the less permanent methods used, the pill is most successful, followed by the IUD. Clients should be informed of any risks associated with some of the most effective contraceptive methods. Effectiveness does not equate safety. There is risk involved in surgery and in use of the IUD. Undesired side effects of long-term pill use are still being studied.

The diaphragm and condom are moderately successful, especially when used in combination with foams and jellies. The rhythm method and the use of foams and jellies alone are the least successful methods of contraception (Hubbard, 1973). As with other matters of personal choice, the nurse must be careful not to impose her values. "Do you plan to practice birth control?" is a less biased question than "What kind of birth control do you plan to use?"

## Abortion

Induced abortion is interference with pregnancy after conception has occurred by removing the fetus from the uterus. A spontaneous abortion, or miscarriage, is the unaided expulsion of the fetus by the uterus. We use the term *abortion* to refer to induced abortion which, on a worldwide basis, is considered one of the chief methods of birth control (Hubbard, 1973). This procedure is prohibited by law in some countries, although the number of illegal abortions indicates that the law is unable to control abortions. Since the United States Supreme Court ruled that abortion could be legalized in most instances in this country, there have been heated, emotional debates and demonstrations among persons with opposite views on this issue. It is unlikely that a woman would become pregnant for the purpose of having an abortion. This procedure is usually seen as an alternative that is more desirable than the continuation of the pregnancy rather than as a desired end in itself.

The polarized views toward abortion seem to be those in favor of allowing the individual woman to choose this alternative, and those in favor of making abortion illegal. To those who believe that life begins at conception and that interference with that life for any reason is morally wrong, abortion can never be considered an acceptable alternative to pregnancy, regardless of the reasons. To those who believe that life does not really begin until birth, or at least until there is movement in the uterus, early abortion is seen as a back-up method of birth control when other methods of contraception have failed, or were not used. In those circumstances where the life or health of the mother is jeopardized by the pregnancy, there arises the ethical question of whether the life and health of the mother is justification for terminating the life and health of the unborn child.

Clients who are considering abortion as an alternative need counselling before deciding. Alternatives to abortion must also be explored, and the pregnant woman deserves accurate information regarding the procedure, any possible complications, and the irreversible nature of her decision as it affects the fetus. Women who are coping with the problem of an unwanted pregnancy are in a crisis. The resolution of that crisis and the coping skills developed have implications for their future mental health.

During the first trimester of pregnancy, an abortion can be performed by sucking the uterine contents out through the vagina via a vacuum-like instrument. If the pregnancy is beyond 12 weeks, surgical procedures or the introduction of saline solution to induce uterine contractions and delivery of the fetus are needed.

## Infertility

Family planning is sometimes equated with limitation of births in families. It can also be used to describe the process whereby couples who have difficulty producing children work to overcome their problems. Fertility clinics are filled with couples who are unable to conceive children due to organic difficulties (infertile) or who are unable to produce the needed sperm or ova (sterile).

A number of methods, including the "ovulation method" of natural family planning (Elder, 1978) are used to assist couples with fertility problems. Artificial insemination, inserting the spouse's or another's sperm into the uterus, is used when sperm motility or hostile vaginal environment is the diagnosed problem. The success of the "test tube baby" opens up another possible solution to infertility and sterility, as well as raising a number of ethical and human considerations.

# PROBLEMS RELATED TO SEXUAL FUNCTIONING

## Problems of Sexual Response

Problems interfering with sexual functioning may be related to basic sexual response, disease, or trauma. Problems of sexual response, or functional problems, occur when there is an attempt to engage in sexual activity with a partner. Common functional problems of the male are impotence, premature ejaculation, and retarded ejaculation. Dysfunction in the female is usually identified as sexual unresponsiveness, orgasmic dysfunction, and vaginismus (McCary, 1979). Treatment of these sexual dysfunctions is best implemented by a qualified sex therapist. The nurse may be the first health professional to whom the person turns and since discussion of sexual functioning is a very personal matter, the client may need some support and encouragement in seeking needed sex therapy.

## Sexually Transmitted Diseases

Diseases which are communicated through sexual contact have long been called venereal disease, or VD. There were negative judgmental connotations of the term "VD" and the term was historically limited to the so-called traditional diseases, such as syphilis, gonorrhea, and a few others. Epidemiologists now use the term *STD* (sexually transmitted diseases). This term categorizes diseases that are transmitted through sexual contact, including viruses and insects (Judson, 1976). It is beyond the scope of this chapter to describe specific sexually transmitted diseases. Such descriptions are readily available to the interested student (Keith and Brittain, 1978).

It is important for the beginning nursing student to be aware that any sores, discharge, itching, or other signs and symptoms specific to sexual organs in males or females should be further evaluated by a physician. Direct contact with a sexual partner is to be avoided until any suspected disease is diagnosed and treated. Signs and symptoms of disease are more readily observable in the male than in the female, since most of the male sexual organs are external.

The anatomical design of the female genital organs allows a higher incidence of undetected infection in the reproductive tract. An unfortunate and potentially dangerous result of this is acute pelvic inflammatory disease (PID). This is an inflammatory process throughout the female reproductive organs. The term PID is often used synonymously with *salpingitis*, or inflammation of the fallopian tubes leading from the ovary to the uterus (Thompson and Hager, 1977). Scarring following such infections is a common cause of female sterility, since resultant strictures in the fallopian tubes prevent the movement of ova and sperm toward each other for fertilization. Rupture of the tubes and resultant peritonitis are severe complications. If a student encounters a female client with fever, chills, malaise, nausea, and abdominal pain, it is essential to investigate the possibility of PID and suggest immediate referral to a physician. This problem is often caused by sexually transmitted diseases, but can also be the result of infection following childbirth, abortion, or other surgical procedures.

## Trauma

Trauma is a third cause for problems with sexual functioning. Perhaps the most gross, and unfortunately one of the most common sexual traumas, is rape. Forcible rape usually means sexual intercourse forced on a person without consent. It is primarily a crime of violence, but since it involves violence to anatomical parts primarily used in sexual expression, and is often perpetrated with actions that outwardly resemble those of normal sexual activity, it often has strong sexual connotations as well. The most common occurrence of rape is that of an adult male forcibly raping an adult female, although young and elderly females are also raped. Gang rape (rape by two or more people) accounts for a high percentage of reported rape cases (McCary, 1978).

Homosexual rape of a man by another man, or group of men, is a well-known occurrence, especially in prisons. All rape victims suffer an experience that is humiliating and damaging psychologically. They may need assistance in working through the grief process (see Ch. 19) as they attempt to resolve the loss of their bodily integrity and possibly their self-esteem and sense of security. Telephone "hot lines" and rape centers now exist in most communities to assist victims by offering crisis intervention.

Woods (1975) has described the biological, psychological, and sociological consequences common among female victims of sexual assault. Biological consequences include physical injury, disease, and pregnancy. Anger, fear, depression, and loss of confidence in relationships with men are the psychological aftermath often found in female rape victims. The social consequences of rape to the victim vary with the reaction of those close to the victim, and the prevailing norms of the community. Attitudes which reflect the victim as being somehow "tainted" by the experience, or that infer her willing participation in the act, are particularly devastating.

For the nurse or other health professional who may be in contact with the rape victim, it is important to remember that a thorough physical assessment is crucial to establish the actual occurrence of the rape from a legal standpoint. Since this should be done as soon as possible, it is an especially traumatic occurrence for the victim as it tends to recall the actual experience. The nurse can provide emotional support and acceptance for the victim. It is important to evaluate what the assault has meant to the victim, and plan for nursing intervention based on the client's perceptions rather than on those of the nurse.

Realistic follow-up and psychological support to the victim and her family should be offered and the adjustment progress of all concerned should be carefully monitored.

## SUMMARY

Sexuality includes feelings and behavior as a sexual being and as a male or female. Throughout the life cycle, identifiable physical and psychosocial sexual characteristics can be observed. Adult sexual functioning and response is continually being researched and therapists in this field are trained to assist in maximizing the individual's potential for sexual functioning. Self-examination of sexual organs is a known help in the early diagnosis and treatment of diseases of the reproductive system.

Reproductive aspects of sexual functioning include pregnancy, childbirth, and family planning methods. Since values in this area of human behavior are often controversial, the nurse must identify her personal values, be aware of alternative value systems, and function in a professional manner.

Problems related to sexual functioning include functional difficulties, sexually transmitted diseases, and rape. The student nurse needs to be aware of the normal in all areas related to sexuality and to be prepared to appropriately refer clients with deviations from the normal.

## LEARNING ACTIVITIES

1. How would you describe the difference between sexuality and sexual intercourse?

2. What would be your response to the statement that sexuality is of concern only to the sexually active adult?

3. What type of sexual activity is likely to occur among elderly men and women?

4. You have been asked to teach a class on breast self-examination to a group of teenage girls. What would you include in this class?

5. Describe the commonly used methods of contraception and comment on factors that will affect the client's choice of methods.

## REFERENCES AND SUGGESTED READINGS

Bardwick, J. M., 1971. *Psychology of women: a study of biocultural conflict.* New York: Harper and Row.

Barnard, M.; Clancy, B.; and Krantz, K., 1978. *Human sexuality for health professionals.* Philadelphia: W. B. Saunders.

Butler, Robert and Lewis, Myrna, 1976. *Sex after sixty.* New York: Harper and Row.

Cohen, Stephen; Beebe, Joyce; and Duperret, Martina. Patient assessment: examination of the female pelvis. *American Journal of Nursing*, October, 1978, pp. 1717–1744.

Elder, Sister Natalie. Natural family planning: the ovulation method. *Journal of Nurse-Midwifery*, Fall, 1978, pp. 25–30.

Feeley, Ellen and Pyne, Helen. The menopause: facts and misconceptions. *Nursing Forum*, 1975, pp. 74–86.

Ford, C. S. *A comparative study of human reproduction.* New Haven: Yale Publications in Anthropology, 32, 1945.

Himes, Norman E., 1970. *Medical history of contraception.* New York: Schocken Books.

Hite, Shere, 1976. *The Hite report.* New York: Dell.

Hubbard, Charles W., 1973. *Family planning education.* St. Louis: C. V. Mosby.

Judson, Franklyn. Update in sexually transmitted diseases. *Journal of the American Medical Women's Association,* January, 1976, pp. 11–19.

Keith, Louis and Brittain, Jan, 1978. *Sexually transmitted diseases.* Colorado: Creative Informatics.

Kinsey, Alfred C., et al., 1955. *Sexual behavior in the human female.* Philadelphia: W. B. Saunders.

————., 1948. *Sexual behavior in the human male.* Philadelphia: W. B. Saunders.

Liu, Yuen Chou. Effects of an upright position during labor. *American Journal of Nursing,* December, 1974, pp. 2202–2205.

Lubic, Ruth W. The impact of technology on health care—the childbearing center: a case for technology's appropriate use. *Journal of Nurse-Midwifery,* January-February 1979, pp. 6–10.

Lubic, Ruth W. and Ernst, Eunice K. The childbearing center: an alternative to conventional care. *Nursing Outlook,* December, 1978, pp. 754–760.

McCary, James L., 1978. *Human sexuality.* 3rd ed. New York: D. Van Nostrand.

Masters, William H. and Johnson, Virginia E., 1966. *Human sexual response.* Boston: Little, Brown.

Murray, Barbara and Wilcox, Linda. Testicular self-examination. *American Journal of Nursing,* December, 1978, pp. 2074–2075.

Otto, Herbert A., ed., 1978. *The new sex education.* Chicago: Follett.

*Our Bodies, Ourselves.* 2nd ed. Boston Women's Health Book Collective, New York: Simon and Schuster, 1976.

Oxorn, Harry and Foote, William, 1975. *Human labor and birth.* 3rd ed. New York: Appleton-Century-Crofts.

Pedersen, Bonnie and Pendleton, Elaine. Menopause: a welcome or dreaded stage of development. *Journal of Nurse-Midwifery,* Fall, 1978, pp. 45–51.

SEICUS. *Sexuality and man.* New York: Scribners, 1970: p. 3.

Sheehy, Gail., 1974. *Predictable crises of adult life.* New York: E. P. Dutton.

Thompson, Sumner E. and Hager, David W. Acute pelvic inflammatory disease. *Sexually Transmitted Diseases,* July–September 1977, pp. 105–113.

Woods, Nancy F., 1975. *Human sexuality in health and illness.* St. Louis: C. V. Mosby.

# 4

# Loss, Grief, and Dying

### Behavioral Objectives

Upon completion of this chapter, the student will be able to:

1. Describe four types of loss.
2. Describe the features of the management of grief.
3. Describe the three stages of a child's perception of death.
4. Describe the five stages of the dying process.
5. Explain the relationship of loss and grief to chronic illness.
6. Describe the nursing implications for any type of loss.

### Key Terms

| | | |
|---|---|---|
| anticipatory grief | denial | personification |
| bargaining | grief | preparatory depression |
| bereavement | loss | reactive depression |
| | "pangs" of grief | |

## Introduction

The concept of loss can be viewed on a continuum from simple—to lose an article of clothing or a book—to the most complex—to lose some part of oneself or one's life. This chapter will introduce the student to the implications of loss along this continuum for both the self and the client. It will be necessary to look at the complexities of loss, especially in an emotional sense. The student will be involved in the physiologic and psychologic aspects of loss, as in the care of the mastectomy client, in progressively more depth as the program of learning unfolds.

## LOSS

Loss may be defined as being deprived of or without something one has had or been used to having. Considering this broad definition, the student can see that a variety of losses occur in any individual's lifetime. Erikson (Ch. 2) talks of the losses experienced through the life cycle. For example, children lose teeth, adolescents lose dependence when they grow older, and the old person eventually loses life as death occurs. Within each of these broad life span examples, the student will find many more losses occurring that affect the lives of the persons involved.

## Types of Loss

**Normal Aging.**    Since aging begins with conception, the individual experiences losses throughout life which are often viewed in either a positive or negative manner. In this process losses are usually balanced by gains. An individual may note physiologic declines by age forty-five, for example, while intellectual and emotional development continues. The elderly person gains the ability to see life in a way not available to the younger person. Enjoyment of children and grandchildren can become a positive developmental experience. Pride in good health at any point on the age continuum is also a positive aspect of normal aging.

Most often aging is a positive concept for the individual growing into adulthood. There is then a plateau of several years (ages 30 to 45) when the person notices very little physical change. At the peak of middle adulthood losses become more noticeable: children leave home, parents die or become ill. At this time persons are more apt to perceive their losses in a negative fashion. It has been suggested in sociological theory that western cultures emphasize youth to the despair of the aging person.

*Nursing Considerations.*    The student will want to pay close attention to the client's age, stage of life, and the implications these will have for the individual. For example, the 45-year-old woman who has a hysterectomy may not grieve over the fact that she cannot have children since she is beyond the normal child-bearing age. However, she may respond to her loss as evidence of her loss of womanliness and femininity. At age 45 most women are beginning to experience the loss of their children to young adulthood, the loss of the 24 hour-a-day mothering role, the loss of some physical stamina, as well as changes in their body contour. It is a time when some women are extremely concerned about their relationships with their husbands (friends, lovers) who are themselves experiencing similar losses.

The adolescent client who is nearing adulthood may develop ulcers or asthma attacks as a response to the loss of childhood. The assurance of security and dependence and the prospect of losing these may cause ambivalent feelings for some adolescents.

The student will also encounter elderly persons who are fighting to keep their independence. They resist the security, dependence, and isolation of some types of elderly care, i.e. leisure villages, hotels for the aged, and nursing homes.

Self-Image.    When there is a threat to one's self-image, as in alterations of the size, function, structure, or shape of the body, a person copes with the changes through adaptation. Depending on the intensity of the threat, past experience, and present support systems, the individual will adapt in a positive, growth-producing manner or in a manner leading to no new growth and no reinforcement of positive coping styles.

Certain situations occur in the lifespan, other than the normal changes in body image brought about by aging, which constitute a loss for the individual. Examples of these might be:

1. changes in body contour due to pregnancy or edema
2. the loss of a limb or the loss of the use of a part of the body
3. loss of one of the senses, hearing or sight
4. loss of an internal body organ
5. changes in body appearance of a temporary nature such as loss of hair with chemotherapy
6. changes in body image as a part of a continuous debilitating condition, as in multiple sclerosis or wasting with certain malignant diseases

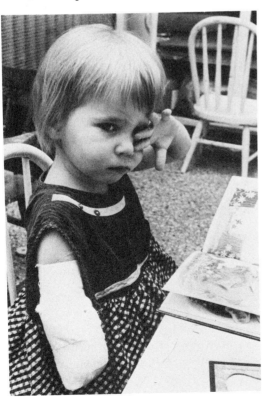

Figure 4-1.    *Body-image alteration necessitates adjustment in self-image at any age. (United Press International photo)*

The way in which an individual copes with self-image losses can be facilitated by the nursing response to the loss, i.e. facial expression and attitude.

*Nursing Considerations.*    Any time an individual enters the health-care system there is a sense of threat and possible loss of self-esteem. The nurse who is aware of this at the most basic level will be able to assist any client in coping with the threat. For example, a client who enters a clinic or private physician's office for a routine physical suffers a loss of privacy and at some level a loss of dignity just because of the necessary routine procedures requiring that all clothing be removed and some kind of gown be worn. When an individual surrenders those things that make him feel secure and comfortable, the anxiety and fear over loss of self cannot be denied.

On the other end of the continuum is the client who must give up all personal belongings and at times even the right to consent to treatment (a next of kin or guardian may give treatment consent). This kind of situation arises in intensive-care units, recovery rooms, and emergency rooms during a serious crisis. Between the two poles, there exist a number of situations which require assistance with coping with loss.

The nurse needs to be aware of the fact that most persons begin dealing with loss that can be anticipated prior to the actual occurrence and, therefore, begin the adaptation process. An example of this is the woman who has a lump in her breast and must have a biopsy. At some adaptive level she begins to consider the possible outcomes the moment the lump is detected.

In considering body image and body integrity, the nursing assessment should include the client's cultural values, spiritual orientation, and beliefs about attractiveness, wholeness, and independence. One's philosophy regarding these will influence the adaptation to the change in body image. The support system of family and friends become important resources for the nurse and the client.

The alteration of body image also may produce challenges or threats to life roles, as in the person who must have a colostomy, or feelings of depersonalization or detachment, as seen in persons who have lost a limb and view that part of their body as "not me." The nurse may note that the client is able to discuss impending surgery or the diagnosis of a debilitating disease in an informed manner. This kind of intellectualization is often necessary as a type of initial denial of the threat.

The response to threat to one's body image may be rage, denial, and grieving. These are normal reactions to a serious loss. The question of abnormal response is usually considered as a matter of degree and duration of the reaction.

The nursing care plan should include support of the family so that positive coping mechanisms will be strengthened and consequently will benefit the client. The nurse will also need to give positive feedback to the client when he is experimenting with effective ways of dealing with the alteration in body image. For example, when a client has a new colostomy and requests a visit from a representative of the Ostomy Society, the nurse might say:

**Nurse:** Mr. B, I understand that you would like to talk with Mr. R from the Ostomy Society.

**Mr. B:** Yes, the doctor is sending me home in two days.

**Nurse:** You are giving yourself all of the opportunities possible to help with getting used to your changes.

**Mr. B:** I think I am ready to begin my adjustment now.

**Loss of Person.**   The loss of a person may include one's own impending death or the loss of a significant person in one's life through death, divorce, choice of vocation, relocation to another part of the world, ending a friendship, or disruption of a family relationship.

*Nursing Considerations.*   It is important for the nurse to be continuously alert to the process of grieving that occurs whenever there is a loss; this is especially true in circumstances involving the loss of a significant person. The student will find it helpful to recognize personal losses as a way of better understanding those of her client. This experience will help in more clearly formalizing a personal philosophy of loss, grieving, and dying. The ways in which people cope with these losses depends upon past experience and support systems. The grieving and the stages of dying will be discussed more fully later in this chapter.

**Loss of External Objects.**   The loss of possessions or objects is not always considered to be as important as those of body image, person, or normal aging. In a technological era where support systems are weakened by the mobility of individuals or by disruptions of family, and where possessions are considered by many to be highly valued, status and position may be closely linked to external objects. The nurse needs to validate with the client how important the lost object was to him in order to assist in the adjustment to the loss.

The continuum of loss from simple to complex is most evident with possessions or objects. For some persons the loss of a family heirloom, although of little monetary value, would be upsetting and a cause for grieving. Families subject to loss of their homes through a natural disaster, for example, flood or fire, or through society's imperatives as seen in urban renewal or eviction, experience extreme reactions to the loss.

*Nursing Considerations.*   When illness causes families to incur debts beyond their ability to manage, possessions often must be given up. There is usually a strong sense of rage, guilt, and blame involved when those kinds of stresses exist.

The nurse who is aware of the financial implications when a family member is chronically or acutely ill can be of assistance as a resource person for referral to community agencies. For example, the person with multiple sclerosis can be referred to the Multiple Sclerosis Society or the person who has suffered a stroke can become a member of the Stroke Club. Awareness of community resources, then, is a nursing responsibility that originates in the beginning levels of nursing education and builds throughout one's professional life.

The examples are endless and each student can cite personal and professional experiences of loss. It is important that each person's loss or sense of loss be viewed as a genuine experience. Caution must be used against judging a person's loss on the basis of one's own personal experience or values. The loss of one's lecture notes may be cause for serious panic in one student while another may treat it lightly. The death of a loved one may cause a severe grief reaction on one person, while another may deal with this loss through a less severe or prolonged reaction. The nurse, then, is a facilitator for the client who needs to express feelings freely without concern of being judged.

## GRIEF

Bereavement is the direct result of a loss. Thus, to be bereft of a person or thing is to be deprived of it. Grief is the feeling or emotion experienced as a result of bereavement.

Although a person may respond to bereavement in many possible ways: anger, flight, depersonalization, or even psychosis; grief is the most universal response.

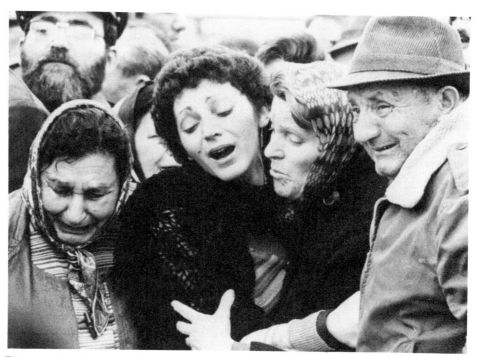

**Figure 4-2.** *Grief may be manifested in many ways—crying, grimacing, holding, touching. (United Press International photo)*

How then can it be recognized? Grief encompasses the total person. It is especially manifested by certain psychological and physical responses to the loss. In general, the grieving person is thrown into a state of disequilibrium. There is difficulty in concentration, insomnia, poor appetite, and forgetfulness. Physiologically the person may manifest symptoms of panic such as shortness of breath, fear of choking, severe tension, lack of muscular power, and a feeling of emptiness in the abdomen.

Most authors consider the stages of grief only in respect to the death of a loved one. Parkes (1972) in his book on bereavement, however, raises the question of the importance of considering grief as a reaction to other types of loss i.e. divorce, employment, a body part. The student should consider the grieving process as applicable to any kind of loss in the life cycle.

## Management of Grief

Parkes (1972) cites seven major features of most grief reactions.

**The Process of Realization.** The bereaved person moves from denial or avoidance of the loss to an acceptance of the pain incurred because of the loss. Since this is the first step in the grieving process, it usually occurs fairly soon after the loss. If there has been an anticipatory period, time before the loss when the bereaved were aware that the loss was going to occur as in terminal illness, the process of realization is sometimes shortened. The nurse can assist the persons involved by being aware of the need to come to the stage of acceptance. Being available to listen or sit quietly with the bereaved person is helpful to the process.

**An Alarm Reaction.** The grieving person manifests the somatic and psychological symptoms described above. Restlessness and anxiety are most noticeable. This feature generally occurs soon after the loss and is of short duration (about one month). The nurse can assist family members in their understanding of the grieving person's behavior.

**Searching.** Prolonged depression is not as characteristic of the grieving process as is acute episodic "pangs" of grief. A "pang" of grief can be defined as an episode of severe anxiety and psychological pain. The bereft person experiences strong feelings of loss and sobs or cries aloud for the lost person or object. These periods occur less often as the grieving process continues, until finally they only occur when something happens to strongly remind the person of the loss, i.e. seeing a picture of the lost one, visiting the old neighborhood, seeing a picture of oneself when health and intactness were present.

**Anger and Quiet.** Anger is a normal part of the grieving process and becomes diminished with the passage of time. The anger generally is not expressed toward the lost object or person, but instead is directed at other loved ones or family. It often involves trivial matters not normally considered worthy of one's anger. The nurse who is aware of this process will be less apt to personalize outbursts of anger directed at her, the staff, or the hospital in general.

The guilt the bereft person feels is manifested in a searching or "going over" of the events leading up to the loss. There is a need to try to place blame for the loss and therefore somehow make things all right again. At this time the nurse will hear statements beginning with "I should have . . . ," "If only I would have . . . ," "They never should have. . . ." The person needs to experience this process and a supportive, nonjudgmental person who listens without comment is a source of comfort.

Feeling of Internal Loss of Self or Mutilation.  During the process of anger and blaming, the grieving person may feel an emptiness inside that could be described as having had something "wrenched from one's guts."

Identification.  The bereaved person has had various roles which have helped to define self. With a serious loss, the individual may have to take on new roles that alter the self-image: from spouse to widow, from active young man to amputee, from concert cellist to multiple sclerosis victim. These changes demand that the individual redefine certain life roles and responsibilities. The way a person handles this process is related to past experience in role definition and to existing support systems.

Pathological Variants of Grief.  Some persons respond to loss in ways not considered to be within the "normal" limits of the grieving process. Some examples of this are delayed grieving of two weeks or more followed by prolonged depression, isolation, and suicidal ideation; an inability to begin the re-identification process; and a prolonged process of guilt and blame.

### Determinants of Grief

Parkes' book (1972) discusses grief reactions and some possible predisposing factors to explain individual differences in the degree and duration of the grieving process. As can be seen from Table 4-1, the bereaved person's grief response is intricately intertwined with life experiences, stages of development, social and cultural expectations and relationships within one's social network.

The nurse who has an understanding of these relationships will be able to anticipate grief responses and assist in the reestablishment of equilibrium for the grieving person.

## DYING AND THE DYING PROCESS

The concept of death is with us from the moment of conception. It is the final stage in the life cycle. The way in which we cope with death and dying is related to environmental, cultural, religious, and traditional influences. The nurse and the client each bring these influences with them into a relationship

Table   4-1    Determinants of the Outcome of Grief

**Life Cycle**

Early childhood losses of significant persons
Later experiences with loss especially of significant person
Previous mental illness, especially of the depressive kind
Other life crises prior to the loss

**Relationship with the Deceased or Lost Object**

Kinship (spouse, child, parent, etc.)
Degree of reliance, need
Strength of attachment
Intensity of feeling about person/object

**Mode of Death**

Timeliness
Previous warnings
Catastrophic
Anticipatory

**Individual Factors**

Sex
Age
Personality
Socio-economic status
Nationality
Religion
Cultural and familial factors influencing expression of grief

**Support System**

Family and friends
Other stresses
Options for role adjustment

Adapted from Colin Murray Parkes, *Bereavement Studies of Grief in Adult Life.* New York: International
Universities Press, 1972, p. 121.

or interaction. For this reason it is important that the nurse be aware of
personal feelings and prejudices regarding the dying process and death.

Responses to death differ depending on where a person is in his life cycle.
For example, society considers the death of a child, adolescent, and young or
middle-aged adult as a tragedy or terrible loss. The closer one gets to late
adulthood the more acceptable death becomes. So a parent may mourn the loss
of a child openly and with great emotion, but the expectation is that this same
person will restrain mourning and grief when the death is of an older aged
mother or father.

The way in which an individual understands the concept of death is also to
some degree based on age and life stage. Nagy (1948, 1959) in a classic study of

children's understanding of death used developmental levels as a measure of the comprehension of death as a concept. She identified the following:

Stage 1 (until about 5 years). The child displays great curiosity about death—where the body goes, why it is buried. There is little emotional realization of a loss, rather the dead are regarded as less alive and there is no grasp of the finality of the occurrence.

Stage 2 (from 5 years to about 9 years). The child appreciates the finality of death but gives it a magical quality. Death is seen as a personification: a mysterious figure that comes in the night or a frightening monster. Children in this age group believe it possible to be lucky and clever and therefore to elude death.

Stage 3 (9 or 10 years and up). The child understands death as final, inevitable, and universal. There is a realization that one's mortality is a condition of life.

These stages are guides for understanding a child's perception of death. The student may recognize that the ability to comprehend death in an abstract manner is directly related to the stages of cognitive development (see Chapter 2). It is important to remember that in times of intense stress adults also regress to more comfortable coping patterns. It is, therefore, not uncommon to observe adults coping with death at the initial moment by utilizing behaviors depicted in Stages 1 and 2.

Ritualistic behavior at the time of a death is considered to be important for adding structure and responsibility to the grieving person's life. Funerals, wakes, family gatherings, and time spent talking about the deceased all contribute to the grieving process in a positive manner.

In our society today more and more people are reaching middle adulthood without ever having experienced the death of a significant person. If someone close has died, it is generally a sudden death or one that has taken place in an unreal setting devoid of recognizable stimuli, i.e. an intensive-care unit. The opportunity to experience the dying process is often interrupted by these settings and both the dying person and those to be left behind have difficulty in working through the dying process.

The study of dying and death has become very popular in the past few years. Universities offer courses in philosophy, medicine, religion, and the humanities which focus directly on dying. One of the most influential persons in the study of dying has been Elisabeth Kübler-Ross (1969). Her stages in the dying process have given needed structure for persons who must understand the emotional stresses of the dying person and the bereaved. The stages of the dying process and their importance to the professional nurse are:

## Denial and Isolation

The denial is usually in the form of such statements as "No, not me." Denial is a buffer against overwhelming news. After the initial period of shock, the client will begin to look more realistically at the facts about impending death. The isolation which occurs is often due to an unspoken conspiracy between client and staff. At the time when the client most needs support and comfort the shock of the news causes hurt, withdrawal and sometimes angry outbursts. Staff are confused by this behavior and may respond by withdrawal themselves.

### Nursing Considerations

a.  Timing in telling a client his diagnosis is important to ultimate acceptance. Denial is almost always an immediate adaptation to the news.
b.  Although the initial denial is worked through, there are periods of time when it is necessary for the client to deny the reality in order to rest from the burden.
c.  Even though the client says that he wants to be left alone, this does not mean total isolation.
d.  The client needs a caring person who is there to offer comfort, support, and talking if desired.

## Anger

This emotion encompasses feelings of rage, resentment, and envy. When the person begins to realize that denial is no longer working, the anger begins. This is often a very difficult time for staff because of the tendency to personalize the anger directed at them. So when the client is irascible, quick to find fault with care, unkind to family members, and critical of the staff in general, the response may be one of further isolation, or labelling him as a "difficult ungrateful person."

### Nursing Considerations

a.  The stage of anger is an important realization stage.
b.  Feelings of resentment and envy are for what will be lost or missed: for example, envy over the potential for life that you and others like you still possess.
c.  The anger is not usually personal. Since it is really against the unknown or higher power (in a spiritual sense), it would be too dangerous for the client to "damn God."
d.  The continued acceptance of the client, along with support and concern, will help lessen the feelings of guilt and remorse which may otherwise result.

## Bargaining

This stage is less clear to the observer and is more private for the dying person. There is a magical quality to bargaining in that the client thinks that there might be a chance of prolonging life by being extra good or doing some special good deed. Most of the bargaining is between the person and some higher power (in a spiritual sense).

### Nursing Considerations

Most importantly, the nurse should be cautious in her responses to the discussions of bargaining that may occur. Respect for the client and supportive responses are important. Hope must be respected.

## Depression

This stage can be subdivided into reactive depression and preparatory depression.

*Reactive depression* can best be defined as the person's response to past losses, such as the deaths of close family or friends or loss of a part of the self through surgery or normal aging. Since this kind of depression generates unrealistic feelings of guilt and shame, it is important to be supportive of the positive aspects the client possesses.

*Preparatory depression* is similar to anticipatory grief in that it is a preparation for the things that will be lost to the dying person. Since this kind of depression is helping the client to prepare for the sad fact that all love objects including life will be lost, it is necessary for the sorrow to be expressed. Cheering statements and admonishments for being so sad are contraindicated. Supportive acceptance by the nurse will be a welcomed comfort to the individual.

### Nursing Considerations

a.  Depression is not always a negative experience. This may be especially true in this stage of dying.
b.  Preparatory depression is a silent, meditative time when touch and nonverbal communication of other types become important parts of the nurse-client relationship.

## Acceptance

This stage is reached when the person has had the time and appropriate assistance in working through the anger, rage, resentment, and depression. It is a time almost void of feeling—neither a happy state nor one of resignation. It is a time of lessened strength. There is a desire to have more quiet, fewer visitors, a wish to spend time with the significant persons in one's life.

### Nursing Considerations

a.  Persons achieve this stage when they have been encouraged to express their feelings of rage, anger, and depression.
b.  Usually the stage of acceptance has some relationship to the life stage of the person. An older individual who has successfully achieved ego integrity (see Chapter 2) may be more ready to accept the finality of death.

A person in the earlier stages of life may need more help in working through the grief.

c.  In nearly all instances of terminal illness, the individual maintains hope for cure or sudden remission. This is not the same as "fooling one's self" but rather the opposite of resignation.

This discussion of the stages of dying is presented in a step-by-step manner. However, in most situations where grieving occurs, the person moves back and forth between stages. Grieving is a cyclical process with continuing overlap. This may cause difficulty in recognizing specific stages unless the nurse is able to assess the client's emotional status accurately. A short assessment guide for use in all situations where loss will occur or has occurred appears in Table 4-2.

## CHRONIC ILLNESS

When considering this discussion of loss, grieving, and death, the student is asked to translate the stages of these emotional experiences into similar stages that must be experienced by a person with a chronic debilitating disease. Conditions such as multiple sclerosis or cystic fibrosis, spinal injuries that leave a person paralyzed, or the residual condition following a cerebral vascular accident (CVA) all constitute serious losses. In any situation where an individual's health is altered and a loss occurs, grieving for this loss must also occur.

The stages of dying and the grieving process are so similar that in certain areas they overlap. In fact, the dying person must grieve for the impending losses, so one becomes a part of the other.

It is very important that the student recognize that dying is not the only reason for grieving; all persons experience losses in their lives, and all persons grieve. The more the nurse is able to relate to these feelings in a personal way, the more able she will be to recognize the feelings of the client.

Table  4-2    Questions to Guide in Assessing Client Behavior in Situations of Loss.*

### Self-Concept

How does your client view himself? Does he like himself? Does he have pride and confidence in himself? Or does he have feelings of failure and insecurity?

What impression about himself does the client project to others? Does he take pride in his appearance? Or does he have careless grooming habits? Does he make deprecating statements about himself? Is he apathetic about his surroundings?

How does he express his identity? Does he see himself as a provider? An authority figure? A marriage partner? A child? A parent?

Table 4-2    Questions to Guide in Assessing Client Behavior in Situations of Loss.* Continued

### Perception

How does your client perceive his illness? Can he describe it and its symptoms?

What is his perception of the meaning for his illness or condition? Does he see it as a punishment? An escape from responsibility? An inconvenience? A vacation?

How does he perceive the persons caring for him? Does he feel they are trustworthy and supportive? Or authoritative, frightening, and inept?

### Stress

What is the nature of the stress your client faces? What does it mean to him?

Does he have to cope with several stresses simultaneously, such as illness and loss of job, or biopsy and surgery?

Is the stressful event temporary or permanent?

Has the client experienced similar stressful events in the past? If so, how has he coped with them?

What resources are available to help him cope? Family, friends, community, religious or professional help?

### Loss

What kind of loss is your client experiencing? Loss of strength? Privacy? Mobility? Independence? Status? Bodily function?

What is the actual loss which he will experience? Appendectomy? Amputation? Laryngectomy? Colostomy? Loss of life?

*Reprinted with permission from the September issue of *Nursing 77*. Copyright © 1977 Intermed Communications, Inc.

## SUMMARY

The concept of loss over the life cycle includes:

1. normal aging
2. self-image
3. loss of person
4. loss of external objects.

The responses to loss can be seen by considering the grieving process and the stages of dying. These two have been recognized for the similarities in the process: denial, anger, and acceptance.

Management of grieving can be facilitated by understanding the major features of the grief reaction: the process of realization, alarm, searching, anger and quiet, feelings of loss of self, and identification. Some important determinants of the final resolution of grief are based on former life experiences and coping behaviors.

Dying is discussed as a form of loss. Kübler-Ross's suggested stages and children's awareness of death are seen as a part of the grieving process. Nursing assessment of client behavior is important when assistance with loss, grief, and dying is needed.

## LEARNING ACTIVITIES

1.  Considering the types of loss discussed in this chapter: Can you recall some of your reactions to your aging process? What object or possession have you recently lost? What was your response to the loss?

2.  How have you experienced the grieving process? Can you identify specific stages?

3.  Choose someone you know (parent, spouse, relative, close friend) who has been bereaved and will feel comfortable talking about it. Ask them to discuss the loss and grieving process with you. Can you identify the stages?

4.  Talk with three children whose ages fit each of Nagy's stages. Discuss death as a concept with each child. Do they appear to visualize death in the ways identified by Nagy?

5.  In your clinical assignment observe your client for expressions of loss or feelings of impending loss. Were you able to detect expressions of grieving? Were these expressions anticipatory in nature? Could you recognize specific stages?

## REFERENCES AND SUGGESTED READINGS

Breuer, J. Sharing tragedy. *American Journal of Nursing*, May, 1976, pp. 758–759.

Burnside, I. M., 1976. *Nursing and the aged.* New York: McGraw-Hill.

Busse, E. W. and Pfeiffer, E., eds., 1969. *Behavior and adaptation in late life.* Boston: Little, Brown.

Carlson, C., ed., 1970. *Behavioral concepts and nursing intervention.* Philadelphia: J. B. Lippincott.

Encounters with grief. *American Journal of Nursing*, March, 1978, pp. 414–425.

Feifel, H., 1977. *New meanings of death.* New York: McGraw-Hill.

Kastenbaum, R. J., 1977. *Death, society, and human experience.* Saint Louis: C. V. Mosby.

Kennerly, S. L. What I've learned about mastectomy. *American Journal of Nursing*, September, 1977, pp. 1430–1432.

Kübler-Ross, E., 1969. *On death and dying.* New York: MacMillan.

————. What is it like to be dying? *American Journal of Nursing,* January, 1971, pp. 54–60.

Lidz, T., 1976. *The person: his and her development through the life cycle.* Rev.ed. New York: Basic Books.

Martinson, I.  Parents help each other. *American Journal of Nursing,* July, 1976, pp. 1120–1122.

Morrison, R. S., 1975.  Death: process or event? In *Life: the continuous process,* ed. Freda Rebelsky.  New York: Alfred A. Knopf.

Murray, R. and Zentner, J., 1975.  *Nursing assessment and health promotion through the life span.*  Englewood Cliffs, N.J.: Prentice-Hall.

Nagy, M., 1948.  The child's view of death. Rpt. in H. Feifel, ed., *The meaning of death.*  New York, McGraw-Hill, 1959, pp. 79–98.

Parkes, C. M., 1972.  *Bereavement: studies of grief in adult life.*  New York: International Universities Press.

Shneidman, E. S., 1974.  *Deaths of man.*  Baltimore: Penguin Books.

Sloboda, S. B.  Understanding patient behavior. *Nursing 77,* September, 1977, pp. 74–77.

Ufema, J. K.  Dare to care for the dying. *American Journal of Nursing,* January, 1976, pp. 88–90.

Wentzel, K. B.  The dying are the living. *American Journal of Nursing,* June, 1976, pp. 956–957.

# 2

# Nursing Care and the Social System

The Family
Groups
The Community
Cultural Implications in Nursing
The Environment

Part 2 moves from consideration of the nursing care of individuals at various life stages to discussion of the larger systems within which an individual functions. A study of the nature and functions of families, groups, and communities within which the individual functions helps identify the systems that support him and in turn expect his support. Cultural and environmental influences that have implications for nursing are described.

# 5

# The Family

## Behavioral Objectives

Upon completion of this chapter, the student will be able to:

1. Describe the concept of a family.
2. Identify various family structures within our society.
3. Describe basic family functions.
4. Describe family developmental stages and the appropriate family tasks for each stage.
5. Identify health-related tasks of the family.
6. Identify social and cultural factors that influence the family's behaviors relative to health.
7. Assess the nursing needs of a family at a beginning level.
8. Describe crisis intervention as it might be applied to a family.

## Key Terms

blended families
communal families
crisis
developmental stages
developmental tasks

extended families
family
family structure
family function
family health tasks

living-together-
  arrangement families
nuclear families
single-parent families

## Introduction

The family has long been identified as the natural and fundamental unit of society. Recent years have witnessed many changes in the structure of families as mobility, technology, and other social and economic factors pressure the traditional unit and require increasing adaptive measures to cope with a multitude of stresses.

Nursing of multiproblem families and family-centered therapy will probably not be the primary responsibility of beginning nursing students. However, providing support and anticipatory guidance to the relatively well family is the responsibility of nurses at all levels of practice. It is important that a family-centered orientation of care be understood for the nursing of the individual as well as the family in which the individual functions. Whether the nurse encounters the client in the hospital, clinic, school, home, or job setting, his care may well depend, at least in part, on the nurse's ability to perceive the client as a unique individual who is also part of a family group.

## FAMILY DEFINITION

There are many definitions of the word *family*, some describing blood or legal relationships, others focusing on the expected roles and responsibilities of the family. Common to all definitions is the idea that a family consists of two or more persons. For purposes of this chapter, Burgess's classic definition of a family as a unity of interacting personalities will be used (Burgess, 1926). This old concept of a family readily encompasses the many "new" relation-

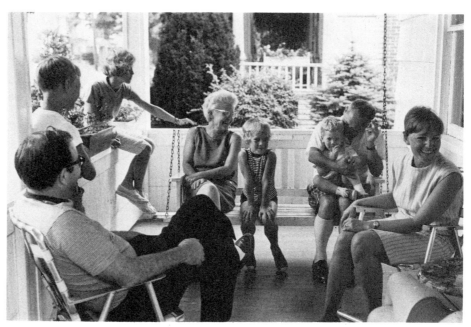

Figure 5-1. *A family gathering.* (Heron/Monkmeyer Press Photo Service)

ships that exist today between people who care for each other and choose to share their living in special ways.

## FAMILY STRUCTURES

The nurse encounters many types of families in her dealings with clients. There is the traditional nuclear family consisting of parents and their children, and the extension of this which includes other relatives and grandparents of the nuclear family and is often called the extended family.

The single-parent family is an increasingly common phenomenon today. This type of family consists of one parent—father or mother—and children. In addition to the single-parent family that results from death and divorce, there is also the single parent who has never married and is living with natural or adopted children.

Blended families (Satir, 1972), which consist of parents and the children of former marriages as well as the present marriage, are a result of the many divorces, deaths, and remarriages that occur.

Group or communal families consist of more than two adults. The group may contain all married couples, all unmarried persons, or a mixture of both. There may or may not be children present. If children are present, the parenting may be done by the natural parent(s) or by the entire group.

Unmarried couples, with or without children, are a growing family unit in our society. This arrangement is sometimes identified as a "living-together arrangement" (LTA) in health records.

Couples of the same sex also live together with or without children. The relationship of these couples may or may not include a physical sexual component.

Being sensitive to possible family structures, and not imposing stereotypes on families and individuals, is essential professional behavior for the nurse. She needs to be aware of her own values and past experiences and to realize how these are influencing her ideas about family structure.

When encountering a client for the first time, the nurse would do well to ask nondirective questions to ascertain the family structure. Rather than opening the interaction with stereotypic questions such as "What is your husband/wife's name?" or "How many children do you have?" the sensitive interviewer asks "Do other persons live with you?" Clients will usually indicate the actual family structure and their feelings about this if the interview is sensitive and nonthreatening. The nurse can then ask for any specifics and obtain a structural guideline about the family. Such an approach prevents unnecessary embarrassment or pain from asking the newly widowed or divorced about their spouse, or quizzing the grieving childless about their children.

Understanding family structures can assist the nurse in making her assessment about the needs of an individual or family. Family functioning, rather than family structure, is the basis for assessing needs. Single-parent families are sometimes referred to as broken homes or incomplete families, even though the family may be functioning well as a close and caring group. The reverse of this discrimination is also true when nuclear families, especially those with sufficient economic resources, are overlooked when they need guidance because their structure seems to be "intact."

In assessing families, and the needs of the group and the individuals, the nurse will want to be aware of special factors that deserve consideration in specific family situations. In assessing the single-parent family, the nurse will want to identify any added stress that the family may be encountering such as the reason for the single parent (choice or not) and the available resources outside the immediate family. Community- and church-related groups can often assist single-parent families in meeting family needs, especially those related to the growth and development of children. Parents Without Partners (PWP) is a well-known group established for this purpose. It has local chapters in all parts of the country. These groups can provide social opportunities for the children and the parents plus allow a discussion of common problems and solutions with others in similar situations.

In the blended family, as in the formation of any new group, it is important to allow for open communication and group process. Interrelationships between children and the step-parent, children and the natural parent, and children from different marriages present a challenging series of stimuli that require orchestration if harmony is to be achieved and conflicts to be worked out constructively. Styles of functioning in previous family situations may need modification and the nurse may be approached for suggestions and guidance as well as support.

A man and woman living together often function and interact similarly to their married counterparts except for legal status. Some of these couples plan to marry at a later date, while others choose not to make a permanent or legal contract. If one of these people is hospitalized, it is very important for the nurse to ascertain the nature of their relationship to assure that they can be visited by the other member of their family despite their lack of legal or blood ties. The nurse can ask the client if the partner is to be notified or informed regarding the client's condition and proceed according to the client's wishes. Similar consideration is given to persons living in communal families or with partners of the same sex.

## FAMILY FUNCTION

The function of a family is described by identifying the appropriate activities of the family in meeting the needs of its members and its responsibilities to the community. Duvall (1962) identified nine family developmental tasks that concern a family at all stages. These include:

1. Establishment of a home to provide shelter, food, clothing, and other physical necessities including health care.

2.  Satisfactory allocation of resources such as money, space, material possessions, and affection.

3.  Acceptable division of labor such as breadwinning, household management, and care of family members.

4.  Socialization of family members to assure acceptable patterns in areas of sexual drives, elimination, food intake, aggression, and sleep.

5.  Communication patterns that provide means of conveying norms for intellectual and emotional behaviors.

6.  Workable policies for inclusion of relatives and new family members into the group.

7.  Mechanisms to assist in the placement of members in the larger society, including participation in community, school, church, political, and economic systems in which persons will function.

8.  Acceptable reproductive patterns including both the bearing and adopting of children, and the release of these children at maturity.

9.  Motivation and morale among members—this includes establishment of a philosophy of life, mutual support and affection among family members, and recognition of achievement.

These family roles and responsibilities are seen as common to all families regardless of their structure or stage in the life cycle. In addition to general family functions, the nurse is especially concerned with family functioning as it relates to health and illness. Freeman (1970) has identified the following health tasks of the family to provide guidelines for nursing assessment:

1.  Recognizing the interruptions of health development such as illness or a child's failure to thrive.

2.  Making decisions about seeking health care.

3.  Dealing effectively with health and nonhealth crises.

4.  Providing nursing care to sick, disabled, or dependent members of the family.

5.  Maintaining a home environment conducive to health maintenance and personal development.

6.  Maintaining a reciprocal relationship with the community and its health institutions.

Utilizing these criteria in assessing family functioning enables the nurse to focus on specific areas to reinforce or to suggest improvements. The reinforcement of existing strengths in family functioning is very important. Such reinforcement not only gives the family needed and deserved recognition, but also serves as a foundation on which to build behaviors that will improve family functioning and the ability of the family to assist its members in achieving their potential.

# DEVELOPMENTAL TASKS AND FAMILY LIFE STAGES

A developmental task is seen as a responsibility that arises at a specific period in an individual's life. Satisfactory accomplishment of this task leads to happiness and success with later tasks. Failure to accomplish the task leads to unhappiness, difficulty with later tasks, and often the disapproval of society (Duvall, 1962). Family developmental tasks are the growth responsibilities that a family needs to accomplish at a given stage in its development.

The concept of family developmental tasks to be done within the life cycle of a family was developed in the context of families being committed to permanent relationships and to the nurturing of children and other family members for a lifetime. Families that are not involved with child-rearing tend to focus mainly on the growth and development of the adult members at various individual stages. Whether these families consist of married couples, unmarried couples, or adults in some type of communal arrangement, criteria for family developmental tasks of these families would correlate with a framework based on understanding of individual developmental tasks as described in Chapter 2.

In families who are raising children, the dependency of the children upon the parents, combined with the parents' needs to be responsible for their own developmental tasks, usually requires that parents avail themselves of existing community resources especially for the social, educational, and health needs of the family. As one of the health professionals working with families and their members, the nurse may find a framework for the life cycle of the child-raising family to be a helpful tool in assessing family and individual health needs. Duvall (1972) has described the following stages in the family life cycle:

**Stage I**     Beginning families (married couple without children).

**Stage II**    Childbearing families (oldest child is between birth and 30 months).

**Stage III**   Families with preschool children (oldest child is 2½ to 6 years old).

**Stage IV**    Families with schoolchildren (oldest child is 6 to 13 years old).

**Stage V**     Families with teenagers (oldest child is 13 to 20 years old).

**Stage VI**    Families as launching centers (first child gone to last child leaving home).

**Stage VII**   Families in the middle years (empty nest to retirement).

**Stage VIII**  Aging families (retirement to death of one or both spouses).

It is obvious that there is an overlapping of two or more of these stages in many families and that the length of the cycles will vary with the number and spacing of the children and the ages of the parents. Recognizing the stage(s) of family development and the shifting tasks of the various stages in the family life cycle can serve as a guide to the nurse in assisting the family in setting mutually agreed upon health goals for its members.

## SOCIAL AND CULTURAL INFLUENCES ON FAMILY HEALTH

Families exist within the social and cultural norms of the larger community. In the United States we have the acculturation of many ethnic family groups into a common society. These groups may maintain their ethnic identity while functioning within the common social structure, or they may strive to move away from their ethnic family customs and identity. Chapter 8 describes some of the cultural beliefs held by individuals and families and the effect of this as it relates to nursing.

Religion and spiritual beliefs can be an important factor in dealing with families. Controversial issues such as contraception, abortion, surgery and blood transfusions for minors, and dietary restrictions are often decided within an existing value system that reflects the values of the family rather than those of health professionals. The nurse needs to be aware of her own system of values and be able to separate these from family beliefs that may contradict these. Nurses working with families and individuals need to strive for mutually acceptable health goals or they can anticipate resistance and lack of family participation in meeting health needs.

## NURSING CARE OF FAMILIES IN CRISIS

A crisis is a temporary situation that requires the reorganization of a person's psychological structure and behavior. Crisis occurs when there is sudden alteration in expectations and the usual coping mechanisms are not sufficient for the task (Kaplan, 1965). Crises in families occur when a problem arises that the family cannot cope with. When a crisis occurs in an individual family member, the entire family group is affected. Such an occurrence requires changes in family functioning to resolve the crisis.

There are two types of crisis: developmental, or maturational; and situational, or accidental. A developmental crisis is one which is seen as part of growth during the normal life cycle. Occurrences which cause changes in families such as the birth of a child, children leaving home, or retirement are times of increased family stress within the normal life cycle. If the family has the resources to adapt to these changes, it is able to cope. When adaptive mechanisms fail, the family is in crisis and may need help in developing new resources. A situational crisis is the result of an external happening, often unexpected and painful, such as the serious illness or death of a family member, divorce, or loss of job (Robichon, 1967).

The phases in crisis for an individual or a family are identified as: shock, defensive retreat, acknowledgement, and resolution. Factors influencing reaction to crisis include actual perception of the crisis, emotional and physical status of those involved, adaptive capacity, past experience with crisis resolution, objective seriousness of the crisis, social and cultural expectations, and the availability of a support system. In assessing a family in a state of crisis, the nurse needs to be aware of both the phase of crisis for the family and its members, and any crisis-related factors that are affecting the family. It is also important to realize that when a large number of normal stresses of family life are occurring at the same time, the cumulative effect of this clustering of stresses can cause a crisis in an ordinarily adaptive family. An example of this can occur when a developmental event such as the birth of a child and a situational problem such as loss of a job or a serious illness happen simultaneously.

Numerous formats and tools have been developed and used to assess families. Table 5-1 illustrates a framework for organizing needed assessment data for families.

The nurse can sometimes assist families in preventing a crisis by anticipatory guidance in preparation for expected developmental events. Such guidance aims at assisting the family in maintaining and preserving its existing resources, and discussing possible alternatives that may need to be considered when a life-changing event is expected. Early recognition of crisis when it does occur, and assistance in needed adaptation, can shorten the duration of the crisis. The nurse often works with other health professionals in the field of

**Table 5-1   Suggested Guide for Collection of Data for Family Assessment**

### 1. Structure of Family
Members by name, age, and relationship to each other

### 2. Functioning of Family
a. Ability to provide for physical necessities (shelter, food, clothing)
b. Allocation of resources (space, money)
c. Division of labor among members
d. Socialization of members
e. Communication patterns
f. Relationship with extended family
g. Relationship with larger community
h. Reproductive patterns (if applicable)
i. Mutual support among members

### 3. Social and Cultural Influences Affecting Health
a. Economic resources
b. Spiritual and religious beliefs
c. Ethnic identification (if applicable)

### 4. Existing or Potential Health Problems
a. Developmental crises (expected life changes)
b. Situational crises (unexpected changes, illness)
c. Anticipatory guidance (especially for high risk situations)

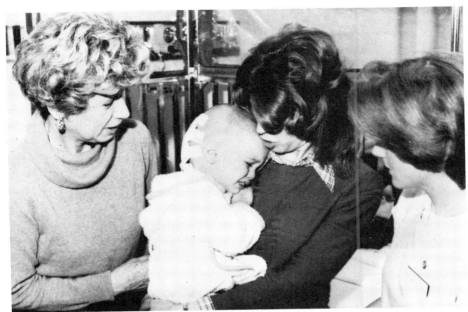

**Figure 5-2.** *The nurse can often assist a family in preventing or working through a crisis.* *(Photo by Frank R. Engler, Jr.)*

mental health and family counselling. Various types of group therapy, as well as individual counselling, are available to assist families in rehabilitation when needed to restore functioning following the disequilibrium that accompanies a family crisis.

Some of the specific measures which the nurse utilizes in assisting families in crisis include:

1. Accepting the family and all of its members in whatever stage they happen to be.

2. Assisting with identification of the problem and the reality of the situation as seen by the family.

3. Suggesting ways of dealing with the crisis in manageable doses while remaining realistic about the magnitude of the crisis (This "one-day-at-a time" approach can be very useful in surviving the acute phases of a crisis).

4. Allowing ventilation of feelings which will help the family to comprehend the reality of the situation.

5. Identifying, with the family's help, the existing strengths and sources of support within the family, among relatives and friends, and in the community.

6. Encouraging individuals or the family to accept responsibility and beginning problem-solving for short- and long-range goals.

7. Reinforcing any behaviors and attitudes that are effective in the situation and using these as a basis for exploring alternative behaviors appropriate to the changes that have occurred.

Crisis is a time of change or a turning point for an individual or a family. The successful resolution of a crisis leads to a level of functioning and integration that is higher than that which existed prior to the crisis. When a crisis is not resolved in a constructive way, it can resurface at a later date and it may contribute to physical and somatic illness.

## SUMMARY

The family is a unity of interacting personalities. Its structure varies and includes many family types. Some of these are the nuclear family, the extended family, the single-parent family, the blended family, the communal family, and the living-together arrangement family.

Functions of a family include providing for the physical, psychological, and social needs of its members. It is also a family concern to maintain the health of its members.

Families exist in identifiable developmental stages and there are developmental tasks associated with each of these stages. Successful achievement of developmental tasks at each stage of the life cycle is important as a foundation for achieving the tasks in later stages.

Social and cultural factors influence families in their health practices and utilization of health services. Family health goals need to be mutually identified by the family and the nurse.

Crisis occurs in a family when a situation arises that is beyond the scope of the family's resources and coping abilities. The nurse needs to understand the stages of crisis and the factors that affect a family crisis. Appropriate nursing intervention can assist families in the resolution of crises.

## LEARNING ACTIVITIES

1. Give your definition of a family and describe one family that you know that conforms to your definition.

2. List three possible family structures. Describe the differences among them and tell why it is important for the nurse to understand these differences.

3. List the developmental stages of a family according to Duvall and identify at least one important task for each stage.

4. What health tasks can a family be expected to accomplish for its members?

5. List four social, cultural, or religious values and describe how each might affect the health functioning of families.

6. Identify a family crisis situation and describe in outline how you would use the nursing process to assist the family.

# REFERENCES AND SUGGESTED READINGS

Ackerman, Nathan, 1958. *Psychodynamics of family life.* New York: Basic Books.

Bell, Norman and Vogel, Ezra, eds., 1960 *The family.* Glencoe Ill.: The Free Press of Glencoe.

Burgess, E. W. The family as a unit of interacting personalities, *The Family,* 7 (1926), pp. 3–9.

Caplan, Gerald, 1964. *Principles of preventive psychiatry.* New York: Basic Books.

Duvall, Evelyn, 1971. *Family development.* 4th ed. Philadelphia: J. B. Lippincott.

Freeman, Ruth B., 1970. *Community health nursing practice.* Philadelphia: W. B. Saunders.

Hall, Joanne and Weaver, Barbara, 1974. *Nursing of families in crisis.* Philadelphia: J. B. Lippincott.

Leahy, Kathleen; Cobb, M; Jones, Mary, 1977. *Community health nursing.* 3rd ed. New York: McGraw-Hill.

Murray, Ruth and Zentner, Judith, 1975. *Nursing concepts for health promotion.* Englewood Cliffs, N. J.: Prentice-Hall.

Parad, Howard and Caplan, Gerald, 1969. A framework for studying families in crisis, in *Crisis intervention: selected readings,* ed. H. Parad. New York: Family Service Association.

Reinhardt, Adina and Quinn, Mildred, 1973. *Family-centered community nursing: a sociocultural framework.* St. Louis: C. V. Mosby.

Satir, Virginia, 1972. *Peoplemaking.* Palo Alto, Cal.: Science and Behavior Books.

Sobol, Evelyn and Robischon, Paulette, 1975. *Family nursing: a study guide.* St. Louis: C. V. Mosby Company.

Toffler, Alvin, 1970. *Future shock.* New York: Random House.

# 6

# Groups

## Behavioral Objectives

Upon completion of this chapter, the student will be able to:

1. Define a group.
2. Describe various group structures with which the nurse may need to work.
3. Describe basic group functions.
4. Describe factors in group leadership.
5. Describe selected nursing implications in the study of groups.

## Key Terms

| | | |
|---|---|---|
| antigroup functions | group norms | secondary groups |
| formal group structure | group structure | self-actualization groups |
| group | informal group structure | self-help groups |
| group consensus | maintenance functions of | task functions of a group |
| group function | a group | teaching/learning groups |
| group leadership | primary groups | therapy groups |
| | reference groups | |

## Introduction

The formation of groups occurs in all societies. In primitive societies, groups were primarily defined by geographical location and by traditional relationships, such as blood and marriage. Today's technology has eased the barriers of distance in maintaining group membership. The same technology has developed distance in the traditional relationships. Job mobility and available options to relocate sever or at least weaken some of the group affiliations to

94

which individuals might cling. New groups form—strangers become friends or at least cooperating acquaintances in new groups.

As a health professional, the nurse needs to be aware of the existence of various types of groups and of the way in which they function. This will enable her to act more effectively as an individual and to judiciously refer her clients to groups that will be helpful to them. Further study of group theory and group phenomena is found in advanced nursing courses. This chapter will introduce some general ideas about groups that are considered by the authors to be fundamental to nursing practice.

## GROUPS

The broadest dictionary definition of a group is "any collection or assemblage of persons or things" (Random House, 1967). The literature on group process generally includes the concept that these persons or things are related in some way.

Sampson and Marthas (1977) describe three bases for interdependent relationships within a group: a common task, a common characteristic, or a pattern of interaction. Examples of all three are frequently encountered in nursing situations. The nursing staff in any agency shares responsibility for the common task of providing nursing care to clients. Common characteristics such as age, needs, or interests, exist in most groups as a major motivation for membership. Patterns of interaction, such as those seen in a family or classroom group, are observable.

## GROUP STRUCTURE

The structure of a group refers to the internal organization and arrangement of relationships that exist. Among the most common factors affecting the structure of a group are membership criteria, size, purpose, and interrelationships among group members.

Criteria for membership describe the persons who may be group members. It is important to know if membership is voluntary or required, stable or changing.

Another important factor in the structure of a group is size. Small groups are those with between 2 and 15 members. Cartwright and Zander (1968) have described group processes for small groups which do not differ substantially within the range of membership for small groups.

Large groups (over 15 members) usually have less participation by the total membership on any given issue. A big group may contain more potential resources than a small group, but the interaction of its members may be less cohesive and more prone to the formation of subgroups than a small group would be.

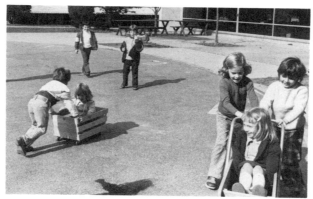

Figure 6-1. *(Mimi Forsyth/ Monkmeyer Press Photo Service)*

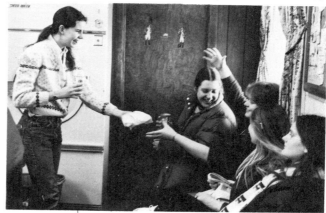

Figure 6-2. *(Sybil Shelton/Monkmeyer Press Photo Service)*

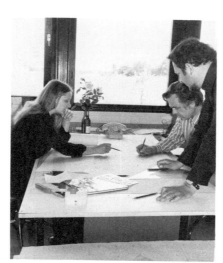

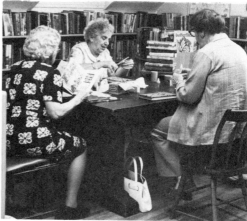

Figure 6-4. *(Sybil Shackman/Monkmeyer Press Photo Service)*

Figure 6-3. *(Edith Reichman/Monkmeyer Press Photo Service)*

*Groups of all ages.*

The structure of a group is also reflected in its purpose. A low structured group, usually few in numbers, where the mutual support of members is seen as more important than achieving tasks, is called a primary group. Secondary groups are those in which there is little attention given to the personal support of individual members. These groups are task oriented, often large, and somewhat rigid in structure, such as a professional organization.

Interrelationships between members of a group are a crucial, though sometimes subtle, indicator of group structure. Berne (1963) has described both a public and a private structure for groups. The public or formal structure is usually well-defined and includes delineation of membership, rights and responsibilities of membership, and the visible relationship of members to each other. The private or informal structure of a group evolves from the needs of the existing members and is often a more powerful operational force than the public structure.

A student nurse beginning a period of clinical experience in a health agency is usually introduced to the staff group with which she will be working. The structure of the group—including identity of members and their respective responsibilities—will be identified. A perceptive student will note not only the public or formal structure that is presented, but also the informal group structure that is operating. Awareness of both of these, and the congruence or lack of congruence between them, is essential to the effectiveness of a newcomer in the group situation.

## GROUP FUNCTION

Group functioning reflects the ways in which a group (a) accomplishes the group tasks; and (b) meets the maintenance needs of its members. To function effectively, a group must consider both these functions.

Picture a group of students assigned to a group project for which they will receive a group grade. They may be very warm and supportive to each other and refuse to set limits on individual group members who are not doing their share of work. This will result in maintaining their friendships but will not result in a group project as planned unless this is done at the expense of the members who do more than their share of the group work.

This group may also choose to define rigid norms for performance in the group and put heavy pressure on some of its weaker members, ignoring their individual limitations. Such measures may accomplish the task at great cost to these individual members. Functioning in a manner that achieves both the task and the maintenance goals is the desired norm for group functioning.

Other issues which affect group functioning are the group norms, the group decision-making process, and the ways which the group chooses to handle conflict. The group norms, or expected behaviors for members, may be defined by outside sources such as a higher authority or a written constitution and bylaws. In less-formal group functioning, the members define the norms and decide how they will handle group members who deviate from these norms. The importance of norms can be seen in professional nursing groups in the peer review process.

Decision-making is also a group process that must be clearly identifiable to all members. In some groups, a majority vote constitutes a decision which binds all group members. Other groups require a consensus—a compromise decision with which all members are comfortable. Some groups do not have an effective process for making decisions and the group may be noted for its nondecisive behavior. Decisions may also be imposed on a group by an outside authority or a recognized authority within the group.

The way in which a group handles conflict is another crucial area of effective group functioning. Conflict is a normal occurrence in a group situation. If it is

Table 6-1    Common Roles of Members in Groups

### Group Task-Related Roles

| | |
|---|---|
| Initiator: | offers new ideas and methods of dealing with group tasks |
| Clarifier: | seeks clarification from the group regarding facts and values |
| Elaborator: | expands on group suggestions and offers ideas for implementation |
| Coordinator: | pulls together suggestions of the group and tries to help subgroups combine efforts |
| Evaluator: | questions the practicality and effectiveness of group plans and offers constructive criticism |
| Recorder: | writes up group decisions and summarizes discussion for future reference |

### Group Maintenance-Related Roles

| | |
|---|---|
| Encourager: | praises and accepts ideas proposed by group members and communicates openness to all group members |
| Compromiser: | seeks ways to resolve conflict between members' ideas by offering alternatives that both sides can accept |
| Gatekeeper: | encourages participation of less active group members |
| Standard Setter: | proposes standards for the functioning within the group |

### Antigroup Roles

| | |
|---|---|
| Blocker: | attempts to thwart forward movement of group by returning group focus to issues that the group has decided not to consider |
| Aggressor: | attacks the ideas and feelings of others in a hostile way |
| Dominator: | tries to manipulate members in order to control group actions |
| Help Seeker: | uses group as forum to express personal considerations in hopes of gaining sympathy for self |
| Playboy: | is uninvolved in group tasks and indulges in inappropriate behavior such as horseplay, cynicism and nonchalance |

handled constructively, it can serve as a positive force in group functioning. When group members are generally supportive of each other, committed to the group task, and able to reach decisions and compromises, there is a good chance that conflict resolution will be open and constructive. When group members are unable to function productively in these other ways, conflict is often destructive and is a serious hindrance to group functioning.

A discussion of group functioning would be incomplete without reference to the roles which are played out within groups. A role is an expected set of behaviors which characterize a person or position. In analyzing roles, we must be careful not to cast an individual solidly into a role and thus limit the way in which we can perceive that individual. Keeping this possible folly in mind, recognition of common roles within groups can be helpful in understanding the structure and function of any group, and in enabling the realistic utilization of the group's potential.

Roles of group members are commonly associated with defined task and member functions (Bales, 1958). A third set of roles is seen in those who are using the group to achieve solely individual aims. These are referred to as antigroup roles (Lifton, 1961). Table 6-1 summarizes some common group roles.

## GROUP LEADERSHIP

Leadership may be seen as a process which moves a group toward its goals. This process can be shared by the group members or it can be centered in a specific person recognized as a leader. Leaders are sometimes assigned in a group, or they may emerge spontaneously from among the group members.

There are three types of leadership commonly observed in groups: autocratic, democratic, and laissez-faire. Autocratic leadership exists when the leader makes all decisions and assumes final responsibility for the group's actions. In a democratic form of leadership, the leader acts as a facilitator in enabling group decisions, but the decision-making is done by the total group. A laissez-faire style of leadership is passive and allows the group to develop with little guidance or input from the leader.

Among the leadership functions which must be handled in the group are: defining of group norms and goals, representing the group to other groups, and administering the resources of the group toward achievement of purpose.

## NURSING IMPLICATIONS IN THE STUDY OF GROUPS

With the proliferation of groups in our society today, most people belong to several groups. For the nurse, this has implications for her own behavior as well as for that of her clients. As a professional, the nurse will be a member of her own professional nursing group and of interdisciplinary groups with other health professionals. Most nursing positions require participation in a group with others in a work situation. The nurse needs to be aware of her own behavior and its effect on group process. In addition to those situations where the nurse is a group member, she may also be expected to provide leadership to groups of people in various hospital and community settings.

Groups have been found to be effective in health education, counselling, and therapy. Reference groups—groups to which one turns for reinforcement of identified values and a sense of identity—may have a large effect on an individual's behavior related to health and illness. A diabetic adolescent will be supported in his efforts to maintain needed diet habits if his peer group values health and good eating habits. Conversely, if his closest friends snack continually on junk food and ignore healthy eating patterns, he may be unwilling to attempt behaviors that would differ from the norms of the group with which he is identified.

The nurse who is assisting this adolescent in assuming responsibility for his health, needs to be aware of the importance of the reference group, and prepared to assist the client in the process of changing undesirable behaviors. Lewin (1958) has described the influence of group process in effecting change. Change is seen to occur in three stages: (1) "unfreezing" old behaviors; (2) defining new behaviors; and (3) "refreezing" the newly acquired behaviors. To "unfreeze" old behaviors, it is usually necessary for a person to decrease his association with or dependence on people who support the undesired behavior. Newly defined behaviors then need "refreezing" by forming new associations which are supportive of the newly acquired behaviors. The success of many health-related community groups such as Alcoholics Anonymous, Weight Watchers, and Smoke Enders is based on the idea of providing new reference groups for people who are attempting to change undesirable behaviors.

Coping groups, which emphasize self-help, are another group community resource. These groups are formed to assist people who are attempting to adapt to changes which have occurred in their lives, usually beyond their individual control. Group members share a common problem such as a specific illness (stroke, heart disease, cancer, chronic lung disease) or a major life crisis (loss of a loved one through death, divorce, or serious illness). These groups are usually led by a qualified professional who assumes responsibility for keeping the group focused on its task of being supportive to the members and initiating and facilitating the exchange of helpful suggestions for ways to deal with the identified problems.

Teaching/learning groups are another source of support offered within the broad field of health care. Group classes teach needed knowledge and skills in a wide variety of areas such as childbirth, parenting, nutrition, and physical exercise. These classes often focus on health maintenance behaviors.

Self-actualization or encounter groups are another group phenomenon of today. These groups are aimed at providing an environment in which individual members can develop themselves in relation to others in a variety of ways. Members experiment with each other in practicing ways of expressing themselves spontaneously.

Therapy groups also seek to provide an environment for personal development and improved functioning. Members of therapy groups have usually identified behavioral or attitudinal patterns within themselves that are not satisfactory in their present situation and, therefore, need change. These groups require the leadership of a therapist skilled in group work as well as in psychiatric treatment. As a nurse develops her professional skills, she may be expected to lead some of the types of groups described.

## SUMMARY

A group is a collection of two or more people who are related in some way such as having a common task, a common characteristic, or a pattern of interaction. The structure of a group reflects its internal organization and the interrelationships of its members. Groups need to accomplish their tasks and, at the same time, consider the needs of the individual members. Leadership in a group is the process of moving toward the group goals. Leadership may be shared by the members or vested in an identified group member.

The nurse's understanding of group process is important to her own professional development since she will often be working in a group situation. Her understanding of available community groups, what they offer, how they function, and who is eligible to join, will enable her to refer clients to appropriate groups for help.

## LEARNING ACTIVITIES

1. What characteristics of group structure are important to the nurse in working with groups? Give a rationale for your answer.

2. What are the two major areas of group functioning and what roles are commonly identified in carrying out these functions?

3. You have been asked to lead a group to teach new mothers how to care for their infants prior to discharge from the hospital. What aspects of group leadership should you consider? How would you plan to implement such a task?

4. What types of health-related groups exist as resources in communities?

5. What do you, as a nurse, need to know about community support groups in order to use them for referrals?

## REFERENCES AND SUGGESTED READINGS

Bales, R. F., 1958.  Task roles and social roles in problem-solving groups. In E. E. Maccoby, T. M. Newcomb, and E. L. Hartley, eds., *Readings in social psy-*

*chology.* 3rd ed.    New York: Holt, Rinehart, and Winston.

Berne, Eric, 1963.    *The structure and dynamics of organizations and groups.*    New York: Grove Press.

Cartwright, D. and Zander, A., 1968.    *Group dynamics.* 3rd ed. New York: Harper and Row.

Knowles, M. and Knowles, H., 1969.    *Introduction to group dynamics.*    New York: Association Press.

Lewin, Kurt, 1958.    Group decision and social change. In E. E. Maccoby, T. M. Newcomb, and E. L. Hartley, eds., *Readings in social psychology.* 3rd ed. New York: Holt, Rinehart, and Winston.

Lifton, Walter M., 1961.    *Working with groups: group process and individual growth.* New York: John Wiley.

Marram, Gwen, 1973.    *The group approach in nursing practice.*    St. Louis: C. V. Mosby.

Mills, Theodore, 1967.    *The sociology of small groups.*    Englewood Cliffs, N. J.: Prentice-Hall.

*The Random House dictionary of the English language.*    New York: Random House, 1967, p. 625.

Sampson, Edward E. and Marthas, Marya S., 1977.    *Group process for the health professions.*    New York: John Wiley.

# 7

# The Community

## Behavioral Objectives

Upon completion of this chapter, the student will be able to:

1. Define the concept of a community.
2. Describe the basic functions of a community.
3. Do a community assessment at a beginning level.
4. Describe selected health-related community resources.
5. Describe selected nursing roles and responsibilities within the delivery of community health care.

## Key Terms

ambulatory health-care facility
community
community health center
extended-care facility
free clinics
health maintenance organization
home health care
official health agency
residential health care facility
voluntary health agency

## Introduction

The study of communities is common to many disciplines. In nursing, the specialty area of community-health nursing has historically combined the practice of nursing with the practice of public health. It is not the purpose of this chapter to address community health nursing in depth. Rather, we wish to introduce the beginning nursing student to the concept of the community and its functions as they relate to nursing practice.

In studying the structure and dynamics of a community, the nurse will notice that its characteristics develop and change as a community grows. Rapid change within our society has resulted in stress and sometimes in major upheavals in communities. Values have shifted in many areas from material concerns to those of self-actualization. Approaching crises of energy and environment further threaten ecology and community stability.

As a health professional concerned with all the factors that influence a client's ability to care for himself, the nurse needs to be aware of the community in which the client functions. Its resources and its limitations will be major determinants in the status of the client's health.

## CONCEPT OF A COMMUNITY

A community is generally defined as an aggregate of people who live in a defined location and share common values and beliefs. To study a community, it is important to look beyond the apparent characteristics and consider the interrelationships that exist as a result of the people and systems involved. For purposes of this chapter, a community is defined as "people and the relationships that emerge among them as they develop and use in common some agencies and institutions and a physical environment" (Reinhardt and Quinn, 1977).

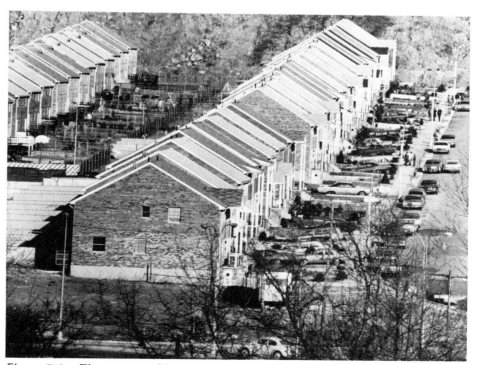

**Figure 7-1.**   *The resources and limitations of the client's community are major determinants of the client's health status.   (United Press International photo)*

In addition to interrelationships within themselves, communities sit in relationship to organizations outside themselves. The small neighborhood group is also part of a city, state, national, and international community. All of these levels, however remote they seem, can impinge on the character and resources of a community. An example of this is the effect which legislation on National Health Insurance will have on services available to residents of even the smallest communities.

## COMMUNITY FUNCTION

The major functions of a community are generally considered to be:

1.  the production, distribution, and consumption of services and goods
2.  the socialization or transfer of values to members
3.  the social control of members to protect conformity to norms
4.  the social interaction between members
5.  the mutual support of members in times of crisis (Warren, 1973).

These functions have implications for nursing and other health professions. The production and distribution of services and goods becomes a major source of employment in a community. Health maintenance considerations, such as industrial safety and mental health of workers, must be considered. Consumer reactions within a community reflect the level of awareness among residents regarding the quality, as well as the quantity, of goods being produced. Health education regarding these is often one of the nurse's responsibilities.

Socialization, or transfer of values to community members, is especially visible in reference to the raising of children. The curriculum of the public school system generally reflects the prevailing community attitudes. Families with a close sense of community identity are often very active in the educational system and in other community affairs in an effort to assure that their children are taught values acceptable to the families. Newcomers to a community may have to take some time to validate values before participating in active community projects that reflect socialization. The nurse who wants to introduce or reinforce health-related values in a school or a community will also have to consider the prevailing norms of the community group and its attitudes toward health-related issues.

Social control of community members includes more than police policy. Regulation of health-related matters, such as those pertaining to communicable disease, air pollution, and traffic safety, are examples of social control that directly concern standards of health.

Social interaction among community members can be seen formally in many forms of communicating, such as media, public forums, and planned recreational programs. Less formal social interactions are seen in neighborhood cliques, special interest groups, and small voluntary groups. Health-related issues are often subject to the influence of these groups.

The mutual support of community members in times of crisis is also seen in both formal and informal levels. Death, sickness, and natural disaster, which highlight human need, also provide opportunity for community members to share resources with other members. A sense of community, or lack of this, can be seen in times of disaster.

## COMMUNITY ASSESSMENT

As nursing students increase their assessment skills and the scope of their practice, they are able to assess the health needs and resources of communities. They can then plan, in collaboration with other health professionals and community members, for appropriate measures to meet selected health needs within communities. A comprehensive community assessment for major health planning would be beyond the scope of this book. The type of community assessment considered here is limited to identifying easily available community data. This will enable a beginning student to understand the community where her clients live and thus be better able to understand the environmental context in which they function. It is important to be aware of the community resources available to support and supplement needed nursing care.

One of the best ways to get the "feel" as well as the "facts" about a community is to walk through the neighborhood and observe. See the physical characteristics—listen to the sounds—speak with the residents—smell the air. Census data and historical information for communities is available at local government offices and libraries. Health-related facts are found at local health departments. The strengths of a community are at least as important as its problems. A suggested guide for community assessment is presented in Table 7-1.

In assessing a community, it is helpful to have a systematic framework. It must be remembered that, although such a framework serves as an organizational guide, a community is an ever-changing phenomenon and thus the assessment process is ongoing. It is also important to define why the community is being assessed. Defining the purpose of the assessment gives a focus to the data collection, allows a highlighting of relevant information, and screens out that which is unnecessary. Examples of ways in which a nurse would use data from a community assessment are described in the following paragraphs.

Environmental data would be a major influence in a family with children afflicted with allergies. House structure and age, the presence of pollen and molds, and the general air quality would need careful analysis in relation to the allergy problems. The type of housing available for the elderly and handicapped of all ages is another environmental reality with which the nurse in the community must be concerned, especially in planning for home care.

Table 7-1    Suggested Guide for Collection of Data for Community
             Assessment

**1. Physical Environmental Data**

    a. Geography (land description, natural resources)

    b. Housing (types and numbers of dwellings)

    c. Pollution indices (water, air, solid waste disposal)

**2. Population Characteristics**

    a. Demography (statistics on marriage, divorce, births, deaths, disease)

    b. Age and sex distribution

    c. Socioeconomic characteristics (levels of education and income, job opportunities, size of families)

    d. Cultural patterns (ethnic groups, historical data, community heritage)

    e. Patterns of wellness and illness (values, health and illness roles, lifestyles)

**3. Agencies and Institutions**

    a. Educational facilities (pre-school through college, continuing education, special education)

    b. Health care services (private, official, voluntary)

    c. Libraries (references, media, mobile facilities)

    d. Spiritual facilities (churches, prayer groups)

    e. Social services (welfare programs, day care)

    f. Recreational facilities (private and public)

    g. Protective services (police, fire)

**4. Community Relationships**

    a. Political system (power bases, political process)

    b. Channels of communication available (newspapers, radio, and TV stations)

    c. Decision-making process: how do members of community accomplish goals?

Population characteristics can give the nurse a general profile of community character. A client who is being treated for heart disease in a clinic may need considerable guidance and support in adjusting his dietary habits and physical activity to cope with the limitations of his illness. If his income is limited, and the eating habits of his family and cultural group include many items that are high in sodium and fat, needed changes in lifestyle will be very difficult. This may cause added stress to the client by making him "different" from the people he needs to be close to, and an added financial "burden" because of his dietary needs. In assisting a client with these problems, the nurse's awareness of his cultural and economic background, as well as his health-related values, will be important to planning appropriate behavior changes with the client and making him aware of available and acceptable community resources.

The agencies and institutions within a community represent the community's organized efforts to help members maintain a desirable standard of living. Of primary interest to the nurse, as a health-care provider, are the health-care services. These may be residential or ambulatory and will offer many levels of health care. Although only 5 percent of health care is provided by hospitals, this is the agency most frequently identified as an expected setting for nurses. Hospitals do employ a larger portion of available nurses than any other type of health-care agency. In addition to the well-known general hospital, there may be hospitals specializing in specific types of health problems such as orthopedics, mental illness, or chronic illness. Extended care facilities and nursing homes also provide residential nursing care.

Nonresidential facilities, such as community health centers, outpatient clinics of hospitals, health maintenance organizations, and "free clinics" may be found in communities. A high percentage of health care is given in the offices of private doctors. A relatively new community service is developing in the surgical centers, where minor surgery is done on a daily basis and the client is discharged by evening.

In addition to knowing what health services are available, the nurse needs to be aware of the needed referral system to utilize services. Understanding the dynamics of a specific health care delivery system, its criteria for eligibility, and its appropriateness for specific patients, is a basic nursing skill in any setting.

Community agencies that are not specific to health care nevertheless are important to persons concerned with the maintenance of health. Social, spiritual, and recreational facilities are crucial to maintenance of mental health, while educational and library resources stimulate and assist in the maintenance of intellectual development. Protective services work closely with health services, especially in times of disaster.

Fragmentation of community services has been an undesired result of increasing specialization of services. A well-organized and visible referral system can counteract this fragmentation. Understanding and utilizing the community's interagency referral system is essential to planning and implementing the nursing process in the community.

Identifying relationships within a community is perhaps the most challenging aspect of a community assessment. Yet, it is essential that the nurse understand where the power and decision-making centers of a community are located. These functions may be done by key people, or groups of people. Knowledge of group functioning and leadership (Ch. 6) enables the nurse not only to influence health-related policies but also to identify for clients ways in which they can make the existing community system work for them.

## NURSING ROLES AND RESPONSIBILITIES IN COMMUNITIES

Nurses practicing in community settings may be found in many and varied roles. However, the nursing process remains basically the same regardless of setting. Freeman (1970) describes the process of nursing in communities as beginning with the establishment of a relationship, including an outreach on the part of the nurse towards the client, prior to beginning the nursing assessment. In contrast to the client in a hospital or residential facility, the ambulatory client has more freedom to leave—or stay away from—the health-care system if he is not comfortable with the nursing interaction and other health-related services. Although it is always desirable to work on an interpersonal relationship prior to making a nursing assessment, it becomes imperative to do this in many community situations.

In addition to functioning in the health agencies previously mentioned, the nurse in the community is also found in schools, places of work, and in homes. Home visiting is a substantial part of the work of most public health nurses and visiting nurses. Home visits can provide actual nursing care—the "laying on of hands"—or provide health education and anticipatory guidance to individuals and families. The nurse making a home visit also assumes responsibility for casefinding—the recognition of health problems that are not yet being treated.

An introductory description of nursing roles in the community would be incomplete without mention of the emergence of the independent nurse practitioners, practicing alone or in a group practice. There are many legal, economic, and political issues that remain to be resolved in different locations before the independent practitioner is fully incorporated into the health-care system (Zahourek *et al.*, 1976). But this nursing resource is on its way to becoming an asset to the delivery of nursing in communities.

## SUMMARY

A community is an aggregate that includes people, physical environment, agencies and institutions, and the interrelationships of all of these. The functions of a community are the production, distribution, and consumption of services and goods; the socialization and social control of members; the social interaction between members; and the support of members in times of crisis. Assessment of a community enables the nurse to utilize the existing community forces, its assets, and its liabilities, to better plan for nursing interventions.

Health-related community resources may be residential or ambulatory, official or voluntary, and provide a variety of health-care services to community residents. The role of the nurse in a community setting includes an outreach to the client in the community as a preliminary step in the nursing process. Knowledge of the community is crucial to implementation of the nursing process and understanding of the client's frame of reference.

## LEARNING ACTIVITIES

1.  What are the essential elements included in the concept of a community?
2.  What functions are communities commonly expected to achieve? Give some examples of how these functions could relate to health concerns.

3.  With a fellow nursing student, investigate a community of your choice. Based on your investigation, prepare a simple assessment of this community, using the guide suggested.

4.  Describe five health-related community resources in the community of your choice. Include in your description any specific criteria necessary for utilization of each resource.

5.  Identify considerations applicable to the nursing process in a school setting, an occupational health setting, and a home.

## REFERENCES AND SUGGESTED READINGS

Brownlee, A., 1978.  *Community, culture and care.*  St. Louis: C. V. Mosby.

Freeman, Ruth, 1970.  *Community health nursing practice.*  Philadelphia: W. B. Saunders.

Futrell, M. and Kelleher, M., 1973.  *The nurse's guide to health services for patients.* Boston: Little, Brown.

Hall, J. and Weaver, B., 1977.  *A systems approach to community health.*  Philadelphia: J. B. Lippincott.

Reinhardt, A. and Quinn, M., 1977.  *Current practice in family-centered community nursing.*  St. Louis: C. V. Mosby.

Tinkham, C. and Voorhies, E., 1977.  *Community health nursing: evolution and process.* 2nd ed. New York: Appleton-Century-Crofts.

Warren, R. E., 1973.  *The community in America.* 2nd ed. New York: Rand McNally.

Warren, R. L., 1965.  *Studying your community.*  New York: The Free Press.

Zahourek, R.; Leone, D.; and Lang, F., 1976.  *Creative health services: a model for group nursing practice.*  St. Louis: C. V. Mosby.

# 8

# Cultural Implications in Nursing

## Behavioral Objectives

Upon completion of this chapter, the student will be able to:

1. Define the concept of culture.
2. Describe the effects of cultural diversity on health-care delivery.
3. Describe the health attitudes of the major cultural groups.
4. Discuss the role of time, family, and religion in the specific culture groups.
5. Discuss general nursing considerations for health care in a culturally diverse society.

## Key Terms

| | | |
|---|---|---|
| attitudes | ethnic | Shintoism |
| beliefs | ideal culture | stoic |
| Confucianism | indigenous | subculture |
| cultural | ritual | Taoism |

## Introduction

An understanding of cultural diversity is basic to quality health care in the United States today. Nursing is the pioneer health profession in taking a

111

position regarding inclusion of ethnic and cultural content in its education programs, both in schools of nursing and in the clinical settings.

Early in the twentieth century, nursing's focus was on the physical well-being of the client. Nurses functioned as "handmaidens" to the physician, carrying out orders regarding the comfort, cleanliness, and physical care of the person. During this phase in nursing history the health practices of the client were not considered important. A "good patient" was one who followed the orders of the medical team. The doctor-nurse health representatives knew what was best for the client.

After World War II, new ideas began to emerge concerning the needs of individuals seeking to enter the health-care system. The growing field of psychology placed importance on the nonphysical needs of the individual. Nursing began to emphasize these identified psychological needs and became concerned with the psychological as well as the physical parts of the person.

In the 1960s political unrest, concern for the social welfare of persons in this country, and both violent and peaceful racial protest caused professionals in the health-care system to look again at the most important and often least considered element of the health-care hierarchy—the client.

Nursing identified the fragmentation of the client which had occurred through: the use of the medical model for diagnosing and treatment planning; the isolation of the client from his family and social group once he entered the system; and the belief that the professional person always knew what was best for the client.

Social change within the larger cultural system led the way to changes in subsystems of the culture. Nursing began to move into an era of self-identification, a time when it became important to define nursing, state professional beliefs, and delineate specific behaviors that belong to nursing.

One of the outcomes of this era in nursing was the identification of nursing's roles and responsibilities with respect to the client. Nursing defined itself as a humanistic profession, seeing the client as a whole person and not some fragmented part. However, making statements or taking positions does not make changes occur. In the past few years, it has become necessary for nursing to identify certain areas which have not been included in nursing education and practice and that have thwarted the effort to consider the "holistic" approach to nursing. Cultural diversity, as one of the most important elements of any nurse-client relationship, was missing in nearly all forms of the nursing profession: literature, education, and practice.

This chapter will introduce the student to the concept of culture, as an umbrella under which such subconcepts as ethnicity, religious beliefs, and ritualism are contained.

## CULTURE DEFINED

Most anthropologists and sociologists have a similar but not identical definition of culture. Some essential ingredients seem to appear in all definitions:

1. Culture is a universal experience.
2. Each culture is unique to its particular group.
3. Culture is stable but not static.
4. Culture encompasses and largely determines one's life, yet is rarely consciously noted (Leininger, 1970).

From these four ingredients it is possible to derive a definition suitable to nursing and health. Culture is a way of life for any designated group's values, attitudes, and beliefs utilizing the heritage of the people to maintain stability. When referring to a group's values or value system, one is generally talking about the group norms or group conception of how people should behave in certain situations and what kinds of goals they should pursue. For example, the American middle-class culture values college education and certain professions such as doctors and lawyers. Attitudes speak to the position the group takes regarding values and beliefs. Beliefs of a cultural system are convictions the group has regarding its members. These convictions are handed down through generations as traditions: for example, teaching a child to trust his parents.

The larger cultural system may have subsystems or subcultural groups. A subgroup is usually comprised of persons who have a distinct identity in some area of their lives but still are related to the larger culture in many ways. Such a group generally cannot maintain its existence without reference to the larger cultural system with its values and practices. Examples of subcultural groups in the United States are: Afro-Americans, feminists, nurses, physicians, persons of the same socioeconomic status or with similar occupations or goals.

## EFFECTS OF CULTURE ON THE HEALTH-CARE SYSTEM

Certain characteristics are true of all cultures. If nursing is to be effective in its delivery of health care then there must be a basic understanding of man and why he behaves as he does. Culture and behavior are closely related.

All cultures have a language by which persons communicate to and with each other and with persons from other cultures. Language includes the spoken word, art forms, games, and rituals. This language is the key to knowing and learning about the needs of the divergent cultural groups who enter the health-care system.

In the United States today, there are distinct cultural groups whose values and beliefs the nurse needs to know about. This section will attempt to discuss these groups based upon certain common divisions: time, group orientation, religious or spiritual beliefs, and health practices. Because generally there is not a conscious awareness of the dominant American cultural group, it will be discussed first and serve as a frame of reference for the others.

## AMERICAN MIDDLE-CLASS CULTURE

This is the main cultural reference group in the United States. All other groups take their value and belief orientation from this larger group. Many persons in the lower socioeconomic group seek to be like the major reference group, while those in the upper socioeconomic group rely upon this group for position and identity. The ethnic groups attempt to assimilate the dominant cultural mores (Papajohn and Spiegel, 1975).

### Time

The American is concerned with time in several ways: future is more important than past or even present; time is to be used productively for future goals, not to be wasted; it is important to be on time and to do things by a timed schedule. Americans have more clocks and watches than any other culture. Everyone has at least one clock, most persons wear watches and radio announcers give the exact time regularly. In personal life meals are eaten "on time," children fed by a timed routine, and some persons organize their entire lives by a definite schedule. Medicine and nursing is a prime example of time importance. Hospitals and clinics have specific times for appointments, tests and procedures, medications and treatments. The nurse finds herself living by a very organized, timed schedule day in and day out. But what of the client who does not understand this time orientation? The Latin American person, for example, who values relationships and the present more than time and future, does not share this concern for time. There is the possibility of conflict when a person of this culture enters the health-care system.

### Group Orientation

Americans pride themselves on being individualists. Independence and self-identity receive priority over the group. Thus, such notions as terming the 1970s the "era of the self" enter into everyday thinking. What about this concept of individuality? It has its history, no doubt, in the early trail blazers of this country who were lauded as rugged individualists. There is a certain amount of ambivalence in this belief, however, since Americans feel they must be independent and belong at the same time.

Fromm (1956) wrote about the person's need to belong, not to be separate. He said the following about the individual in a democratic society such as this one:

> Most people are not even aware of their need to conform. They live under the illusion that they follow their own ideas and inclinations, that they are individualists, that they have arrived at their opinions as the result of their

own thinking—and that it just happens that their ideas are the same as those of the majority. (Fromm, 1956, p. 14)

In nursing, the culturally diverse client who must consult the family or larger community before coming to a decision may be seen as lacking in character and strength because he cannot make his own decision. The nurse who understands the importance of the larger group to other cultures will not be as apt to misjudge this person.

The family is a type of group. In middle-class America the family is usually comprised of mother, father, and children under the age of 18. Kinship ties and extended family are not valued as highly as in some cultures (Asian, Latin, Indian). Since the future is more important than the past, one sees the tendency to devalue opinions and experiences of older persons. The American nuclear family is an independent, isolated unit dependent upon itself for social and economic sustenance. There are no binding relational rules that make it necessary that relatives accept one another and get along.

When the family consists of a husband and wife, the husband is considered responsible for the welfare of the wife and children, even though the wife may work. The father usually works away from the home and is isolated from his family for the greater part of each day. Emotional isolation from relatives, for both husband and wife, seems to increase with age. By middle adulthood it is not unusual to find that persons are closer to friends and co-workers than to siblings or cousins.

The mother in the middle-class culture is expected to place the interest of the group (family) above her own. She is not to be too autonomous or too individualistic. This is changing, but not rapidly.

This is a culture where rewards are given to the successful people who are viewed as goal-oriented, forward-moving, doers and achievers, interested in personal advancement and success.

Certain values characterize the society in general. Cleanliness is a dominant value closely related to optimal health and physical well-being. Physical health is to be sought after and cherished. Thus the government, a middle-class bureaucratic organization, involves itself in health matters such as physical fitness, anti-smoking, and clean air.

## Religious or Spiritual Beliefs

The middle-class American culture is comprised mainly of Protestant denominations, Roman Catholics, and persons of the Jewish faith. In most instances the church or religion is an integrated part of the individual and family life. Persons are more concerned with how their religion can assist them today and in the future than with past history.

## Health Practices

In the American middle-class culture health is another dominant value. Optimal health is considered to be a prescribed right and value for all

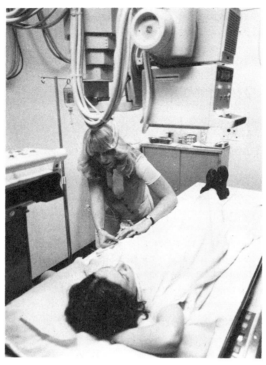

**Figure 8-1.** *In the middle-class culture, optimal health is maintained through regular health checkups. (Paul S. Conklin/Monkmeyer Press Photo Service)*

Americans. This could be considered one of the elements of the *ideal* cultural beliefs for Americans. The ideal culture comprises beliefs, values, practices, and feelings the people consider desirable, but these are not always practiced in reality. Thus, it is believed that all persons have the right to optimal health, but the means for achieving this are not available to all members of the culture. Some major attitudes toward health are:

**1.** Mastery of the environment is more important than adjusting to it. Thus, illness and disease are seen as challenges to be mastered through research, scientific study, formation of foundations and funds, and bureaucratic control through agencies for protection of the citizen. Examples of these are the Cancer Institute, the March of Dimes, the Food and Drug Administration, Easter Seals, and the Jerry Lewis Muscular Dystrophy Telethon.

**2.** Illness is a challenge to be overcome. The general attitude is that the weak (sick) are to help themselves as much as possible. The strong will help the weak only if their problems are caused by circumstances beyond their control. If the illness or problem is due to lack of "will power" or "inner strength" the person is devalued. Thus, an injury suffered from an industrial accident will receive more support than the illness of a "skid row" alcoholic.

**3.** Ill persons are expected to want to get well. Persons who are ill are less likely to be kept within the family. They are often sent away to some health institution to "get better." Isolation from the family is a general practice as shown by the emphasis on hospitals, sanitariums, and nursing homes. Dependency and illness are discouraged at all times (Murray and Zentner, 1979).

The belief in optimal health is exemplified by the demand for total health insurance coverage for the middle-class American. Health facilities are modern and readily available in areas of the country where the largest representations of the dominant cultural group are located—cities, large university/medical complexes, and suburban counties. Americans place great emphasis on physical exercise, vitamin ingestion, and regular health check-ups. One irony in these beliefs about health is the difficulty the health-care system has in convincing persons that prevention is the best route to optimal health. Americans overeat, overdrink, and smoke to dangerous excess, and then expect the medical personnel to cure the ills. In other cultural orientations one sees persons practicing prevention through careful control of excesses in diet, drink, and emotional outbursts. These persons are often viewed by Americans as lacking in ability to enjoy life or to recognize the "good things in life."

It is important for the student to recognize that Americans within the poverty range, although they are said to have the right to optimal health according to the cultural ideal, are not given avenues for achieving this ideal. Thus, the orientation toward health of ethnic persons of color and poverty groups, such as residents of Appalachia, are often different from those of the dominant culture.

## SPANISH-AMERICAN CULTURE

This cultural specification includes the three main subcultural groups in the United States: Mexican-Americans, Spanish-Americans, and South Americans. The majority of the persons in this cultural group are located in New Mexico, Arizona, Texas, Southern and Central California, Southern Colorado, and the coast of Florida. Some larger cities on the east coast attract smaller subgroups, for example, metropolitan New York and Washington, D.C. have Spanish-American populations.

Although each subcultural group has its own unique cultural mores, there are certain values and beliefs fundamental to the larger cultural group. These will be discussed here. The student is encouraged to research more specifically those subgroups indigenous to her geographic area.

### Time

In general the culture emphasizes the present. Little attention is paid to the past (it cannot be changed) and the future is seen as vague and unpredictable (it cannot be manipulated, what will be will be). People do not plan for the future, but only hope it will be better than the past or present. There is a belief that man does not have control over his own destiny.

## Group Orientation

The extended family and the church are important socializing systems. Individualism is devalued and dependence on the group is bred into the person from birth. Respect for the elderly is seen in the dominant role of grandparents, aunts, and uncles as rulers of the family.

It is a patriarchal system where the father has responsibility for guidance, leadership, and decision-making. In Spanish-American communities, the kinship network is evident in the sharing of responsibility for child-rearing and discipline. The relationship lines between cousins are unclear and everyone is like a brother or sister to everyone else.

The woman is expected to bear children and care for the home and family. Only the eldest son is allowed to have any authority or control and this is usually in the absence of the father through death or debilitating illness.

## Religious or Spiritual Beliefs

Most Spanish-Americans are Roman Catholic. However, the ties to the church are less powerful than in the past. There is less ritualism and less

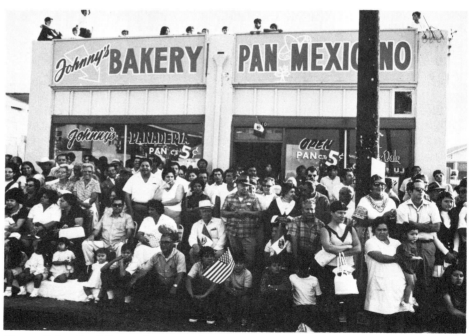

**Figure 8-2.** *For Mexican-Americans, the group is an important cultural foundation.* (Batzdorf/ Monkmeyer Press Photo Service)

idolization of the clergy. The health beliefs and practices of this culture are strongly influenced by the religious heritage.

## Health Practices

The Spanish-American is not concerned with the concept of "better health." He views man as basically bad and normal health as always subject to attack. The attack is caused by unknown external forces. Illness is considered a part of life, and man has little control over nature and God.

Health is seen as a state of balance between mind and body. If a person is sturdy, able to work, and can maintain normal activities with an absence of pain, he is healthy. The ill person is cared for by the family. Since illness is believed to be caused by external natural forces such as cold, heat, storms, water, or sinning, indigenous health practitioners are the first to treat the illness.

Some examples of beliefs about disease causation are:

**1.** Evil eye, *mal ojo,* (măl oho) a disease caused by a person looking admiringly at another's child. To break the spell the person must pat the child's head. Children are not directly admired in the Spanish-American culture, so unlike the extremes of admiration Americans heap on all children. A nurse who admires a Spanish-American child will be giving the child *mal ojo,* if she is not aware of this belief.

**2.** *Susto* is a common illness with symptoms of agitation and depression. It is believed to be caused by a frightening experience, and can result in death.

**3.** *Empacho* is a gastrointestinal upset caused by overeating, eating disliked foods, or eating hot bread.

The head of the house, usually the oldest man, decides if illness is present and what treatment is necessary. Very little attention is paid to minor aches, pains, colds, or stomach upsets. Being ill brings no special considerations. Usually folk remedies are tried first: wearing of healing objects, medals, special jewelry or articles of clothing, and ingestion of specific preparations. Indigenous practitioners administer herbals, poultices, infusions, and topical cures. Massage and manipulation are also used. Some of the names for folk practitioners are *sobador,* a massage specialist; *partera,* a midwife; *medico,* a general specialist in folk medicine; *curandero,* a specialist with the gift to cure given by God; *albolario,* a specialist in the treatment of victims of witchcraft.

The Spanish-American must be gravely ill to seek professional medical care. Operations are seen as a threat to body wholeness and are to be avoided at all cost.

**Nursing Considerations**   The nurse who is concerned with health-care delivery in a Spanish-American community will need to give full consideration to the role of the family and the community in health delivery. Advice and suggestions are more acceptable than directions and orders. The inclusion of the indigenous health practitioners in planning and implementing care will build trust between the nurse and the clients.

Ritualism is an important ingredient in the culture. Therefore, when the nurse is involved in health teaching, ritualistic plans will be learned and practiced more readily. Rituals offer one a sense of security and provide guidelines for specific actions.

Finally, the nurse must consider local social and cultural practices and their relationship to stress and illness. One important way to gain this knowledge is to visit the homes of clients on a regular basis.

From this discussion the nurse can recognize certain important cultural differences which have implications for health delivery:

1. surgical procedures cause extreme anxiety because of the threat to body wholeness
2. the wholeness of the body is related to external forces, especially of heat and cold (e.g. if one's feet get wet it is important to wet the head to create a balance and prevent a sore throat)
3. illness may be viewed as a punishment from God
4. additional special situations: e.g. during the 40-day post partum period a woman should not expose herself to any situation where bad air (*mal aire*) might enter the vagina. Thus, bathing in a tub or shower is not done.


## ASIAN-AMERICAN CULTURE

In this discussion Asian-Americans include Chinese, Japanese, and Vietnamese cultural influences.

### Time

The major emphasis in this cultural orientation is on the past. Ancestors and tradition are very important to the culture. This can be seen in the strong relationship of ancient religious beliefs which influence present lifestyle, such as Confucianism, Shinto practices, and ancestor worship.

### Group Orientation

The family and kinship network is all important. The elderly and the father are traditionally given the authority positions in the family. In the Vietnamese family, honor of father and mother is the foundation of all family relationships. The family is the main unit of ownership, production, and management. Thus, the Asian cultures encourage dependence on the group and discourage individualism. Tradition is the key concept.

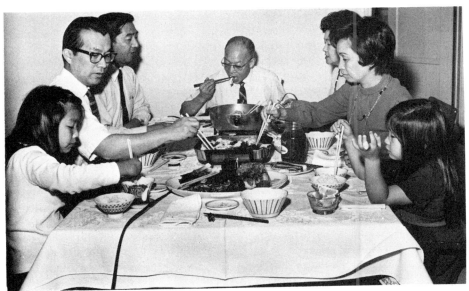

Figure 8-3.   *Tradition helps to maintain the family and kinship network important in the Asian-American culture.   (Fujihira/Monkmeyer Press Photo Service)*

## Religious or Spiritual Beliefs

Ancient religions are still the basis for most spiritual beliefs. Japanese believe in a body-mind-spirit relationship strongly tied to magicoreligious teachings of Shintoism, the state religion of Japan until 1945. Shintoism worshipped Emperor, ancestor, ancient hero, and nature. Those who follow this belief have intense loyalty and devotion to nature's gifts—lakes, trees, and blossoms—and a great concern for cleanliness, a reflection of ancient ideas surrounding dread of pollution in the dead (Murray and Zenter, 1979).

The Vietnamese reflect the strong influence of Confucianism with its emphasis on the family unit. The Chinese are influenced by the teaching of Confucius as well as by Taoism. More representative of Taoism than Confucianism is the yin/yang belief. Yang is represented by light or red and yin is dark. The belief is that everything exists in these two interacting forces with each representing specific qualities. Yang is positive or masculine—dry, hot, active, moving, and light. Yin is negative or feminine, wet, cold, passive, restful, and empty. The combination of the two represents all possible dualisms: day/night, summer/winter, health/illness, etc. (Murray and Zentner, 1979).

## Health Practices

In general the Asian cultures stress physical fitness and discipline in daily habits. Highly valued are the mental, spiritual, and esthetic aspects of the person. It is the duty of each person to maintain an even temper and to be fair to all persons.

From early childhood the individual is taught not to show emotion. This is especially true in minimizing responses to sickness or injury. Many Americans see the Asian person as stoic because of a lack of emotional display in times considered appropriate for such behavior—crying in pain, yelling in anger. In reality, this is a culturally prescribed (learned) behavior. What the individual may feel inside is not shown.

The Asian culture stresses respect for the individual and reverence for the body. Health practices and beliefs are often a mixture of ancient customs and religious beliefs.

**Nursing Considerations** In contacts with a person from the Asian-American culture the nurse will want to remember that it is a cultural imperative that a person does not show emotion such as reactions to pain, fear, embarrassment, or indignities caused by misunderstandings between the client and the staff. Tradition and family are very important. Often when a person of an Asian culture is ill, a female member of the family will want to care for the client and even prepare food at home to bring to the client. Males are not accustomed to having females tell them what to do nor are they prepared for the businesslike curtness of a hospital routine.

From this discussion then the nurse can anticipate certain needs of the Asian-American client that would enhance the planning and implementation of nursing care. Some of these needs are:

1. respect the individual and family
2. always address the client and adult family members by their given names
3. knock before entering the room of the client
4. attempt to discuss plans with the client rather than give directions or orders
5. be aware of times when the client (or family) might be under extreme stress but would not show it, and therefore, would not ask questions or lodge a complaint. For example, the client may not ask for pain medication, the nurse would have to assess the need by questioning the client.

Some of the above needs are ones that nursing should always practice with all clients. Although this is always desirable, in the case of the Asian-American it becomes imperative to ensure against offending the dignity of the person. Extra concern for the self-respect of the individual is appropriate here.

## AMERICAN-INDIAN CULTURE

The American Indian has the only culture that is truly indigenous to the continent of North America. Due to circumstances of war, occupation, and eventual disinheritance, the American-Indian tribes have become isolated subcultures of the larger cultural system. All Indians share beliefs and values of the dominant culture; however, each tribe is unique in its language, customs, and rituals. The nurse needs to have a general knowledge of Indian culture which can then be focused on a specific tribe should the need arise.

## Time

The American Indian is not generally future oriented; instead, each day is taken as it comes. Many Indian homes have no clock as time is relative and individuals focus on what needs to be done. The Indian lives each day to its fullest, not concerned with tomorrow. Since time is a continuum with no beginning and no end, this concept can present problems for the nurse. For example, the Indian does not eat meals according to a schedule; today he might eat two meals and tomorrow four. If a medication is prescribed to be taken with meals this can present a problem to the nurse who does not understand the time concept.

## Group Orientation

The family and the tribe are of the greatest importance to the Indian. Relatives are involved in all aspects of child-rearing and family care. For

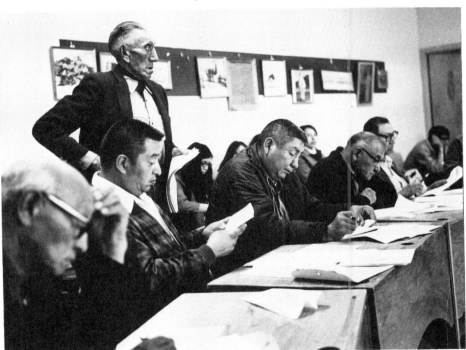

**Figure 8-4.** *A tribal council meeting epitomizes the group organization of the American Indian culture. (Michal Heron/Monkmeyer Press Photo Service)*

example, Indian grandmothers occupy positions of great importance in child-rearing. In some tribes the grandmother must grant permission for a child to be hospitalized for health care.

The Indian kinship system often involves aunts, uncles, and cousins being labelled as brothers and sisters. A child may have several sets of grandparents if they have all been involved in the rearing and care of the child.

Child-rearing is different from that of the dominant American culture too. Indian children are considered assets and the child is encouraged to be independent, and adept in self-care and in the care of others, especially other family members. Respect and courtesy are fundamental concepts to the Indian and are often misinterpreted as indifference by the Anglo person.

## Religious or Spiritual Beliefs

There is little distinction between medicine and religion for the Indian. Rituals and elaborate "sing" or healing ceremonies are prevalent practices in some tribes.

The Indian sees death as a natural part of the life cycle and, therefore, does not protect children from the experience. Death is the time for going to the other world of long-ago ancestors. Funerals usually take place in the home with elaborate feasts and gift-giving. Some tribes still prepare the body according to tribal tradition. It is important for persons from other cultures to be aware of the need for body integrity even after death. An amputated limb, for example, must be properly buried so that later when the individual dies he can be buried with his limb.

## Health Practices

Central to Indian health practices are the medicine man, the use of ritual "sing" and healing ceremonies, and the presence of family members in the room with the sick person. The nurse who is aware of Indian practices will respect them and make certain that time and space are provided for the specific ceremonies. For example, in most tribal cultures there are sacred foods often used in healing ceremonies. Corn is one of these foods, and cornmeal may be sprinkled on the floor in the hospital room. The nurse needs to respect this ritual and inquire from the family regarding the disposition of the cornmeal. In some instances it can be discarded, but in others it must be collected and placed in a proper container at the bedside.

Nursing Considerations   Although generalizations are possible regarding American-Indian cultures, each nurse must become familiar with the unique tribal practices in her geographic area. The Navajo, for example, places great importance on modesty. The nurse must ask permission before carrying out any bathing procedure, because disrobing in front of strangers causes great discomfort.

From this discussion, the nurse can anticipate the need to become familiar with tribal customs and rituals if health-care and teaching are to be effective:

1. health teaching or treatment involving the concept of time should employ sunrise and sunset, seasons, and monthly cycles as well as clocks

2. the use of an indigenous dietary aide for special diet-teaching is very important

3. there must be side-by-side cooperation of Anglo medical practitioners and the medicine man

4. there must be recognition of the necessity for body integrity at all times. For example, the hair cleaned from a brush of a Navajo Indian must be saved for proper disposal by the Navajo.

## PUERTO RICAN AND AFRO-AMERICAN CULTURES

For each area of the country there are specific subcultures, all of which cannot be discussed in this chapter. An interesting phenomenon that occurs is the relationship between social class and ethnic groups of color. In the United States, this relationship is obvious to the student of sociology or anthropology, particularly in relation to Afro-Americans and Puerto Ricans. The Appalachian is a subculture distinguished on the basis of social class. However, should an Appalachian individual leave his area and succeed in dominant middle-class culture, it would be difficult to distinguish him from another middle-class American. If a person is of a different color from the dominant cultural group, the distinction is made before social class can even be established. Branch (1978) has stated that America is a racist society because of continuous subtle and not-so-subtle learned attitudes and behaviors about ethnic groups. In this society the great separator is color.

With these thoughts in mind, the student will be able to begin an examination of her personal attitudes and beliefs as they relate to ethnic groups of color, persons considered within the parameters of poverty, and groups who, because of seemingly positive values and beliefs, are differentiated on this basis (i.e. Jewish or Arabic persons).

### Puerto Rican Culture

This section will be concerned with the Puerto Rican who resides in the United States. It is necessary to understand some basic political information in order to fully appreciate the confusion some Puerto Ricans feel regarding their personal rights in the United States. Puerto Rico is a territory of the United States. Although the people are citizens of the United States, those who live on the island do not vote in federal elections of pay federal income taxes.

In Puerto Rico, the social structure for the average person is not as strong or as well-supported as some of the other cultures discussed. Time is of a present, here-and-now orientation, and there is little conception of future. The person does not generally feel pressed for time. The family is an extended one, but it is easily strained by disagreements between the relatives of the wife and the relatives of the husband. The fragility of this network seems to be the result of the great size of the extended family and the lack of a definite and stable line of authority.

The male authority line has been weakened over time by an historical lack of support for legal (binding) marriage. Thus, the male may have a consensual (common-law) marriage with a wife and children, and also maintain at least one mistress and children. The financial stress of such an arrangement may be one reason that Puerto Ricans began to migrate to the large cities of the United States. New York City is the most outstanding example.

The migration to large cities led to the development of subcultures of poverty-stricken Puerto Ricans shocked by the vast differences in values, attitudes, and beliefs of themselves, of the dominant culture, and of the Black subculture with which they competed for survival. One of the outstanding consequences of this migration was the further breakdown in the family. Along with this was the inner feeling of desolation and isolation. In order to survive, future orientation would have to be learned. Health-care personnel who recognize the signs of culture shock or culture depression are in a position to begin teaching so that a community network of support can eventually evolve.

## Afro-American Culture

Branch (1978) adeptly made the point that this is the only culturally diverse group in the American melting pot that did not choose to come to this country. This may have something to do with the problem of assimilation, although one would be naive to discount the obvious difference in color. Historically, the status of the Afro-American, that of a slave, and the numerous myths about his intelligence, body differences, and origins have compounded the existing prejudices.

It is true that legislatively and legally great strides have been made to protect the rights of all minorities, specifically ethnic groups of color. As has been previously noted, legislation cannot change what a person has learned and believes from his culture.

The Black person in America occupies positions at all socioeconomic levels. In health-care delivery the nurse will be in contact with Black persons from many countries and ethnic backgrounds—African, West Indian, Bahamian— and all socioeconomic levels. Each of these groups is unique in values, beliefs, and mores. It is important for the nurse to respect differences among persons and to find out from them their particular needs and beliefs.

Some diseases or illnesses seem to be more prevalent in one group or culture than another. Sickle-cell anemia is indigenous to Mediterranean persons and persons from tropical areas. One disease that seems to be of particularly high incidence in the Black population in the United States is hypertension. It is believed that this is closely related to the stresses of poverty—poor diet, lack of exercise, crowding, inadequate leisure time, and continuous feelings of low self-esteem.

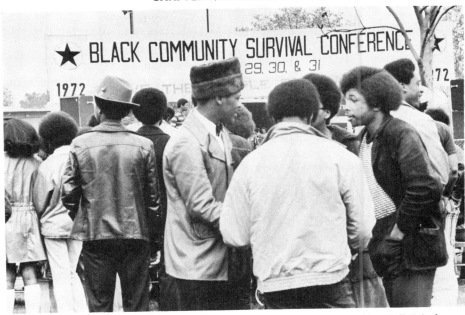

**Figure 8-5.**   *Black Americans work to increase cultural unity and power.*    *(Sam Falk/Monkmeyer Press Photo Service)*

Time orientation for the Black culture is predominantly present-oriented. This is mainly due to the fact that upward mobility is so difficult, and the future, therefore, holds little that is different.

The family is generally a kinship network with internal structure. Religious and family activities are closely tied together. The elderly person occupies a position of status within the subculture. For example, often the grandmother or an aunt is in charge of child-rearing. The Black person has historically suffered many indignities that have persisted into the present time. Thus self-esteem has been greatly affected.

## RELIGIOUS BELIEFS

Throughout this chapter, religious beliefs have been incorporated into the discussions of various cultures. It is appropriate to focus briefly on the overall concept of religious belief as it may affect the health-illness concept.

Almost all persons have some religious or spiritual belief that affects the way in which sickness, pain, and death are perceived.

In most instances, formalized religions are based on scripture or sacred word. They have a basis of authority or some source of power, e.g. the Roman Catholic pope. Religion offers the individual membership in an identifiable group, as well as providing guidelines for distinguishing between right and wrong, and offering some ideas of what one can expect after death.

Religion is usually a consolation to the sick and dying, since it offers hope. However, there may be times when sickness is seen as punishment from God, and thus becomes a source of increased anxiety for the client.

Some religious practices or restrictions may influence the client's care. For example, in Judaism there are dietary restrictions regarding the eating of pork, shellfish, and many other foods not properly prepared. Baptism before death is an imperative for Roman Catholics and for some Protestants. Some religions forbid the drinking of any stimulants including coffee and tea, and others forbid such treatments as blood transfusion.

It is not practical to enumerate in depth the tenets and practices of each denomination. The student is encouraged to consult some of the references at the end of the chapter for further reading on specific religions. It is especially important to have knowledge of the religious beliefs and practices of the groups to be served in one's particular health-care area.

## NURSING IMPLICATIONS

There are some important points that can assist the student in a humanistic approach to relationships with clients of cultural difference.

**1.** Approach all clients openly as if you are each newborn and ready for any relationship needs.

**2.** Rely on knowledge learned about signs and symptoms, not just visual assessment. What if you were blind or deaf? How would you assess a client then?

**3.** Find out from the client exactly what his needs and preferences may be.

**4.** Include the family, but remember that the client's family composition may be different from your orientation.

**5.** Religion and its role in health care and teaching is important to most cultures.

**6.** Nearly every culture, other than the dominant American culture, puts the group before the individual. This means that group decisions and authority lines are respected over and above the individual. This orientation is alien to most health-care workers in this society.

Early in this chapter reference was made to nursing as a subculture. Many authors write about the hospital and the health professions as subcultures in this society. Recalling that a culture is a way of life for any group of persons, one can see that it could be argued that the hospital is a sociocultural system. The members of this system—health care providers—understand the attitudes, values, and beliefs of their system. The persons entering the hospital view it as alien and frightening and often do not speak the subculture's language.

The nurse who is able to contemplate this scene as a client might view it can better understand the feelings of persons entering the system. Security of family, personal belongings, and familiar foods are imperative in decreasing the stress factor. A question for each nurse to ask might be, "What do I take with me to college, school, vacation, or the hospital to make me feel better?" The answer might suggest the reasons why all persons need familiar things around them.

## SUMMARY

Culture is a way of life for any designated group's values, attitudes, and beliefs utilizing the heritage of the people to maintain stability. The larger cultural systems, such as the American middle-class, have subsystems or subcultures. These subcultures rely upon the larger culture for their referent values and attitudes while maintaining many of their own beliefs, values, and rituals.

All cultures have a language by which they communicate within their culture and to other cultural groups. Time, group orientation, religious or spiritual beliefs, and health practices are all important parts of most cultural groups. Differences occur in the emphasis placed upon one or another of these important divisions.

The nurse can establish relationships with persons of different cultures by maintaining an open and interested manner. It is of utmost importance that all health-care workers increase their knowledge of the predominant subcultures in the American society. With the increased emphasis on self care and holistic health care, the nurse must be knowledgeable of cultural mores.

## LEARNING ACTIVITIES

1.  Identify one culturally diverse group in your community. Can you find specific areas of difference based on time, group orientation, religious or spiritual beliefs, and health practices?

2.  What is your cultural group? How does it compare in values and attitudes with others discussed in this chapter?

3.  In your clinical experience, interview a client of a different culture regarding attitudes toward hospitalization. What did you learn about differences in perception between you and the client regarding: the environment, time, nursing care, specific illness, dietary needs?

4.  Do you have enough knowledge about the dominant religions in your community? Can you discuss restrictions, dietary beliefs, basic tenets? Seek an interview with at least one member of a religion with which you are unfamiliar.

## REFERENCES AND SUGGESTED READINGS

Auger, J. R., 1976.  *Behavioral systems and nursing.*  Englewood Cliffs, N. J.: Prentice-Hall.

Branch, M.  Cultural components in nursing education. Nurse Education Conference, Second National Conference, New York. 1978.

Brownlee, A., 1978.  *Community, culture and care.*  St. Louis: C. V. Mosby.

Davitz, L. J.: Sameshina, Y.; and Davitz, J.  Suffering as viewed in six different cultures. *American Journal of Nursing,* August, 1976, pp. 1296–1297.

Fromm, E., 1956.  *The art of loving.*  New York: Harper Brothers.

James, S. M.  When your patient is Black West Indian. *American Journal of Nursing,* November, 1978, pp. 1908–1909.

Kniep-Hardy, M. and Burkhardt, M. A.  Nursing the Navajo. *American Journal of Nursing,* January, 1977, pp. 95–96.

Leininger, M. M., 1970.  *Nursing and anthropology: two worlds to blend.*  New York: John Wiley.

McMahon, M. A. and Miller, P.  Pain response: The influence of psycho-social-cultural factors. *Nursing Forum,* 17 (1978), 58–71.

Mead, M., 1970.  *Culture and commitment.*  Garden City, N. Y.: Doubleday.

Mitchell, P. H., 1977.  *Concepts basic to nursing.*  New York: McGraw-Hill.

Montagu, A., ed., 1974.  *Culture and human development: insights into growing human.*  Englewood Cliffs, N. J.: Prentice-Hall.

Murray, R. B. and Zentner, J. P., 1979.  *Nursing concepts for health promotion.* 2nd ed.  Englewood Cliffs, N. J.: Prentice-Hall.

Orque, M. S.  Health care and minority clients. *Nursing Outlook,* 24 (1976), 313–316.

Papajohn, J. and Spiegal, J., 1975.  *Transactions in families.*  San Francisco: Jossey-Bass.

Primeaux, M.  Caring for the American Indian patient. *American Journal of Nursing,* January, 1977, pp. 91–94.

Pumphrey, J. B.  Recognizing your patient's spiritual needs. *Nursing 77,* December, 1977, pp. 64–69.

Skipper, J. K. and Leonard, R. C., eds., 1965.  *Social interaction and patient care.*  Philadelphia: J. B. Lippincott.

Tamez, E. G.  Curanderismo: folk Mexican-American health care system. *JPN and Mental Health Services,* December, 1979, pp. 34–39.

Tsuda, S.  Vietnamese evacuee camp: a learning environment. *Nursing Outlook,* 24 (1976), 313–316.

# 9

# The Environment

### Behavioral Objectives

Upon completion of this chapter, the student will be able to:

1. Describe relationships between environment and health.
2. Identify the physical, biological, and psychosocial dimensions of the environment.
3. Describe environmental implications for nursing.
4. Identify common hazards to health in the environment.
5. Describe the process of infection.
6. Describe the role of the nurse in prevention and control of infection.
7. Describe nursing implications of communicable disease.

### Key Terms

| | | |
|---|---|---|
| antiseptic | disinfectant | nosocomial infection |
| asepsis | ecology | pathogen |
| barrier technique | entry portal | reverse isolation |
| carrier | environment | reservoir |
| clean technique | host | sterilization |
| contagious disease | infection | surgical asepsis |
| contamination | immunization | susceptibility |
| | medical asepsis | |

## Introduction

Recent years have witnessed a growing concern for prudent use of the environment as we become more aware of the interdependence between people and the world in which they live. René Dubos (1965), long recognized as an expert in the field of environmental science and health, has written of the challenge of using the environment to maximize man's potential. Dubos perceives health as meaningful only when it is understood in terms of the person functioning in a given environment. Dunn (1961) has also written extensively of the inevitable relationship between environment and health.

As a health-care provider, the nurse is constantly confronted with environmental conditions that either support or undermine her efforts to assist clients in promoting and maintaining their health. This chapter will discuss some of the important environmental considerations that have implications for nursing.

## ENVIRONMENT

### Dimensions of the Environment

Environment is generally defined as the aggregate of surrounding things, conditions, or influences, especially as affecting the existence or development of someone or something. In its broadest sense, the environment is seen to include not only the planet earth, but the universe beyond. Studies of environment are found in many disciplines since the environment is an essential back-up to life and its activities. The overall concept of an environment includes physical, biological, and psychosocial dimensions. Physical factors such as elements and temperature influence the type of measures needed to produce maximum health. Air conditioning to control

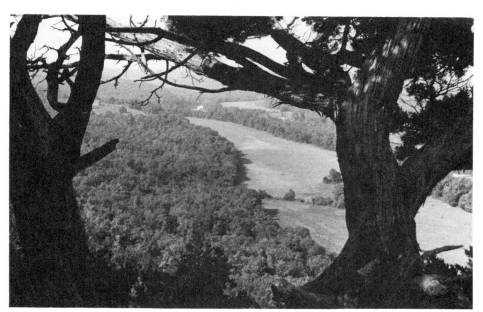

Figure 9-1. *The natural environment.* *(Godsey/Monkmeyer Press Photo Service)*

excessive heat and pollen contamination in hot, damp regions is an example of this. Other physical or external factors to be considered for health include availability of adequate food and water supplies, open space, housing, and sanitation facilities.

The biological factors in the environment, especially as they relate to the spread and control of disease-producing organisms and individual resistance to disease, are another aspect of the environment that is important in the consideration of health.

Some psychosocial dimensions of the environment are job opportunities, economic resources, and government laws that reflect attitudes toward health care, provision for health-care delivery systems, and available opportunities for education and recreation.

## Environmental Implications for Nursing

It is essential that nurses understand the ecosystem, especially as it relates to health and illness. One of the first nurses to write on the effects of the environment on health was Florence Nightingale, who stated that "symptoms or suffering generally considered to be inevitable and incident to the diseases are very often not symptoms of the disease at all, but of something quite different—of the want of fresh air, or of light, or of warmth, or of quiet, or of cleanliness, or of punctuality and care in the administration of diet, of each or all of these" (Nightingale, 1860).

In addition to meeting the environmental responsibility incumbent on all citizens, the nurse is often in a position to serve on planning boards or as a consultant for community agencies focused on health concerns. Through professional nursing organizations, nurses can be heard as a collective voice concerned with environmental health.

The following Policy Statement of the International Council of Nurses (1975) summarizes the interest of the nursing profession in the environment:

The preservation and improvement of the human environment has become a major goal of man's action for his survival and well-being. The vastness and urgency of the task places on every individual and every professional group the responsibility to participate in the efforts to safeguard man's environment, to conserve the world's resources, to study how their use affects man and how adverse effects can be avoided. The nurse's role is to:

—help detect ill-effects of the environment on the health of man, and vice-versa;

—be informed and apply knowledge in daily work with individuals, families, and/or community groups as to the data available on potentially harmful chemicals, radioactive waste problems, latest health hazards, and ways to prevent and/or reduce them;

—be informed and teach preventive measures about health hazards due to environmental factors, as well as about conservation of environmental resources to the individual, families, and/or community groups;

—work with health authorities in pointing out health hazards in existing human settlements and in the planning of new ones;

—assist communities in their action on environmental health problems;

—participate in research providing data for early warning and prevention of deleterious effects of the various environmental agents to which man is increasingly exposed; and research conducive to discovering ways and means of improving living and working conditions (RNAO News, 1976).

Nursing is directly involved in the control of disease, as well as the promotion of health within the environment. Although we have made great strides in the prevention and control of communicable diseases, we continue to be plagued by strains of bacteria and viruses that are resistant to currently known agents. The continued development of these organisms within our environment represent an ongoing threat to our well-being. The increasing incidence of chronic disease invites continued scrutiny of the patterns of living we choose which lead to chronic illness. Patterns of health-care delivery which emphasize the curative and rehabilitative aspects of treatment, rather than prevention, deserve close attention.

The nurse's potential to influence the environment will obviously vary with the setting. In a hospital or other inpatient type of facility, the nurse may have maximum control over the environment. In a home setting, the nurse can use her skills in health education to attempt to effect change in an unhealthy environment, by making the family aware of the consequences of the existing environment and offering information on how this can be changed. The success of this type of influence is dependent to a large degree on factors beyond the direct control of the nurse. In a work setting, the occupational health nurse can work with management to strive for a safe and healthy environment. She can also use health education processes with workers in an attempt to produce behaviors that contribute to health rather than to illness.

Overall environmental factors such as air quality, clean water, and solid waste disposal are usually controlled by the community in which a person resides. Measures to assure that these factors are adequately policed are under the law. The more personal aspects of an individual's environment, which can be influenced directly or indirectly by the nurse, include factors of both safety and comfort. Safety includes freedom from known hazards as well as aids such as ramps or handrails and other needed adaptations to a setting, to accomodate the special needs of any age person. Comfort measures which affect health include appropriate temperature and humidity; adequate ventilation, space, and lighting; provision for privacy; the opportunity to provide for one's self-care as far as possible in areas of eating, sleeping, and elimination; and a psychologically supportive environment in which there is respect for individual differences. It is especially important for the nurse working in a hospital to remember that the client has relinquished the control he usually has over his environment. This can be an added source of stress since the burden of adaptation is on the client. The nurse who is sensitive to this, and allows the client to exercise some choices when this is possible, can help lower the client's anxiety level in the hospital.

## Common Health Hazards in the Environment

The United States Department of Health, Education, and Welfare has identified a number of environmental pollutants and exposures that have a definite effect on human health. These are categorized as: **1)** community air pollution, **2)** food and water contaminants, **3)** land pollution, **4)** thermal exposures, **5)** radiation and microwaves, **6)** noise and vibrations, and **7)** housing and household agents. Air pollutants, especially those from cars and industrial wastes, have caused increasing problems with air quality in the United States today (HEW Statistics for Determining the Effects of the Environment on Health, July, 1977). These agents affect pulmonary function and aggravate symptoms of chronic obstructive pulmonary disease (COPD) such as emphysema, asthma, and bronchitis. Changes in the heart and lung function of healthy individuals occur in the continued presence of these pollutants. It has become a sadly commonplace experience in many large metropolitan areas to have days of pollution "alerts" where those with heart and lung problems are advised to stay indoors while persons in better health experience less serious but bothersome symptoms such as sore throats, running noses and eyes, and increased allergic reactions to the general air pollution.

Food and water contaminants include bacteria, viruses, metal, and other chemicals which spoil our food and water supply. Gastrointestinal infections, hepatitis, and poisoning by metals such as lead are among the more common manifestations of this pollution.

Land pollution encompasses the lack of efficient methods of human and industrial waste disposal, and increased use of pesticides. Hookworm and other infections are transmitted by improperly treated excreta. Increased intake and storage of heavy metals in the human body produce systemic toxic effects.

Thermal exposure is another factor in illness. Increased respiratory disease and frostbite occur in extremes of cold, while aggravation of renal and circulatory disease and heatstroke are dangers in localities where temperatures are consistently high.

Radiation is found in sunlight, diagnostic x-rays, therapeutic radiation, and industrial-related radiation. Burns are a hazard from radiation, and exposure to these rays has a definite effect on the occurrence of skin cancer. The potential effects of nuclear power and reprocessing plants, and microwaves, remain under investigation.

Noise and vibrations affect hearing and contribute to permanent hearing losses. The quality of life, especially for those living in cities, is substantially affected by the many sources of noise. By disturbing sleep and interrupting rest, noise is one more contributor to the many causes of stress in the urban environment.

Housing and household agents which have a definite effect on health include defective appliances which explode or give off fumes, dust which aggravates asthma and allergies, structural factors such as wiring or stairs that contribute to fires, falls, and other accidents, faulty household equipment, and toys that do not meet safety standards.

## Cigarette Smoking as an Environmental Hazard

In addition to the environmental hazards that have evolved as a result of community and national lifestyle choices, there are hazards in the immediate environment due to individual behavioral choices. Smoking is one of these. A Federal survey on adult uses of tobacco conducted by the National Clearinghouse for Smoking and Health in 1975 indicated that 39.3 percent of men and 28.9 percent of women are smokers in the over-21 age category. Between 70 and 80 percent of these smokers feel smoking is harmful to their health and could lead to disease and death. Ninety percent of these smokers expressed a desire to quit, yet 57 percent of these same smokers feel they will still be smoking in 5 years. These figures speak to an interesting discrepancy between attitude and behavior in the adult population (Fisher, 1977).

There is also a discrepancy between attitude and behavior among health professionals, especially nurses. A 1975 survey of 20,000 physicians, dentists, pharmacists, and nurses showed that smoking among nurses was at a level in 1975 that was similar to what it had been in 1969 (37 percent). Levels for the other groups had dropped between 7 and 11 percent in the same period, following the Surgeon General's report on smoking and health. The members of all these professions were in general agreement that cigarette smoking is seen as a cause of heart disease and oral cancer, and as a contributor to lung cancer, chronic bronchitis, and pulmonary emphysema (HEW, Smoking Behavior and Attitudes of Physicians, Dentists, Nurses, and Pharmacists, 1975).

Since smoking pollutes the air that everyone present must breathe, many locales have adopted policies that allow people to choose smoking and nonsmoking sections in public places. Despite all the available knowledge of its effects, smoking continues to be a habit supported by part of the population. The nurse needs to be aware of her own values and behaviors in this area, and to allow others the freedom of choosing their values without undue pressure from her in her professional capacity.

## PREVENTION AND CONTROL OF INFECTION

### Infectious Process

The control of microorganisms that cause infection is a serious concern in nursing. The infectious process is illustrated in Figure 9-2.

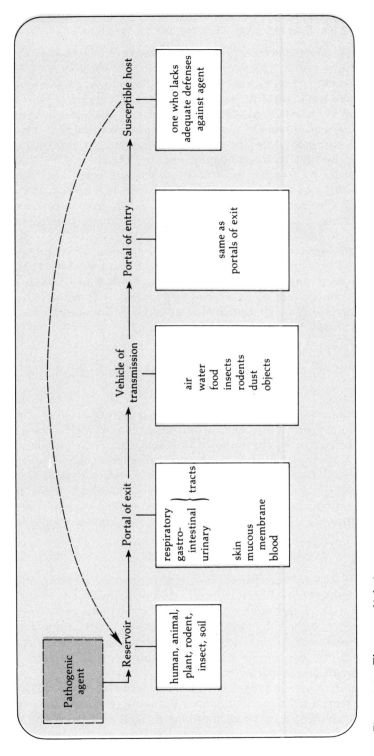

**Figure 9-2.** *The process of infection.*

The key factor in infection is the existence of a pathogenic agent. This agent lives and grows in a location called a reservoir which may be a human, animal, plant, rodent, insect, or section of land. Sometimes people without symptoms can have the disease or pathogenic agent. These people are called carriers.

Agents that live on the soil are easily available, whereas those with reservoirs inside other living things require an exit if they are to spread. Some of the common exits are via the respiratory, gastrointestinal, and urinary tracts; the skin, mucous membranes, and blood.

In order to travel to new destinations, the agent also requires a vehicle. These vehicles include air, water, food, insects, rodents, dust, and inanimate objects. Droplet spray from the nose and mouth onto the skin or mucous membrane of another is a common way of transmitting infection, as is direct person-to-person contact.

Before arriving in a new host, the pathogenic agent must find a portal of entry. These are similar to the portals of exit mentioned above.

The final step in the journey of the agent is into a susceptible host or one who lacks the needed defenses to protect himself against the agent's attack. The susceptibility of the host is strongly influenced by his general health status. Additional protection may be given to potential hosts by immunizations.

## Role of the Nurse in Prevention and Control of Infection

The role of the nurse in interfering with the infectious process is to interrupt the process at some point, and thus prevent the spread of the infectious agent. Both medical and surgical asepsis is utilized in patient care, and both refer to the removal of disease-producing organisms. In medical asepsis, the major focus is on keeping organisms confined within a given area. In surgical asepsis, the major focus is in keeping an area free of organisms.

Specific nursing actions to accomplish infection control include cleaning, disinfection, and sterilization of equipment; handwashing; barrier techniques; proper waste disposal; and the prevention of nosocomial infections.

## Care of Equipment

Care of equipment used for client care is the responsibility of the nurse. Any equipment that has been used is considered "dirty" and must be appropriately cleaned before reuse. This includes removing any remaining organic materials by scraping and rinsing with cold water; washing the equipment in hot soapy water with a stiff brush if needed; rinsing thoroughly; and disinfecting or sterilizing the equipment. Disposable equipment and dishes are preferable when available.

Disinfecting equipment with a chemical disinfectant kills many pathogenic organisms but does not kill spores and some resistant strains of bacteria. This procedure results in "clean" equipment. To sterilize equipment, thus killing all forms of bacteria, spores, fungi, and viruses, sterilization procedures involving heat are generally utilized. These include autoclaving, boiling, or dry heat measures.

## Handwashing

Handwashing is the most important measure for disease and infection control. The preferred equipment for handwashing is a deep sink with running water from foot- or knee-controlled faucets, and liquid soap from a dispenser, also controlled by foot or knee. The essence of handwashing is a combination of chemical (soap) and mechanical (physical energy) means of removing and destroying harmful organisms. The procedure is illustrated in Figure 9-3.

Hands need to be washed between client contacts, before handling food or eating, and after going to the toilet. Lotion on hands can prevent breaks in the skin due to frequent washings. Clients and their families need to be taught the importance of this procedure and shown how to do this properly if they are unaware of the correct procedure.

## Barrier Technique (Isolation)

Barrier or isolation techniques are examples of medical asepsis used when a pathogen is known or suspected to be present. Physical barriers such as space, gowns, masks, and gloves are used to confine the organism. These procedures also isolate the client who is the host. The nurse needs to be sensitive to the client's feelings of being different and "dirty."

Psychological support is important, as is appropriate physical contact to assure the client that he is not an outcast. The distancing by personnel and other clients, and the appearance of people in gowns and masks can be frightening, especially to children. When at all possible, it is important to explain exactly what is being done and why the procedures are necessary. A squeeze of the hand or a leisurely back rub can be very comforting to a person whose illness has set him apart from his usual sources of physical contact and affection.

Gowns are used to protect the nurse and prevent contamination of her clothes. Ideally, disposable gowns can be used, or else gowns can be laundered after each use. If this is not possible in a given hospital or home setting, the gown should be put on so that clothing is covered. The outside of the gown is then considered "contaminated," and the inside of the gown is "clean." For reuse, the gown should be hung in such a way that the clean side is protected from contamination yet is accessible for regowning as shown in Figure 9-4. The nurse washes her hands *before* removing the gown and then carefully slides her arms out through the inside of the sleeves. Masks are another barrier used for protection against pathogens. It is generally accepted that masks are useful only while still dry, and for limited durations such as 2 to 3 hours. A new mask should be used for each client if more than one client is being isolated.

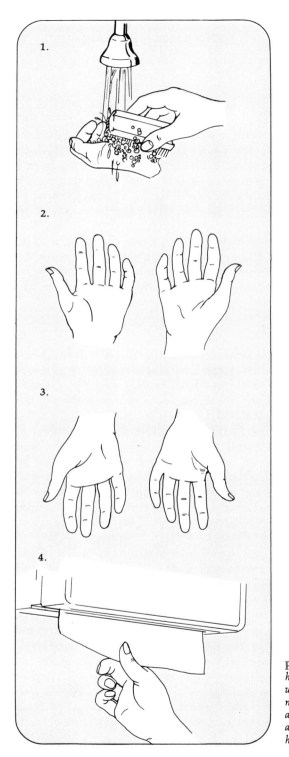

**Figure 9-3.** *Procedure for washing hands: (1) Soap hands well, using running water; soap or brush hands; clean fingernails. (2) Hold hands up for surgical asepsis. (3) Hold hands down for medical asepsis. (4) After rinsing thoroughly, dry hands with paper towels or blower.*

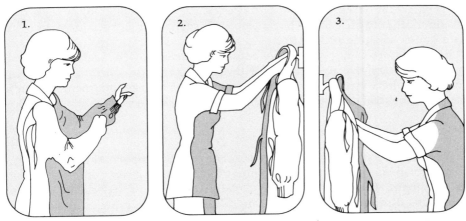

**Figure 9-4.** *Procedure for gowning: (1) Remove gown without touching the outside. (2) Hang gown so that inside can be reached without touching the outside. (3) For reuse, slide hands inside. Do not allow outside of gown to come in contact with your clothes.*

Sterile gloves are sometimes used as a barrier in changing dressings and giving treatments. The gloves are cuffed before sterilization. When the nurse opens the sterile packet, the inside of the glove is considered clean, and the outside is considered sterile. The inside of the first glove is grasped at the cuff and the other hand slides into it without touching the outside of the glove. Using the hand that is now gloved, the nurse slides her fingers under the cuff of the second glove, this time being careful not to touch the inside, and slips it over her second hand. The outsides of the gloves are now ready to work with the wound for treatment and should not touch anything else.

Barrier technique can be used in reverse for clients who are highly susceptible to infection, such as persons with leukemia or extensive burns. To do this, the goal is to keep all pathogens out of the defined area.

Nurses need to be aware of themselves as carriers of organisms from one person to another. Equipment, such as blood pressure cuffs, or toys used in waiting rooms and play areas, can be vehicles that inadvertently break barrier technique.

## Waste Disposal

Proper waste disposal is essential for hygiene at all times. When contagious disease is present, extraordinary precautions are taken. After meals, uneaten food is put into the appropriate flush system and dishes are sterilized before reuse. If an automatic dishwasher is not available, dishes can be autoclaved or boiled. Disposable dishes are a frequently used alternative to dish sterilization.

Laundry is usually kept near the client's unit in a bag until there is enough to send to the large laundry. The client's bag (contaminated) is then put inside another bag (clean on the outside) and marked. This procedure is known as a double bagging technique.

Excreta from clients who have contagious diseases are carefully emptied into the general sewage facilities if these are adequate within a setting. In instances where central sewage is not available, or sewage treatment methods are questionable, disinfectants such as lime chloride are used.

## Nosocomial Infections

Although the prevention and control of infection is important in all settings, it is in the hospital setting that the nurse has the most direct control over the environment. It is estimated that 5 percent of all hospital clients acquire infections during hospitalization. These infections are referred to as nosocomial infections.

Many hospitals have an infection-control practitioner. This person, often a nurse, is concerned with overall policies and procedures that prevent and control infection within the hospital setting. They are available to consult with staff when particular problems arise, and welcome information from staff that will help to anticipate and prevent the spread of infection within the hospital (Darling, 1977).

## COMMUNICABLE DISEASE

## Communicable Disease as a Health Hazard

Communicable disease is defined as a disease which may be transmitted directly or indirectly from one individual to another. It is usually caused by an infectious agent.

The toll in life and health from communicable disease in the United States in recent years has been considerably lessened by a combination of factors. These include the use of sanitation measures at the community level, increased individual resistance due to better nutrition and general living standards, mass immunization against common diseases, and use of antibiotics and other antimicrobial agents when disease does occur.

Although progress has been made, a review of the weekly Morbidity and Mortality Reports from the Federal Center for Disease Control in Atlanta, Georgia, is sufficient to remind even the most optimistic among us that communicable diseases remain with us and require constant vigilance. Occasional outbreaks of polio remind us that some parents see immunizations as unnecessary until an epidemic occurs. Measles outbreaks in persons who were immunized early in the development of the measles vaccine remind us that continued monitoring of existing and developing vaccines is needed.

The care of the person with a communicable disease is governed by the actions discussed earlier in this chapter for control of infection. It is assumed that the nursing student will study specific communicable diseases, with their complications and treatments, in more depth as she progresses in her nursing education. The purpose of the limited discussion here is to bring to the student nurse some awareness of the existing measures of prevention of commonly encountered communicable diseases.

## Nursing Implications for Communicable Disease

When a nurse is caring for a new mother, in addition to the usual teaching of care of the newborn, it is important to make the mother aware of when and how she can protect the infant from the communicable diseases that are common in our environment. This anticipatory guidance is important to the health of the child and the family.

Children are immunized against diphtheria, tetanus, pertussis, polio, measles, rubella, and mumps beginning at an early age (2 to 3 months). Smallpox vaccination was formerly required prior to a child's entering school but this is no longer being done routinely. Childhood immunizations are available through private physicians and public health clinics. In addition to the above-mentioned vaccines, children are screened and tested for tuberculosis during routine physical examinations. Tuberculosis remains a threat to health in this country today, with thousands of new cases reported annually. It is especially important that people working as food handlers, such as in restaurants and school cafeterias, be tested regularly for possible tuberculosis. Chest x-rays and tuberculin testing are available at local health departments.

Adults who plan to travel abroad should contact the U.S. Public Health Service for current information on diseases prevalent in the country of their destination and plan to be properly immunized before obtaining a passport.

Tetanus is one of the immunizations that should be kept up during adulthood. Current practice is a booster dose of tetanus vaccine every 10 years, with closer dosage, at the discretion of the physician, in the event of a deep wound.

Influenza and hepatitis are two common communicable diseases that continue to escape eradication. Viruses that do not respond to existing chemotherapy are also an ongoing problem. Venereal disease has reached epidemic proportions, especially among young adults. This was discussed further in Chapter 3.

The nursing student needs to be aware of the existence and threat of communicable disease to both the individual and the community. Health education by the nurse can greatly help lower the incidence of this unnecessary health hazard.

## SUMMARY

Environment and health are interdependent, with concern for health necessitating concern for the environment. World and community environmental conditions have impact on individuals and families. Management of an immediate environment, such as a home, hospital, or work location, is often a direct concern of the nurse. Awareness of the many factors involved in the safety and comfort of the physical, biological, and psychosocial environment is essential to comprehensive nursing assessment.

Common hazards existing in the environment include pollution, food and water contamination, radiation, and noise. Individual behaviors, such as smoking, can affect the overall environment.

The nurse has a responsibility to prevent and control infection in any setting where she practices. Understanding the nature of pathogenic organisms, and the process by which they spread, is essential. Techniques such as handwashing, care of equipment, waste disposal, isolation, and general disinfection of the environment are used.

Communicable disease continues to plague our society in some areas. Health education by the nurse regarding immunization and methods of disease control can help to alleviate this problem.

## LEARNING ACTIVITIES

1. Describe physical, biological, and psychosocial factors in the environment that influence health.

2. How can the nurse influence the environment to improve and facilitate health behaviors?

3. What are some of the common hazards existing in the environment? What type of changes are needed to improve or remove these hazards?

4. How do individual behavior choices affect the environment?

5. Describe the process of infection. Define agent, host, portal of entry, portal of exit, reservoir, and vehicle.

6. Describe some common techniques used in the prevention and control of infection.

7. What is a communicable disease? Name some of the common childhood communicable diseases for which immunizations are available.

## REFERENCES AND SUGGESTED READINGS

Beneson, Abram S., ed., 1975. *Control of communicable diseases in man.* 12th ed. American Public Health Association, Washington, D.C.

Brown, M. S. What you should know about communicable diseases and their immunization. *Nursing 75:* Part 1, September, 1975 pp. 70–72; Part 2, October, 1975 pp. 56–60; Part 3, November, 1975, pp. 55–60.

Castle, M. Isolation: precise procedure for better protection. *Nursing 75*, May, 1975, pp. 50–57.

Darling, LuAnn; Cox, Cheryl; and Axnick, Karen. Role development: buffers and balance in the infection control team. *Association for Practitioners in Infection Control*, Vol. 5, No. 1, March, 1977, pp. 7–12.

Dubos, Rene, 1965. *Man adapting.* New Haven: Yale U. Press.

Dunn, Halpert, 1961. *High level wellness.* Virginia: R. W. Beatty, Ltd.

Fisher, Lucille. *National smoking habits and attitudes.* American Lung Association Bulletin, September, 1977, pp. 6–9.

Hall, Edward T., 1966. *The hidden dimension.* Garden City, N.Y.: Doubleday.

Henderson, Virginia and Nite, Gladys, 1978. *Principles and practice of nursing.* 6th ed. New York: MacMillan.

Jenny, J. What you should be doing about infection control. *Nursing 76*, November, 1976, pp. 78–79.

Kilbourne, Edwin D., ed., 1969. *Human ecology and public health.* New York: MacMillan.

Nightingale, Florence. *Notes on nursing: what it is and what it is not.* New ed., rev. and enlarged, London: Harrison and Sons, 1860, p. 5.

*The Random House dictionary of the English language.* New York: Random House, 1967, p. 477.

Registered Nurses Association of Ontario, *RNAO News*, 32:19, January/February 1976.

Smoking behavior and attitudes of physicians, dentists, nurses, and pharmacists, 1975. In *Morbidity and mortality weekly report*, U.S. Department of Health, Education, and Welfare; Center for Disease Control, June 10, 1977.

Statistics needed for determining the effects of the environment on health. U.S. Department of Health, Education, and Welfare; Public Health Service, Health Resources Administration, July, 1977.

# The Nursing Process

Communication
Assessment
Planning, Implementation, and Evaluation

Part 3 introduces the means by which care is given—the nursing process. This includes the skill of communication, which is the foundation of the nurse-client relationship, and the four steps of the nursing process: assessment, planning, implementation, and evaluation.

# 10

# Communication

### Behavioral Objectives

Upon completion of this chapter, the student will be able to:

1. Define the basic elements of communication.
2. Describe levels of communication.
3. Identify components of the nurse-client relationship.
4. Describe the relationship of listening and silence to communication.
5. State differences between effective and ineffective communication.
6. Identify techniques for effective communication.
7. Identify barriers to effective communication.
8. Describe the relationship of touch and territoriality to communication.

### Key Terms

| | | |
|---|---|---|
| communication | metacommunication | proximity |
| congruence | mutuality | self-concept |
| listening | nonverbal | territoriality |
| | perception | verbal |

## Introduction

Human beings transmit ideas, thoughts, experiences, and feelings by a process known as *communication*. Understanding this complex process is vital to the success of all interpersonal relationships. In the evolution of nursing, communication has become one of the major facilitators as well as one of the obstacles to the nurse-client relationship, the nurse-nurse relationship, and the nurse-community relationship.

Communication encompasses all possible modes for sending a message to another person and for receiving feedback. Much of our everyday communication is habit and therefore is often out of our conscious awareness. The nurse needs to develop an awareness of her self and her impact on the individual with whom she is interacting. This chapter will involve the student in the dynamics of the communication process. The emphasis will be on communication with an adult client. Reference will be made to communication with children, adolescents, and older adults when relevant. There will be discussion of staff and community relationships as they are affected by communication.

## COMMUNICATION DEFINED

There seem to be as many definitions of communication as there are persons who communicate. Various disciplines define it differently, but in general we in nursing see it as the sending and receiving of messages by use of symbols: verbal and written words, gestures, and body language. It also involves a reciprocal exchange of information and ideas. During communication, one's values, judgments, attitudes, beliefs, and feelings are conveyed both verbally and nonverbally.

Satir (1972) states that communication is "the largest single factor determining what kinds of relationships a person makes with others and what happens to him in the world about him" (p. 30). This statement emphasizes the important idea that all communication is learned. More important is the idea that since communication patterns are learned, they can be changed.

A normal infant enters the world with the capacity to receive and send messages. The persons who care for him are models for the way he will learn to communicate. Since learning to communicate is an ongoing process throughout life, this becomes an important point for nursing. Illness may require that the client change his mode of communicating. Also, the nurse may need to modify her communication patterns in order to function in her role, both in relation to her clients and with her peer interactions. For example, when student nurses practice communication techniques, they will often be very quiet and reluctant to talk with clients, stating that they are the "quiet type" and cannot "pry" into another person's life. Since it is important for the nurse to learn to assess the client's situation by talking with him, the process of communicating for purposes of gathering information and conveying understanding and empathy must be learned by the student.

## BASIC ELEMENTS OF COMMUNICATION

In any communication between two persons there are certain necessary ingredients:

## Proximity

For interpersonal communication to take place, the persons sending and receiving the messages need to be close enough for eye contact and for touch to occur when appropriate or desired. If neither verbal nor nonverbal modes are possible, then interpersonal communication is not occurring. The following is an example of interpersonal communication in which proximity is apparent. A nurse is teaching a new mother how to hold her baby. There is the sending and receiving of messages, both verbal—encouraging words from the nurse, and nonverbal—smiles and eye contact between mother and nurse, and the probability of touching. A communication not considered interpersonal could be a telephone conversation where nonverbal cues are absent, or a letter where the verbal and nonverbal cues are absent and the written word is the message mode.

## Sender

There must be a person who has some information to give, or who wishes in some way to change an idea or feeling of another person or group of persons. The sender then speaks and at the same time conveys the message to the other person(s) through body movements and expressions.

## Message

This is the thought or idea the sender wishes to convey.

## Receiver

This is the person who listens and assimilates the message from the sender.

## Feedback

The receiver must in some way indicate that the message was received and understood.

Figure 10-1 demonstrates the cyclical nature of communication. In effective interpersonal communication, this cycle will occur and recur as often as is necessary within a single communication module. There are a variety of interferences possible in this ideal model. Since no two persons are exactly the same, personal experiences, feelings, ideas, and coping behaviors may influence the way in which communication occurs.

## Congruence

In order to achieve effective communication, it is necessary to have both the verbal and nonverbal messages saying the same thing. A common incongruity in communication occurs when a person says one thing but means or implies another. This is often referred to as a "double-level message" or a "meta-communication." Such an incongruency can be seen in the following situation:

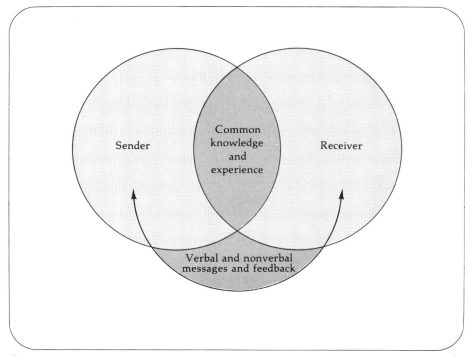

**Figure 10-1.** *Communication is an interactive process.*

**Nurse:**   Good morning Mrs. K, I just saw your lovely new baby.
**Mrs. K:**   (crying softly) Oh yes, Mr. K and I are very happy.
**Nurse:**   You say you are happy but I see that you are crying . . .

The nurse has been able to point out to Mrs. K the incongruity in her verbal and nonverbal messages. The nurse must be aware not only of possible incongruities in her clients' messages, but also in her own communication with fellow workers, friends, and family. A common place to find the nurse saying one thing and meaning another is in communication with young children. This often occurs when an adult does not listen attentively and consequently responds distractedly.

## Perception

All people perceive their surroundings differently. Perceptions are the interpretations we make of the sensory input from messages received. Our perceptions are based on our beliefs, values, judgments, and feelings; they reflect the way we are experiencing our surroundings. The client who has had a previous positive experience with illness and hospitalization will be more apt to perceive the hospital as a helping place. A person who has never been hospitalized but has heard personal accounts of a negative nature will possibly perceive his hospitalization with fear and dread.

The nurse can facilitate communication by being aware of her own perceptions and sharing them with her client. Feedback is the most valuable tool for clarifying perceptions and misperceptions. This can be seen in the following example:

Setting:   Emergency Room of a general hospital. A nurse is just beginning to interview the mother of Tommy, age three, who may have a fractured arm.

Nurse:   Mrs. R, I am Ms. B, a nurse, and I would like to ask you some routine questions.

Mrs. R:   (appears anxious) Yes, of course.

Nurse:   Tommy has injured his arm?

Mrs. R:   Yes, he fell down the stairs.

Nurse:   And did he get the bruises at the same time?

Mrs. R:   Of course! Why are you asking these questions? What are you thinking? We love Tommy!

Nurse:   Mrs. R, we have to fill out this routine Emergency Room admission form. I know you are distraught about Tommy's accident, but we are concerned only with your and Tommy's comfort. You may look at the form if you like.

The nurse perceived that the client was very upset and that the questions were apparently threatening to her. In the course of their discussion, Mrs. R revealed that she was afraid that the nurse would accuse her of not being a good mother. The nurse had perceived this and offered the client support and trust.

## LEVELS OF COMMUNICATION

Interpersonal communication is considered to occur on two levels: verbal and nonverbal.

### Verbal Communication

This is simply the spoken word. At birth infants hear words and begin to recognize their meaning from voice inflection and gestures accompanying the words. The child first uses words because of imitation of a model, not comprehension of meaning. As the child grows older he begins to understand the meaning of words and when to use them. By the age of four a child is able to understand most words spoken to him and to then use these words to express himself.

Words may mean different things to the sender and receiver, depending upon their cultural background. For instance, the word "bloody" is a slang expression to the British, but is used mainly as a descriptive adjective in the

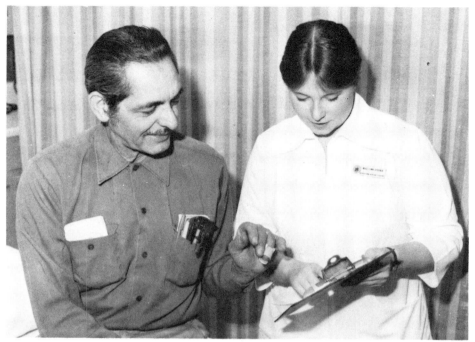

**Figure 10-2.** *Verbal communication is used to relay information and to clarify instructions in the nurse-client relationship. (Photo by Frank R. Engler, Jr.)*

United States. Within a culture there may be regional or geographic differences in word meaning, for example, in a specific region of the eastern United States rubber bands are called "gum bands," and the word "soda" has a different meaning to persons in the midwestern and eastern United States. Cultural implications in communication are very important to nursing since there must be a mutual respect for differences as well as clarification of meaning when necessary.

## Nonverbal Communication

There are many feelings and thoughts that cannot adequately be put into words. The majority of communication, in fact, probably occurs in the nonverbal sphere.

Merriner (1975) speaks of nonverbal communication as accidental or deliberate and states that true feelings are communicated nonverbally. Accidental nonverbal communication is probably not in the person's immediate awareness, as when a person is twisting a strand of hair while listening to a friend speak. If this behavior is called to her attention, she may be surprised to realize she is doing it. However, a person who is bored with a speaker or in a hurry to go may deliberately tap her fingers in agitation.

Whether accidental or deliberate, body movements and positions convey messages through actions.

Signs are another mode of nonverbal communication. Sign language is considered to be the most complex form. Signs for traffic control, prohibition of smoking, and advertising are examples of nonverbal symbols of communication. Objects or possessions are considered by many to be another form of nonverbal communication. Such things as automobiles, boats, furnishings, clothing, and jewelry are examples of ways a person may express feelings and attitudes about himself.

The expression of nonverbal communication is also influenced by learned behaviors during childhood and by culture. The handshake, for example, is a greeting in most western cultures but may be considered an invasion of privacy in some cultures.

The ability to attend to the nonverbal communication occurring with the verbal is an important nursing measure. The nurse must learn to listen with her eyes and ears in order to receive a congruent message. Much of what we perceive nonverbally is colored by personal experience and preconceived ideas. One important point, however, is that there is much more universality in the meaning of nonverbal communication than is found in verbal. Tears and laughter have nearly the same meaning across cultures.

## THE NURSE-CLIENT RELATIONSHIP

The strength of the therapeutic relationship between the nurse and the client will depend in part on whether the nurse is able to assist the client in new, positive life experiences. To accomplish this, the nurse continuously strives to understand the client's expressed behaviors and their meanings. She must also be continually concerned with her own role and its influence on the lives of her clients. To this end she must continuously adjust and readjust her own attitudes, feelings, and approaches. In a sense, then, the nurse must be able to use her personal *self* in positive ways in working with her clients.

### Individual Aspects of the Relationship

In considering the establishment of a relationship between the nurse and the client, communication is the major vehicle in the development of the relationship. There are some important aspects regarding the individuals involved in communicating: self-concept, self-perception, and self-awareness.

**Self-Concept**  Self-concept may be defined as the composite of a person's thoughts, feelings, hopes, strivings, fears, and fantasies. The development of the self-concept is believed to begin in the first year of life when the child begins to differentiate himself from mother, thus "discovering himself." Within the normal growth pattern there is a continuous and evolving process of self-discovery throughout life. Earliest signs of the development of self-concept are usually seen when the child begins to have some control over things in his environment. For example, the one-year-old may decide on what toy to play with or the food he will choose to eat from his plate. With the advent of language, self-awareness is expressed through the use of such words as *I, my, mine,* and the recognition of one's name as an identifying label. Children two to three years old are heard to say "my mommy," "my teddy bear," and the like. Identification may be seen in situations where a child refers to himself in the third person: "Joey wants a drink of juice."

Jersild's (1965) discussion of self includes:

**a.** a perceptual component: the way the individual perceives himself, how he appears, his feelings, attitudes, and what he shows others. Some authors refer to this as the Phenomenal Self or that which is recognizable or observable about a person. To the observant person such things as footsteps and voice tone are recognizable in a given individual

**b.** a conceptual component: a person's own recognition of his assets, liabilities, distinctive characteristics, and abilities; and

**c.** an attitudinal self: a person's feelings about himself as reflected in attitudes of self-esteem and self-reproach, feelings of pride and shame, and aspirations for future success.

**Self-Perception** Self-perception is reflected in the things a person reports about himself. Usually this is a conscious recognition of personal qualities and characteristics of both a positive and negative nature. A client who is in the hospital for tests may have difficulty sleeping. When the nurse talks with him about this, he may say, "I'm okay. I just have difficulty sleeping whenever I am in strange surroundings." The client is aware of his need for safety and security in familiar surroundings in order to sleep. In another example, a nurse may ask a client to refrain from smoking prior to a diagnostic test and suggest removal of the cigarettes from the room. The client may respond with, "Oh, that isn't necessary. I am a person of my word and you can trust me on that point!" The client is recognizing her qualities of honesty and at the same time denying any possibility of being untrustworthy.

**Self-Awareness** Like the first two concepts, self-awareness has equal importance for both nurse and client. The individual must have an awareness of the psychological processes which control behavior: thinking, remembering, and perceiving; and must be able to identify the ways in which these are manifested in one's everyday life. In order to assess the psychological aspects of awareness, the person gathers information based on such questions as, How do I feel? What is going on inside of me? What effect or meaning does this have for me? At the same time the individual must also assess his image, i.e., attitudes, feelings, perceptions, and ideals. In the process such questions as, Who am I? What am I like? What do I think about myself? What do I feel about myself? will need to be considered. If the nurse is lacking in her ability to check on her own awareness, she will have difficulty in assisting the client in recognizing his needs.

The nurse is called upon to cope with many reactions and behaviors on the part of clients, staff, and the community. She will always react to a given situation first as herself in a personal sense. She, therefore, must be able to describe how she feels about the experiences she is having and why she is reacting to them as she is. The nurse must also be able to assess herself in her professional role, i.e. what are her expectations, feelings, and behaviors as a nurse? Once the nurse has dealt with these personal issues, she is better able to understand the client's responses and to assist the client in adjusting to the additional stresses of illness and/or loss.

## Establishing the Relationship

Communication is an integral and inseparable part of any nurse-client relationship. The time the nurse has to spend with an individual client may be limited, but the quality of the interaction is far more important than quantity of time. Certainly the nurse who spends five or ten minutes a day with a client will have less opportunity to establish a trusting relationship than the nurse who has more time to work on establishing the relationship. It is possible, however, to perform all mechanical duties and technical care necessary

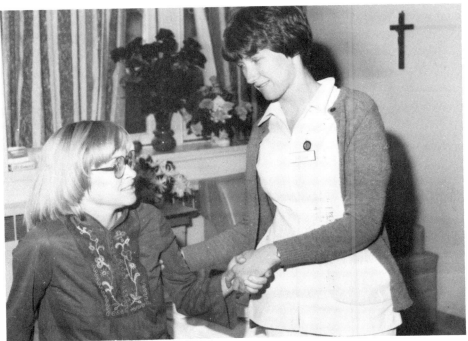

**Figure 10-3.** *Establishing a relationship involves tactile, verbal, and nonverbal communication. (Photo by Frank R. Engler, Jr.)*

without ever talking with the client at all. Some nurses do this. The authors have observed nurses giving total care to a client: bath, bed change, and treatments, without ever communicating on an interpersonal level:

Nurse:    Good morning Mr. W, how are you this lovely morning?
Client:    Well, I don't feel too bad.
Nurse:    Good. You look fine. Well now, I am going to help you with your bath, change your bed, and get you up in the chair.
Client:    Well (looking tired), I just now finished breakfast.
Nurse:    Then we can get started right away. (Nurse brings basin and bath begins) Did you see that hilarious television special last night, Mr. W? . . .

The nurse in this example has failed to respond to the client's nonverbal messages. She has also not included him in the planning and implementing of his own care.

Goals for effective communication in the nurse-client relationship should include:

a.    facilitating the nurse-client relationship
b.    allowing for accurate information-gathering
c.    allowing for participation of the client in the planning, implementation, and evaluation of the care received
d.    encouraging an openness and sharing between nurse and client in all aspects of care.

Facilitating the Nurse-Client Relationship    The nurse who is able to integrate the various influences at play when any two persons meet (self-concept, attitudes, perceptions, preconceived stereotypes,) will be able to approach the nurse-client relationship from an empathic viewpoint. If she is comfortable with herself, she can then begin to help the client to increase awareness and trust. It is easy to become involved in physical care, following of orders, and performance of clerical duties, forgetting the client as a total person. There are times when lifesaving measures take precedence over other aspects of care, but these are exceptions in the normal course of the nurse-client relationship. The nurse who is unhurried and takes time to explain procedures usually will find that the relationship develops mutuality. Mutuality is considered to imply a relationship with give and take, a sharing of responsibility, a participation in the planning. To use the example of Mr. W, again with evidence of mutuality:

Nurse:    Hello, Mr. W. I am Ms. S, a student nurse, and I will be working with you today.
Client:    Hello, what will you be doing?
Nurse:    Well, I will be assisting you with your bath and will help you to the chair.

Client:   Oh, I see.
Nurse:   Did you have a restful night, Mr. W?
Client:   It was not too bad, but I have just finished breakfast.
Nurse:   You sound tired. Do you want to rest for a short time before your bath?
Client:   Yes, thank you. Maybe twenty minutes?

**Allowing for Accurate Data Collection**   Information-gathering has become an important aspect of the nursing process and includes the use of most of the senses—touch, smell, hearing, and sight. Accurate information involves the ability to listen, observe nonverbal behavior, and clarify the information being received. The nurse who is rushed usually is not able to effectively collect accurate information from the client (client's family). If there are preconceived ideas about the person, this too may interfere with information-gathering. The following is an example of problems with data collection.

Situation:   A grey-haired woman arrives on the pediatric unit with a three-year-old child. Ms. S is the nurse assigned to admit the client.

Nurse:   Hello, I am Ms. S and I will be asking you some questions and helping Lori get settled.
Mother:   Thank you, we appreciate it.
Nurse:   Lori is three years old and will be having surgery tomorrow?
Mother:   Yes, that is correct.
Nurse:   And will you be staying with her, or will her mother be coming in?

The nurse in this situation assumed that the grey-haired woman was the child's grandmother on the basis of preconceived ideas about grey hair denoting an older person.
Actually, techniques for interviewing will be addressed in the next section of this chapter; however, our perceptions must be understood in order for the best of interviewing techniques to be successful.

**Allowing for Client Participation in Care Received**   The nursing process includes planning, implementation, and evaluation of care. The success of the nurse-client relationship probably depends most on the client participating in all areas of his care. Since the ultimate goal in the nursing care plan is to promote self-care for the client, it seems reasonable to have the client help in the planning and naturally to follow with implementation to the best of his ability. The area most often slighted in the process is evaluation, which involves feedback from the client and sharing of feelings between the nurse and the client.

Nurse:   Mrs. H, you and the baby will be going home in the morning.
Client:   Yes, we are really looking forward to it. Thanks to your teaching and helpful information, I feel quite relaxed.

Nurse:  You found the information helpful. I'm glad. I would be interested in hearing how things go at home.

Client:  I will be happy to let you know.

The nurse has received some feedback from the client regarding her effectiveness. This is also an example of how nurses can research (not in the strict sense) their impact on the client and the health-care system.

**Encouraging an Openness and Sharing**  When the client feels that he can trust the nurse to understand his fears, concerns, feelings of loss of control, etc., it is possible to share these. The nurse can encourage openness and sharing through her manner with the client and through example.

Situation:  The physician has just left Mrs. M's room after telling her she has some "stones" and will need an operation if conservative treatment does not work. Mrs. M's student nurse has been with her during the doctor's visit.

Nurse:  Mrs. M, I know you were anxious to have the doctor visit. Did he answer your questions adequately?

Mrs. M:  Yes, I guess so.

Nurse:  I know sometimes I get lost when technical words I don't quite understand are used. Should we share our understanding of what he said?

Mrs. M:  (smiling) You have trouble too at times? Well, I know what "stones" are because my mother had them, but "conservative treatment" sounds a little scary.

The nurse had shared something of herself with Mrs. M and therefore set an example, and at the same time helped promote trust in the relationship.

With this understanding of the basis for a nurse-client relationship, we can discuss some of the elements of effective communication techniques.

## EFFECTIVE COMMUNICATION TECHNIQUES

Effective communication and an effective nurse-client relationship are interdependent. Certain techniques or ingredients can be learned to facilitate effective communication.

### Nonverbal Techniques

**The Initial Contact**  There are two important issues in the initial nurse-client contact—the nurse's manner as she enters the room or territory of the client, and the way that the introduction takes place. Since the first issue deals with nonverbal communication, the discussion is included here. In entering a client's territory, the nurse needs to remember that she must respect it in the same way she would if she were entering a stranger's home. (More will be said about territoriality in the last section of this chapter.) The introduction itself

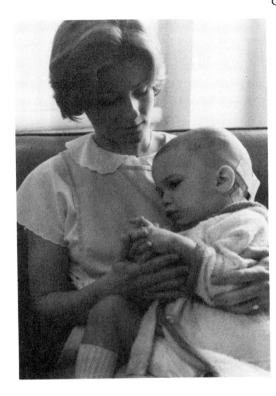

**Figure 10-4.** *Touch is an important source of communication and security for children. (Photo by Frank R. Engler, Jr.)*

appears to be a relatively simple behavior, but has a great influence on the progress of the relationship. Most important here is the overall comfort of the client. The nurse, therefore, needs to find out how the client wishes to be addressed. Some considerations are:

*The Age of the Client* With a small child the nurse would probably introduce herself by her first name and ask what the child's name is ("Hi, I am Linda. What is your name?"). The object here is to minimize threat and authority and meet the child at his own level. If the client is an adolescent, again the nurse may use a similar way of introduction to allow for a feeling of equality and to minimize authoritarianism. With a client of the same age as the nurse, it would be important to be aware of this peer situation. At issue would be the need to help put the client at ease and at the same time maintain a respectful tone, (e.g., "Hello, my name is Linda Boyd. I will be your nurse for today. What would you like me to call you?"). In this example, the nurse has offered the client the option of calling her by her first or last name, while allowing the client to state his own preference. Finally, with persons who are older, the nurse may introduce herself as in the above example. This again allows the client to choose how he will address the nurse and how he wishes to be addressed.

*The Need for Maintaining a Professional Role* Some clients may presume too much familiarity, or may cause the nurse to feel uncomfortable, (for example, "Hello, I am Ms. Boyd . . . ." "Hi, honeybun, just call me Chuckie." "I would prefer that you call me Ms. Boyd. May I call you Chuck or Mr. Jones?") There are times when it is necessary to set limits so that the client's overall care is not jeopardized. As the nurse continues to grow in self-awareness and self-confidence, she is more able to recognize when to set limits and when not to.

*The Nurse's Perception of Her Own Role*   This will influence how she introduces herself. Student nurses often have difficulty thinking of themselves as professional persons and therefore find introductions stilted and uncomfortable.

In the end, the way that we introduce ourselves, and the way we address others, has some relationship to our self-concept and our perceptions. The most important issue is not to decide on only one way to address and be addressed, but to insure comfort and respect for both parties. A person's name is closely related to his identity and self-concept. It is usually unique to him and, therefore, should be respected as his personal property.

### The Art of Listening

Most people think of listening as synonymous with hearing. Listening, however, is an active process and demands the full attention of the listener. Attentive listening is considered to be the key to effective communication. The nurse who wishes to improve her communication skills should consider listening to be as important as speaking. In fact, if listening is absent, speaking become a useless endeavor. Think for a moment of a time when you were talking excitedly to a friend only to realize she was not listening. How did you feel?

To listen completely is to use one's ears and eyes, and at times the sense of touch (as with blind and deaf persons whose sense of touch becomes as keen as our eyes or ears). Listening provides clues to help understand a person, meets emotional needs of the speaker, helps avert and solve problems, and is important to effective leadership (Kron, 1972).

Distractions are the greatest problem in effective listening. It is important to recognize that extraneous noises and sounds, odors, personal thoughts, and general health can interfere with listening. Sometimes just taking a minute to isolate the distraction and become aware of it will eliminate it as a distraction. Take a minute to concentrate on the noises around you—What are they? talking, automobiles, clanking pipes, footsteps, etc. Now that you know them, put them aside and listen to a friend who is talking with you. Your ability to concentrate should be much improved and your attention to outside sounds diminished.

The sounds that are just out of our awareness are the greatest distractors. The student needs to be aware of her surroundings so that she can give her full attention to the client. Merriner (1975), in her discussion of effective listening, emphasizes the importance of concentrating as completely as possible on what is being said; listening between the lines for such things as implied thoughts and indirectly expressed feelings; and checking for congruency—does the nonverbal communication support the verbal?

The art of listening may be affected by reduced hearing ability, as in deafness, congenital defects, and infectious processes. Reduced attentiveness may be due to lack of interest, unfamiliar vocabulary, and often by conditions within the physical surroundings: poor acoustics, extreme temperatures, uncomfortable furniture, or distracting mannerisms of the speaker.

The student nurse can increase listening effectiveness by being aware of the developmental process, too. When communicating with a small child, stooping to get down to his level increases the comfort level and tells him that he is being listened to. With elderly persons, it is often necessary to allow them total face-front view of the listener and to assess their hearing and vision abilities.

**Silence**    The use of silence as a communication technique can be positive when it is comfortable for the client. To the nurse a silence of 30 seconds seems like a lifetime. However, short silences allow the client to organize thoughts, contemplate what has just been said, or possibly to do some reminiscing. The nurse has the opportunity to observe nonverbal behavior and to organize thoughts or direction of the interaction.

Silence may become a negative tool when it lasts too long and consequently produces anxiety in the client. The nurse has a responsibility to break a silence in this instance.

## Verbal Techniques

In the interaction with a client or a client's family, there are specific techniques of effective communication which, when used properly, create an atmosphere of openness and sharing.

**1.**   *Using broad opening statements* allows the client to set the direction and tone of the conversation while beginning to express himself.

Nurse:   Hello, Mr. G. You look concerned about something.

**2.**   *Clarifying* helps to make the meaning of what the client has said clear and hopefully helps to avoid misunderstanding.

Nurse:   Hello, Mr. G. You look concerned about something.
Client:   Well, the doctor just left, but I'm okay.
Nurse:   I'm not sure I understand . . . .

**3.**   *Giving accurate information* helps to correct any misconceptions and possibly helps the client to better evaluate his situation.

Client:   Well, the doctor was listening to my heart and suddenly he looked upset and ran out of the room.
Nurse:   I can understand your concern, Mr. G, but the doctor was responding to an emergency call he just heard on the speaker.

**4.** *Reflecting* as a technique helps the client to consider his remark more carefully and to expand upon it if he wishes.

Client:   Well, that explains everything.
Nurse:   You were saying that he listened to your heart.

**5.** *Validating* allows the nurse to check with the client to see if his need has been met.

Client:   Yes, he does that every day, maybe I have heart trouble, too.
Nurse:   Mr. G, your doctor routinely listens to his clients' hearts. In your case I think your ulcer is the major problem.
Client:   Well, that is good to know.
Nurse:   Are you feeling less concerned now, Mr. G?

**6.** *Sharing observations* allows the nurse to share her perceptions of the client's physical or emotional state, thus increasing awareness on the part of the client.

Nurse:   Hi, Joey, how was your trip downstairs?
Client:   I got to ride on the big bed with wheels (all smiles).
Nurse:   You look like you had some fun for a change.

**7.** *Using general leads* encourages the client to continue to express himself.

Client:   I just haven't felt myself since breakfast this morning.
Nurse:   Oh?

**8.** *Selective reflecting* encourages exploration of some part of a statement.

Client:   I just haven't felt myself since breakfast this morning.
Nurse:   You don't feel yourself?

**9.** *Verbalizing implied thoughts and feelings* is a technique for verifying the nurse's impressions while assisting the client with self-awareness.

Client:   I just haven't felt myself since breakfast this morning.
Nurse:   You feel that breakfast had something to do with it?

This is not an exhaustive discussion of effective communication techniques. However, if the student understands these and is able to apply them, her interactions with clients, friends, and her own family will improve.

## BARRIERS TO EFFECTIVE COMMUNICATION

It follows that if there are techniques for improving communication, there are also blocks or barriers to communication. These are generally ways of expressing feelings, judgments, or perceptions that tend to stop effective communication.

 **1.** *Failure to listen* is a block that the listener is often unaware of. It is a powerful mechanism for stopping communication (see section on the art of listening).

 **2.** *Judgmental statements* tend to make the client feel inadequate or inferior and therefore reluctant to share further feelings.

Client:   I feel as if my husband will think I am ugly now.
Nurse:   Oh, you shouldn't feel that way.

 **3.** *Reassuring cliches* are pat statements that tend to minimize the significance of the client's feelings and imply lack of interest on the part of the nurse.

Client:   It looks as if I am not going to be able to continue in my old job.
Nurse:   That must be difficult for you, but everything will work out in the end.

 **4.** *Expressing approval* tends to focus on the nurse's values and often implies that her concept of right and wrong will be used in judging the client's behavior.

Client:   Maybe I would feel better if I talked with my minister.
Nurse:   I think you definitely would. I consider ministers to be very understanding and helpful.

 **5.** *Expressing disapproval* is an indication of a lack of acceptance of the client's feelings and attitudes. This kind of communication is often used with children and with adults who are being treated as children.

Client:   I don't really want to have my right arm show at all since I cannot use it and it looks terrible.
Nurse:   Now, Mr. C, you shouldn't feel that way about your arm; after all you are luckier than some who cannot use either arm.

 **6.** *Giving advice* has the nurse imposing her own judgments on the client, not accepting the client's feelings and actions.

Client:   Now that my last child has graduated from high school, I don't know what to do.
Nurse:   You should take a course and go into real estate business—that would fill up your time.

 **7.** *Changing the subject* puts the conversation tone and lead in the hands of the nurse, blocking client attempts to discuss necessary things.

Client:   Well, I have been working for the same company since my first was born and now she is in college. It will be hard to retire and leave that life.
Nurse:   What college does your daughter attend? I am thinking of going back myself.

The student may have noted in these examples that more than one block may occur in a single interaction. Becoming aware of one's communication patterns will help to decrease the occurrence of barriers to effective communication.

## TOUCH AND TERRITORIALITY

An important, but often neglected facet of communication in nursing practice, is the concept of touch and territoriality. In contemplating the act of touching another person, two considerations come to mind: **1.** one must not invade or infringe upon that person's territory, and **2.** one must not invade the other person's personal space.

*Territoriality* as a concept refers to a tangible demarcation in its broadest sense. When one thinks of marking one's territory, yards, rooms, and sitting or playing areas come to mind. Certainly it is appropriate to consider a hospital room or part of a room a client's territory when he is occupying it. A knock on the door or a "May I come in" is a sign of respect for the person. In nursing care, we often invade a person's territory, assuming the right because we are "helping." Young children are the most vocal about their territory and would not hesitate to set limits. A ten-year-old may have a sign on his door "Knock before entering or evil things will occur!" Four-year-olds will simply say "Get out of my place!" As we grow into adulthood and become more socialized, we are reluctant to state our wishes quite so openly. This is especially true when illness is present and there is a feeling of lowered self-esteem.

One's personal space is not so easily defined. It is intangible and its boundaries fluctuate with the emotional and personal safety state of the individual. Personal space travels with each individual. There are times when a person invites another into his space, in moments of intimacy, sharing, and camaraderie. Still, at other times, a person has little or no control over his personal space, as in a hospital situation when nursing procedures must be done—dressing changes, baths, taking of vital signs, etc. (Hein, 1972). The nurse can increase the client's comfort level in these situations by clearly communicating her intent.

The issue of personal space revolves around the individual's right to privacy and to a distance factor that allows for comfort. Communication tends to alter in direct relation to distance. Intimate distance is generally considered to be from 0 to 18 inches and is characterized by the unmistakable presence of the other person—smell, position, and the possibility of touch; personal distance of about 1½ to 4 feet still allows for close physical contact—holding, grasping, touching (handshake); social distance of 4 to 12 feet controls the degree of physical domination one person may have over another, but at the same time allows for effective eye contact (sitting across the table from another person); and public distance is anything beyond 12 feet, essentially eliminating the possibility of personal involvement (Hall, 1959).

In the discussion of territoriality and personal space, touch has been

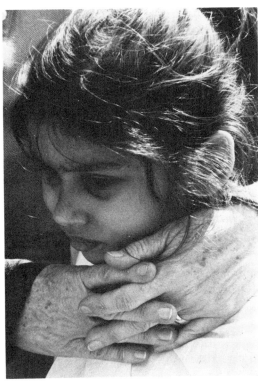

Figure 10-5. *Touch is the essence of nonverbal communication.* (Paul S. Conklin/Monkmeyer Press Photo Service)

referred to repeatedly. There are, of course, various forms and reasons for touch. There is the intimate fondling touch of the mother and father for their newborn, the loving touch of parents for their children at play and at work, the intimacy of lovers, the caresses of loved ones and family members, the smack of a slap, or the feel of a push, to name but a few.

Touch is a form of nonverbal communication. It is generally presumed in the nurse-client relationship. Touch has many cultural determinants which are outgrowths of tradition and taboo. Since it is such an important reaching-out gesture in the nurse-client relationship, the nurse needs to recognize that differences may exist from culture to culture. In some cultures, for example, greetings are extended by kissing and hugging while in others a polite smile or hello is enough. (Culture and care are considered in more depth in Chapters 1 and 2.)

## SUMMARY

Communication is the universal process for conveying one's thoughts and feelings to another. In nursing, it is the most important ingredient of the nurse-client relationship.

Communication includes both verbal and nonverbal signs and symbols. The spoken word is the most popular mode of communicating.

In nursing other dimensions occupy equally important positions: listening, touch, personal space, respect, and openness with the client. Nurses may learn to improve their ability to communicate through understanding techniques which facilitate or block their communication with a client.

## LEARNING ACTIVITIES

1. Observe a friend or family member for about one half hour. Note nonverbal communication, expressions of self-concept, body language.

2. Sitting face-to-face with a partner, each study the other for three minutes. Now look away and state what your partner is wearing, her expression, any body language noted. The partner should then state her observations.

3. Using a tape recorder or videotape, simulate a conversation with a client. Play back and identify effective techniques and blocks to effective communication.

4. Formulate your attitudes and feelings toward helplessness and illness.

5. Take time alone to study yourself in the mirror. What do you look like when you are happy? Sad? Angry? Hurried?

## REFERENCES AND SUGGESTED READINGS

Epstein, C., 1974. *Effective interaction in contemporary nursing.* Englewood Cliffs, N. J.: Prentice-Hall.

Hall, E. T., 1959. *The silent language.* Greenwich, Conn.: Fawcett Press.

Hein, E. C., 1973. *Communication in nursing practice.* Boston: Little, Brown.

Jersild, A. T., 1965. Social and individual origins of the self. In Don E. Hamachek, *The self in growth teaching and learning.* Englewood Cliffs, N. J.: Prentice-Hall.

Kron, T., 1972. *Communication in nursing.* Philadelphia: W. B. Saunders.

Lewis, G. K., 1973. *Nurse-patient communication.* 2nd ed. Dubuque, Iowa: Wm. C. Brown.

McCloskey, J. C. How to make the most of body image theory in nursing practice. *Nursing 76,* May, 1976, pp. 68–72.

Mereness, D., 1970. *Essentials of psychiatric nursing.* 8th ed. St. Louis: C. V. Mosby.

Mereness, D., and Taylor, C. M., 1978. *Essentials of psychiatric nursing.* 10th ed. St. Louis: C. V. Mosby.

Moustakas, C. E., ed., 1956.    *The self: explorations in personal growth.*    New York: Harper and Row.

Petrello, J.    Your patients hear you, but do they understand? *RN, 39,* (1976), 37–39.

Ruesch, J. and Kees, W., 1969.    *Nonverbal communication: notes on the visual perception of human relations.*    Berkeley, Cal.: U. of California Press.

Satir, V., 1972.    *Peoplemaking.*    Palo Alto, Cal.: Science and Behavior Books.

Schwartz, L. H. and Schwartz, J. L., 1972.    *The psychodynamics of patient care.*    Englewood Cliffs, N. J.: Prentice-Hall.

Shubin, S.    Familiarity: therapeutic, harmful, when? *Nursing 76,* May, 1976, p. 18.

Sundeen, S., et al., 1976.    *Nurse–client interaction: implementing the nursing process.*    St. Louis: C. V. Mosby.

# Assessment

## Behavioral Objectives

Upon completion of this chapter, the student will be able to:

1. Identify the important ingredients of the nursing process.
2. Describe the elements necessary for launching the nursing process.
3. Identify the major phases of the nursing process.
4. Define the assessment process.
5. Describe the role of observation, nursing history, and communication in assessment.
6. Describe the major behavioral components of the psychological assessment.
7. Describe the *nursing diagnosis*.

## Key Terms

| | | |
|---|---|---|
| adaptation | displacement | psychotic |
| anxiety | nursing diagnosis | rationalization |
| assessment | nursing history | reaction formation |
| basic human needs | nursing process | repression |
| compensation | physical assessment | stress |
| defense mechanism | process | stressors |
| denial | projection | sublimation |
| depression | psychosocial assessment | |

## Introduction

The practice of nursing is based on the nursing process, and therefore this process is a core concept in nursing education. Most nursing programs introduce the concept of the nursing process in the first nursing course. The actual use of the process in the clinical laboratory is based on learning each phase or step in the process in a building fashion, until the student is finally able to integrate the entire process into the desired holistic approach to client care.

Yura and Walsh (1978) describe the nursing process in the following manner:

> . . . it is central to all nursing actions, applicable in any setting, within any frame of reference, and concept, theory, or philosophy. It is flexible and adaptable, adjustable to a number of variables, yet sufficiently structured so as to provide a base from which all systematic nursing actions can proceed. Phases, or steps, in the nursing process are identifiable. They can be examined, analyzed, and pursued deliberately by nurses as they provide care for clients. Although the exact labels identifying the nursing process may differ among groups of nurses from one geographic area to another, there is a common theme underlying the process: it is organized, systematic, and deliberate (p. 1).

There are several important points from the above quotation for the student to bear in mind:

1. The nursing process is *adaptable.* Some educators add substeps to give more emphasis, some agencies refer to it by other names i.e., Problem-Oriented Records (POR), and some institutions develop forms for each step. The student will find that there are some differences in its use depending upon size of the health agency or institution, geographic location, and philosophy and goals of a given health agency.

2. The nursing process offers enough *structure* to allow for systematic nursing actions. The four main steps of the nursing process are: *assessing, planning, implementing, and evaluating.* Continual discussion goes on in the nursing literature as to the subcomponents of each of these steps. No matter what is added, the student will always be able to identify these four steps.

3. The nursing process is *organized*—one step follows another; it is *systematic*—the steps are arranged in a building fashion characterized by an ordered method; it is *deliberate*—each step is carefully weighed and considered with respect to the care of the client.

This chapter will introduce the student to the *assessment* step of the nursing process. This step is the key to the effectiveness of the entire process. Assessment is complex in that it involves several careful and deliberate substeps. Chapter 12 considers the remainder of the nursing process: planning, implementation, and evaluation.

## THE NURSING PROCESS

A process may be defined as a systematic moving forward toward some goal. It is always considered as a series of actions moving toward a specific end. When one thinks of the developmental process, for example, it can be seen that the life cycle is a systematic process of growth with a moving forward to the goal of completing the cycle. The developmental process includes the ever-important element of change throughout the cycle. So, in the nursing process the student will see the movement toward a goal, revisions or changes necessary along the way, and subsequent adaptations to allow for the process to continue.

The use of the nursing process requires a high level of intellectual skill including such abilities as organization, judgment, decision-making, and the ability to analyze and evaluate outcome. Once the nurse has mastered the basic theory and application of the nursing process, she can tailor the steps to her own individual nursing style.

Areas of emphasis in this text have been on interpersonal, interactional, and technical skills for the practicing nurse. These are the important skills the nurse must bring with her to the nurse-client relationship. Establishing this relationship is necessary to the nursing process. In order to have the nursing process work for both the nurse and the client, certain elements must be present:

**1.** Establishment of a mutually trusting and caring relationship, where the nurse's role in the client's care is clear.

**2.** Establishment of a working relationship with mutual goal-setting; where the client's input is encouraged and expected.

**3.** Inclusion of members of the client's family in the process.

**4.** Maintenance of an environment conducive to goal attainment.

## ASSESSMENT: PURPOSES AND PROCESS

The assessment step has a twofold purpose: **(1)** it is the initial and foundational step in the nursing process; **(2)** it is an ongoing process that continuously overlaps the other three steps.

An assessment is a continuous and deliberate gathering of data which will assist in identification of the client's present and potential strengths. It begins the moment the nurse comes into contact with the client and continues throughout the length of their relationship. Components of assessment used to expedite the process are:

**1.** observation

**2.** data-gathering

**3.** interviewing

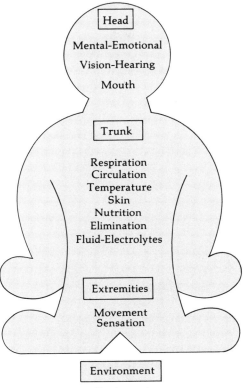

Initial impression

Age-Race-Sex-General state
Anything commanding attention

Head

Mental-Emotional

Vision-Hearing

Mouth

Trunk

Respiration
Circulation
Temperature
Skin
Nutrition
Elimination
Fluid-Electrolytes

Extremities

Movement
Sensation

Environment

Equipment
Significant people
Social-Cultural Influences

| Mental status | Respiration | Nutrition | Sensation |
|---|---|---|---|
| Emotional status | Circulation | Elimination | Equipment |
| Vision and hearing | Temperature | Fluid and electrolytes | People-social-culture |
| Mouth | Skin | Movement | Learning |

**Figure 11-1.** *The assessment man. (Copyright 1977, American Journal of Nursing Company. Reproduced, by permission, from* **Nursing Outlook,** *25 [Feb. 1977], 103, 105.)*

Specific tools have been developed to assist the nurse in obtaining the information about the client necessary to meet his needs and plan for problem-solving. These are usually the nursing-history form, the interview report, and the physical examination. Each institution or agency has its own preference for the types of tools to be used, so that there is a consistency in record-keeping; for example, charting, progress reports, and order sheets. It is the nurse's responsibility to be fully acquainted with the specific practices of her employing institution.

The best tools or methods for data collection can never replace the importance of listening and relaying to the client the notion that he is cared for and respected. It is during these interactions that the nurse and client exchange information: the client gives the nurse important information about his basic human needs; the nurse informs the client (and/or family) about hospital routines and practices, or available community resources should the client not be in a hospital setting.

## Observation

The observation of the client should begin the moment the nurse comes into contact with him. It includes a head-to-toe appraisal of the client (Figure 11-1). A rapid scan of the environment would include such questions as: What has the client brought with him to the hospital or clinic? or What does his home tell you? The nurse would also observe which significant persons were with the client at this time—spouse, parent, sibling, friend.

In some situations the client (or a family member) is given a history form to fill out upon admission. This is considered to be less than ideal as an assessment method. However, if this is the preferred method of data collection, the observational period becomes one of the primary means of establishing the initial relationship.

## The Nursing History

This is the ideal means for gathering pertinent initial data about the client. There is generally a particular form used to collect the data (Table 11-1. See Appendix for complete guide.) Most nursing histories include information about the client in the categories of social data, physiological data, usual patterns of daily living, environmental factors, the client's perceptions of his own health-illness status, his expectations of the health-care system, and his concerns regarding his health and his health care.

There are a variety of approaches that can be used in order to gain this information. The format may be a systems orientation, it may utilize a head-to-toe appraisal, a developmental level, or it may be based on a basic human needs model. The latter model is the one most suitable to the authors' holistic approach to the nurse-client relationship.

The basic human needs theory (Maslow, 1954) proposes that man has certain needs that must be satisfied if he is to reach his maximum level of wellness. These needs are arranged on an ascending continuum (Figure 11-2).

Table 11-1    Portion of Nursing History Guide*

Patient's Name _____ Diagnosis _____
Age _____ Sex _____ Occupation _____
Information obtained from _____ Relationship _____

A. Safety and Security
  1. Do you need help with your bath while in the hospital? Yes _____ No _____
     If yes, describe:

  2. When do you prefer to bathe? Morning _____ Afternoon _____
     Evening _____ No preference _____

  3. Is your skin usually: Dry _____ Normal _____ Oily _____
     What, if anything, do you normally use on your skin?

  4. Do you need help brushing your teeth? Yes _____ No _____
     If yes, describe:

  5. What is the condition of your teeth? Dentures _____ Good _____
     Poor _____

  6. What is the condition of your mouth? Dry _____ Sores _____ Good _____

  7. Does the condition of your teeth or mouth limit your ability to eat?
     Yes _____ No _____ If yes, describe:

  8. Do you have difficulty seeing? Yes _____ No _____
     If yes, describe:

  9. Do you wear glasses? _____ Contacts? _____
     If yes to either, do you wear them all the time? _____ Part of the time _____

*Reprinted with permission of the North Central Technical College Program of Nursing, Mansfield, Ohio.

Physiological needs take precedence over the others because survival is at stake if they are not met—man must have food and water, air, rest, elimination, and freedom from pain. When an individual is suffering from an obstructed airway, for example, the opening of the airway is the only important basic human need at that time.

Safety and security needs involve the environment of the individual. Shelter and protection from the elements are necessary to maintain basic comfort needs. These needs may at times be either real or imagined; for example, fear of attack on a dark city street would be a real safety and security threat. Sometimes, however, persons may experience feelings of threat that are not based on reality, such as a young child's fear of the dark, or a fear of the water.

The need for love and belonging refers to group and family affiliation where most individuals receive approval, affection, caressing, and touching (Ch. 1).

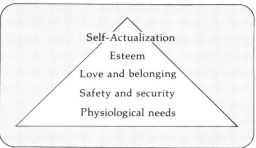

Figure 11-2. *Maslow's hierarchy of needs.*

In discussion of the developmental process (Ch. 2), extensive space was devoted to the importance of self-esteem and self-identity at all stages of life. All persons need to feel respected, worthwhile, and held in high regard by loved ones, peers, and associates. The health-care system is too often a place where esteem needs are given little or no attention. Low self-esteem contributes to more prolonged illness, slower healing process, and increased anxiety.

The highest need category, according to Maslow, is that of self-actualization, or the need to attain one's greatest potential. It includes satisfaction of aesthetic needs—nature, creativity, and knowledge.

In Maslow's theory the emphasis is on the needs of the individual and fulfillment of these needs. In many cultures the needs of the individual are secondary to those of the reference group (Ch. 8). It is then necessary to consider the basic human needs theory in relation to a dichotomous situation of the individual and group.

The taking of a nursing history encompasses observation and interviewing techniques. Communication skills that include attention to verbal and nonverbal cues are very important (Ch. 10). The nursing history should be taken as soon as possible after the nurse and client meet for the first time. Ideally it should be a comfortable, nonthreatening, and respectful interaction for the client. It may be the main activity between the client and nurse, or it may be integrated into the initial care of the client. Since all admissions to the health-care system are not planned or orderly, it may be necessary to begin the nursing history in the emergency room or the intensive care unit.

The setting and type of care may vary. However, there are certain categories that can assist the nurse in gathering data in a systematic, organized, adaptable, and comprehensive manner.

When possible, a standard question format is most helpful in data gathering (Table 11-2). The nurse may also wish to have a quick reference plan that reinforces the orderly, consistent approach to observation. The Assessment Man (Wolff & Erickson, 1977) is an example of this type of initial observation guide (Fig. 11-1). This tool can serve as a short-term assessment guide used to augment the nursing history.

The nursing history, as shown in Table 11-1, is used for planning short- and long-term nursing care. Its elements are:

1.  basic human needs.
2.  perceptions about health status.
3.  attitudes and expectations of the health-care system.
4.  social and cultural influences on health.
5.  plans for self care, discharge planning, community and family resources.

## PHYSICAL ASSESSMENT

The physical examination is a part of the overall assessment step. It can be accomplished in conjunction with the nursing history or it can be done separately. It involves the examination of the client for physical signs that may assist in clarifying his condition. It is usually best to have a systematic method for the physical examination, such as the head-to-toe method.

Each region of the body is examined. The student is reminded to expose only that part of the body being examined, as privacy and self-esteem needs are violated by disregard for the client's body integrity.

The nurse uses her own senses as assessment tools:

1.  sight—inspection
2.  touch—palpation and percussion
3.  hearing—auscultation and voice sounds
4.  smell—odors of the body such as mouth odors and body secretions.

She also applies knowledge of the emotional and psychological status of the person through observation of orientation to time and place, mood, and anxiety level. The physical assessment is a skilled procedure, requiring definitive knowledge of the normal physical appearance and structure of the body.

The usual progression in the physical examination is:

1.  Head: size, shape
    a.  scalp
    b.  hair
    c.  eyes
    d.  ears
    e.  nose
    f.  mouth and throat
2.  Neck
3.  Chest and lung area
4.  Breasts

5. Abdomen
6. Genitals
7. Rectum
8. Extremities
9. Neurological system
10. Endocrine system

Important points to remember in physical assessment are:

1. The body is normally symmetrical and therefore left and right sides can be compared for likeness—arms, legs, ears.
2. Take into consideration underlying organs—the thyroid gland, liver.
3. Consider laboratory reports—urinalysis, blood count.
4. Include temperature, pulse, respiration, and blood pressure.

During the physical assessment the nurse must be keenly aware and respectful of the client's feelings about exposure, intrusion on privacy, and feelings regarding self-disclosure, telling personal or intimate things about oneself.

## PSYCHOSOCIAL ASSESSMENT

The nursing history includes an assessment of the mental health and adjustment of the client, as well as the role of family, religion, cultural diversity and community in the client's life. It is imperative that the nurse consider the client's perceptions of his illness and his needs. The emotional health of the client is as important as his physical health. Very often, attitudes and perceptions influence length of illness, recovery, and desire to interact with the health-care system in the future.

In assessing a client's mental-emotional status the nurse needs to be aware of the levels of anxiety and depression manifested in times of stress, and the adaptation measures used to cope with these stressors. In considering a client's response to entering the health-care system, the nurse should know that: **(1)** all behavior has meaning; **(2)** all behavior is subject to change; and **(3)** all human responses are flexible and adaptable. With these principles in mind, there can be a consideration of the role of anxiety, depression, stress, and adaptation in the process of assessment.

### Anxiety

Generally, anxiety is described as a feeling of dread, fear, foreboding, worry, or uneasiness that is experienced by all people. The degree of the anxiety will help to decide whether it is recognized by the person and what measures will be taken to deal with it.

Anxiety is manifested by physiological and psychological responses. These responses are usually a reaction to a threat to the *self*: a sense of helplessness, a sense of isolation, and a sense of insecurity.

Psychological responses or behavior evoked by anxiety may include anger, complaining, crying, denial, constructive action, defensive behavior, irritation, restlessness, sullenness, quarrelling, panic.

The degree of anxiety may be described as mild, moderate, or severe. This is usually dependent upon the degree of threat to the self and is defined in terms of one's level of awareness.

In *mild* anxiety the individual is able to focus on most of what is happening, as in the anxiety experienced by students about to take an examination. *Moderate* anxiety involves a more limited ability to focus on what is happening. For example, when a student is preparing an injection for the first time, she may become confused in her procedure due to anxiety. The instructor assists her in focusing on her behavior and is supportive of her feelings. She is then able to respond appropriately. *Severe* anxiety is manifested by extreme agitation and an inability to focus on what is really happening. A person in a state of panic best exemplifies this.

**Nursing Considerations**   If the nurse is to intervene in the client's anxiety, she must be able to:

1. Recognize that anxiety is present.
2. Help the client to recognize his anxiety.
3. Help the client gain insight into the causes of his anxiety.
4. Help the client cope with the threat he faces.

Anxiety is usually a response to a stress. Since stress is a part of everyday life, there is generally a level of stress and anxiety ever-present in all persons. It is when the balance is upset that one observes physiological and psychological changes.

## Stress

Selye (1975) has described stress as the usual wear and tear one experiences in life. Stress or stressors would then be classified as both pleasurable (positive) and distressing (negative), depending upon the situation. The stressors are the causative agents of the stress, such as emotional experiences of love, anger, shock, or feelings about disease. Thus, stress could be defined as a state or condition caused by a stressor and manifested by the observable changes within the individual exposed to the stressor.

The main cause of stress is change. The student can readily see that if any change causes increased stress, then any time an individual must enter the health-care system there is stress. Illness of the self or loved ones causes tension and anxiety. Other types of changes important to the nurses's awareness in a holistic approach to health care, are such stressors as a move, a job change, a family difficulty, or the passage from one lifestage to another.

Factors that may affect an individual's response to stress are:

1.   the nature of the stressor, e.g., failure in an exam or loss of a loved one.
2.   the number of stressors to be coped with simulaneously, e.g., hospitalization for illness and loss of a job.
3.   the duration of exposure to the stressor, e.g., a few days snowbound after a blizzard is exciting, but by the seventh day the stresses of being snowbound begin to surface.
4.   one's past experiences with a comparable stressor.

Past experiences with comparable stressors are a very important part of assessing a client's ability to cope or adapt to stress (change). Selye's (1975) general adaptation syndrome explains the response of the organism to the stress. There is first an alarm reaction when the conscious and unconscious perceive the stress and prepare to act. The action, or state of resistance, occurs next and the physiological and psychological forces mobilize to cope. At this point there may be changes in behavior with successful coping with the stress. If this does not occur, one sees the final stage of exhaustion where the individual may succumb without some outside assistance.

Nursing Considerations   In situations where stress is expected to increase, the nurse needs to be aware of the client's past experiences with stress. Some questions need to be asked regarding past coping behavior, perceptions of the stressors, and the plans for present coping. This assessment is necessary for planning care.

## Adaptation

The way in which one alters or modifies behavior in response to stress is considered to be the adaptation to the stress. One school of thought is that one has adaptations and maladaptations, depending on whether the coping style is considered positive or negative, helpful or detrimental. Another viewpoint is that all coping behaviors or responses to stress are adaptations. There has been no definitive agreement on this issue.

Adaptations or coping behaviors may be psychological responses, physiological responses, or a combination of the two. The latter is most often observed. Some examples of adaptation to stress are:

1.   Ritualized behavior such as eating, laughing inappropriately, handwashing.
2.   Hyper- or hypoactivity as seen in alterations in one's activity level—sleep, exercise, leisure activities.
3.   Less-organized behavior such as disorganization, poor attention span, mild confusion.

**4.** A greater sensitivity to one's environment such as increased irritability to normal household noises, and lowered frustration tolerance with loved ones.

**5.** Alteration in bodily functions or physiological activity such as increased pulse, increased blood pressure, diarrhea or constipation.

**6.** A distortion of reality as seen in difficulty with decision-making and/or problem-solving.

The student can see that stress and anxiety appear to evoke similar physiological and psychological responses. The steps necessary for assisting a client with anxiety, therefore, would be applicable to stress, which may be the cause of the anxious feelings.

## Depression

*Depression* is a common adaptation to certain stressors and is characterized by a sense of futility and a loss of self-confidence.

There are a certain group of responses or behaviors that may be observed in any depressed person. The major differences in these symptoms or feelings is in degree. There is always a dysphoric mood characterized by persistent and prominent feelings of hopelessness and emptiness. Other symptoms that may be observed are:

**1.** An appetite disturbance (increase or decrease).

**2.** A sleep disturbance (increase or decrease).

**3.** Loss of energy.

**4.** Alteration and activity level—retardation or agitation.

**5.** Loss of interest in usually pleasurable activities.

**6.** Slowed thinking with a decreased ability to concentrate or remember.

**7.** Self-blame and inappropriate guilt.

**8.** Recurrent thoughts of death or suicide.

The depression may be mild, moderate, or severe in degree.

*Mild* depression may be referred to by some as "blue spells" and is almost always a response to stress. In general, the individual has some idea of the reason for the feelings, and they are of short duration. Disappointments and minor failures are usually the cause. The nurse will observe low spirits, crying, irritability, and lowered self-esteem.

*Moderate* depression is most often related to loss of a loved one. The grief and mourning is characterized by deep sadness, lowered self-esteem, and self-accusations related to the lost one. There is also observable exaggeration of the symptoms of mild depression.

*Severe* depression in an individual not considered to be psychotic (out of contact with reality) is characterized by more drastic and more persistent lowering of self-esteem. It is also known as neurotic depression. Persons who suffer from severe depressions have generally had a history of not learning new functional behaviors from past stress and anxiety experiences.

There is no definitive formula for the management of depression. Some possible nursing approaches may be:

**a.**   Assist the client in bearing painful feelings. The presence of the nurse as a caring person reassures the client that someone is interested in him. If it is difficult for the nurse to spend long periods of time with a depressed person, she can try to designate specific times when they can be together.

**b.**   Assist the client in resolving the conflicts and problems that are causing the depressed feelings. The nurse can use communication skills in assisting the client to reflect. She can validate and clarify, thus helping the client to recognize feelings, both cognitively (head) and viscerally (heart). The client will feel assured that he is not alone in his sadness.

**c.**   Assist the client in dealing with his anger. The depressed person isolates himself from loved ones, who then withdraw from the sadness. There is anger generated by the isolation (even though self-imposed). The nurse can explore with the client the behaviors which have contributed to the social isolation.

**d.**   Assist the client in adopting new behaviors more suitable to a life of higher self-esteem and goal success. The nurse can explore with the client some of the ways in which new social skills can be developed, new relationships established, former relationships revived.

## Defense Mechanisms

*Defense mechanisms* are another form of adaptation to stressors. Thus adaptation is usually defined as an unconscious substitute for more effective problem-solving behavior. The defense mechanism is a psychic activity used to make a feeling or impulse disappear. In general, an individual uses defense mechanisms to avoid uncomfortable or unwanted feelings, to channel feelings into more socially acceptable behaviors, and to resolve conflict. Defense mechanisms were first described by Freud (Ch. 2) and therefore are identified with psychoanalytic theory. They are not, in and of themselves, detrimental or destructive to the individual. They are assessed based upon the extent of their use and the degree of reality impairment they may cause. Denial, for example, as described in the first stage of dying, is considered a necessary and positive defense against overwhelming news. The denial only becomes a problem if it is prolonged and impedes the other steps in the realization process. (Ch. 4).

Some common defense mechanisms are:

**1.   Repression**   unconscious forgetting. Freud believed that much of a person's early childhood experiences are not remembered because of repression.

**2.   Displacement**   the shifting of a feeling or emotion from one object or person to another. A person angry with his supervisor yells at his family when he arrives home.

3. **Projection**   attributing one's own feelings, impulses, or attitudes to another person or object. A student frustrated over receiving a poor grade blames it on the teacher rather than realizing that he did not study the subject.

4. **Reaction formation**   going to an opposite extreme to avoid carrying out an unacceptable impulse. An example is the oversolicitous behavior of a parent for his child, because the child reminds him of his own hated or feared parent.

5. **Sublimation**   channelling the energy of an unacceptable drive or impulse into an adaptive, constructive pursuit. The youth who has impulses to strike out at parents and teachers joins the boxing team.

6. **Compensation**   behavior used to make up for a handicap or limitation. The young woman born into a family of musicians but with no ear for music becomes a physician.

7. **Rationalization**   justification for acts or decisions which are not necessarily rational or logical.

8. **Denial**   blocking the awareness of wishes, impulses, or emotions by disowning them. In the popular television program *M.A.S.H.*, the staff makes jokes and pretends that the war is not there in an effort to keep the emotional reality of war separate from the real situation.

The list of defense mechanisms is not exhaustive, and is meant to introduce the student to one of the adaptation modes that may need consideration when doing the psychological assessment of the client.

## THE NURSING DIAGNOSIS

The nursing diagnosis is the final product of the assessment step of the nursing process. Once the nurse has gathered all of the assessment data, it is necessary to systematically collate the data so that a pattern of needs and problems can be identified. It is from this pattern that the nursing diagnosis is made.

The nursing diagnosis lays the groundwork for the planning phase by identifying client problems amenable to nursing actions. The next phase will begin with goal-setting and planning of nursing interventions.

Validation of the nursing diagnosis is an important part of the process. The nurse needs to be able to have some corroboraion of the problems identified. The usual sources for validation are the client, the family or close friends, medical records, team members, and reference material should there be questions concerning a better understanding of the problem.

## SUMMARY

This chapter has introduced the student to the nursing process. The discussion included principles of the use of the process as well as implementation of the process in nursing care.

Assessment, as the first phase of the nursing process, was discussed in depth. Observation, nursing history, and physical and psychosocial assessment were discussed. The importance of understanding the relationship of anxiety, stress, and adaptations to these were emphasized. Finally, the adaptations of a mental-emotional nature were discussed.

## LEARNING ACTIVITIES

1.  Choose a classmate whom you do not know well and role-play a situation in which you would do a complete assessment of the person.
    a.  What observations were you able to make during the assessment?
    b.  What nonverbal messages did you give to your partner?
    c.  Were your interviewing techniques adequate?
    d.  Were you able to gather all of the data you desired?

2.  Can you arrange the needs of your partner in some kind of orderly, systematic, and concise manner?

3.  How would you proceed with the physical assessment?

4.  What did you note regarding your partner's psychological state? Anxiety, depression, defense mechanisms, adaptations?

5.  Are you able to state and validate a nursing diagnosis?

## REFERENCES AND SUGGESTED READINGS

Anxiety recognition and intervention, programmed instruction. *American Journal of Nursing,* September, 1972, pp. 2–24.

Baer, E. D.; McGowan, M. N.; and McGivern, D. How to take a health history. *American Journal of Nursing,* July, 1977, pp. 1190–1193.

Bates, B. and Lynaugh, J. Teaching physical assessment. *Nursing Outlook,* 23 (1975), 197–302.

Bloch, D. Some crucial terms in nursing: what do they really mean? *Nursing Outlook,* 22 (1974), 689–694.

Blount, M., et al. Documenting with problem-oriented record system. *American Journal of Nursing,* September, 1978, pp. 1539–1542.

DuGas, B. W., 1977. *Introduction to patient care: a comprehensive approach to nursing.* Philadelphia: W. B. Saunders.

Fuller, D. and Rosenaur, J. A. A patient assessment guide. *Nursing Outlook,* 22 (1974) 460–462.

Krozy, R. Becoming comfortable with sexual assessment. *American Journal of Nursing,* June, 1978, 1036–1038.

McCloskey, J. C. The problem-oriented record vs. the nursing care plan: a proposal. *Nursing Outlook,* 23, (1975), 492.

Marcinek, M. B. Stress in the surgical patient. *American Journal of Nursing,* November, 1977, 1809–1811.

Marriner, A., 1975. *The nursing process: a scientific approach to nursing care.* St. Louis: C. V. Mosby.

Maslow, A. H., 1954. *Motivation and personality.* New York: Harper and Row.

Perley, N. Z., 1976. Problems in self-consistency: anxiety. In C. Roy, *Introduction to nursing: an adaptation model.* Englewood Cliffs, N. J.: Prentice-Hall.

Peterson, M. H. Understanding defense mechanisms. *American Journal of Nursing,* September, 1972, pp. 2–24.

Scherer, J. C., 1977. *Introductory medical-surgical nursing.* 2nd ed. Philadelphia: J. B. Lippincott.

Selye, H., 1976. *The stress of life.* Rev. ed. New York: McGraw-Hill.

Selye, H., 1975. *Stress without distress.* New York: Signet.

Wolff, H. and Erickson, R. The assessment man. *Nursing Outlook,* 25 (1977), 103–107.

Yura, H. and Walsh, M. B., 1978. *The nursing process: assessing, planning, implementing, evaluating.* 3rd ed. New York: Appleton-Century-Crofts.

# 12

# Planning, Implementation, Evaluation

Introduction
Planning
Implementing
Evaluating
Summary
Learning Activities
References and Suggested Readings

### Behavioral Objectives

Upon completion of this chapter, the student will be able to:

1. Define the planning phase.
2. Describe the important elements involved in planning.
3. Define the implementation phase.
4. Describe the elements of the implementation phase.
5. Define the evaluation phase.
6. Describe the evaluation phase.
7. Identify the important considerations in recording.
8. Describe problem-oriented medical records.

### Key Terms

| | | |
|---|---|---|
| analysis | motivation | synthesis |
| evaluating | planning | validation |
| implementing | problem-oriented medical records | |

## Introduction

The nursing diagnosis theoretically marks the end of the assessment phase and is the bridge to the planning phase. This chapter will introduce the beginning student to the basic theory and process of planning, implementation, and evaluation. In most fundamental nursing courses the emphasis is placed on the assessment phase and the important intellectual processes and technical skills necessary to assess the client successfully. Mastery of abilities in data collection, interpersonal relations, and communications skills, as well as physical and psychosocial evaluation, are necessary for assessment of client needs. Finally, being able to synthesize, collate, and validate the collected data to use in planning the care serves as the bridge to Phase II of the process.

## PLANNING

A brief review of the nursing diagnosis is appropriate to this discussion of planning nursing care. The nursing diagnosis is the conclusion reached by the nurse following the assessment. There are usually several client problems identified that can be solved or alleviated through some nursing action.

The statement of assessed problems forms the basis for goal-setting and the planning of nursing actions. In most instances this process is outlined by the nursing care plan (Fig. 12-1).

Planning involves deliberate and systematic goal-setting for client care. Some important elements in planning are:

1.  **Goal-Setting**   Working with the client (family) to establish short- and long-term goals for ultimate self-care.

2.  **Priority-Setting**   Based on established goals, some problems will be immediate, some intermediate, and some long-range. The judgment of how to categorize the problems is made by the nurse in collaboration with the client (family). This process involves deliberate and careful consideration of the goals as well as validation of data through continuous assessment.

### The Nursing Care Plan

In most instances the nursing care plan is a formal written plan developed by the nurse in collaboration with the health-care team and the client. This care plan forms the basis for all nursing actions. It is an important source of information and communication among health-care personnel. The formal written care plan is essential to continuity of care. Practical nurses, student nurses, and registered nurses who are newly graduated or inexperienced in practice should expect to be able to work from a well-written and deliberate nursing plan including nursing diagnoses and descriptions of the nursing actions to be implemented (Orem, 1971). The nursing care plans may differ in format and extensiveness of information depending upon the particular health care institution.

## IMPLEMENTING

This phase of the nursing care plan is action-oriented. The implementation involves:

1.  Putting the care plan objectives into action.

NURSING CARE PLAN

| Admission Date 1-13 | Diagnosis Carcinoma of colon | Date | Patient Needs and Problems | Plan of Care |
|---|---|---|---|---|
| Date Procedure 1-17 | | 1/19 | Post-op pain and discomfort | Validate with client, give pain medication |
| Rt. Colectomy, Abd-Perineal | | | | |
| Bath Complete ✓ Ind. ___ Assist ✓ | | | | |
| Showers ___ Tub ___ Bed ___ | | | Promote venous return | Continuous surgical (T·E·D) hose Range of motion exercises. |
| Chair 3 X Day Walk ✓ X Day to BR | | | | |
| Ind. ___ Assist ✓ Bedrest ___ | | | teaching and support in accepting colostomy | Spend time with client allowing for discussion; have visual aids; invite another colostomy person to talk with client. |
| Dangle ___ X Day Brp. ✓ Bsc. ___ | | | | |
| Op Ad Lib ___ | | | | |
| Diet Diabetic 1500 cal soft | | | | |
| Feed ___ Assist ✓ | | | | |
| Abnormal X-Ray/Lab Findings | | | | |
| Flat plate Abd-prominent liver shadow | | | | |
| FBS 218 | | | | |
| Notify in Case of Emergency | | | Short Term Goals | Long Term Goals Teach care of colostomy. |
| wife | | | comfort aseptic technique to prevent infection | Review diabetic diet and hygiene. Discharge Plans Contact local colostomy club. Meet with client and family to discuss home care. |
| Religion Catholic | | | | |

Figure 12-1. One type of nursing care plan. (By permission of Bucyrus Hospital, Bucyrus, Ohio)

2.  Coordinating the skilled care to be given by all team members.
3.  Giving direct nursing care.
4.  Delegating duties and responsibilities as appropriate, including client self-care activities.
5.  Applying intellectual, interpersonal, and technical skills to fulfill goals of the nursing care plan in a holistic manner for each client.

Some important nursing abilities are put into action during this phase of the process. These include teaching/learning methods, recording, and implementing of future goals (discharge planning).

## Teaching/Learning Process

All nurses are continuously involved in teaching and learning. Nurses do client, family, community, and staff teaching. Learning takes place through staff conferences, ongoing educational programs, client feedback, nursing literature, and peer evaluation, to name a few examples. In any situation the teacher is the catalyst or spark bringing the learner and knowledge together with the results being some specific reaction. Learning is the acquisition of new knowledge and a subsequent change in behavior based on this knowledge.

In considering the teaching/learning process as a dynamic part of implementing the nursing care plan certain influencing factors are important to the process:

1.  There must be a need, problem, or dilemma that will serve as the motivator to learn
2.  Information must be available that will allow the person to make realistic decisions about behaviors
3.  Support and direction are necessary while the person is in the process of altering behaviors or conforming to decisions already made
4.  Reinforcement must be given to insure continued adherence to the behavior change (Douglass and Bevis, 1974)

The following example serves to illustrate these four factors: Mr. S has been diagnosed as having diabetes. While he is hospitalized, Nurse N has identified as one nursing problem, "enjoys eating high-carbohydrate diet." Nurse N listed diet teaching as a nursing action. The nurse then made an instructional plan that would include Mr. & Mrs. S in each step. In discussions with Mr. S she found that he was frightened by his diagnosis and did not want to become sickly. Mr. S seemed *motivated* to learn more about diabetes and to change some behaviors.

Nurse N proceeded to make printed and audiovisual material available to Mr. and Mrs. S regarding diabetes. She also invited a diabetic person to talk with Mr. S. Nurse N was giving Mr. S adequate *information* with which to reach a decision.

Mr. S suggested that he begin planning his own menus and deciding on snacks. Nurse N *supported* this activity and invited the health team member expert in special diets to serve as a consultant to Mr. S. Mrs. S participated in this planning just as she had in the previous activities.

Mr. S was very pleased with the number of foods he could include on his diet and still remain within the set limits. Nurse N gave him commercially prepared exchanges for some of his favorite foods. His daily blood sugar levels and urine tests were further *reinforcements* for his managing ability.

Douglass and Bevis (1974) have identified the following ingredients in principles of teaching/learning assessment: formulation of objectives, motivation and reinforcement, establishing the learning environment, learning activities, and evaluation. They go on to state that "assessment is determining the present status of the individual; goal setting is establishing the changes that are necessary; teaching is facilitating changes; and evaluation is assessing what changes occurred and whether they were the desired changes" (p. 33).

The student may note that principles of teaching and learning resemble the phases of the nursing process. It is as if they are juxtaposed in execution and purpose.

Some important considerations can help make the teaching/learning process a positive and successful one.

## Factors Affecting the Learner

**1.** Age, developmental stage, and past experience affect learning and motivation

**2.** Sociocultural reference group influence nature, content, and acceptibility of learning

**3.** Obvious need to learn based on the health-illness perspective determines what will be learned

**4.** Goals that are realistic and include the client are most successful

**5.** Choice of a nonanxiety-producing environment enhances learning ability

**6.** Ample practice time with reinforcement for learning

**7.** Inclusion of family members where appropriate

## Factors Affecting Teaching

**1.** Consistency and trustworthiness

**2.** Enthusiasm and interest in the client and subject matter

**3.** Teaching image: personal appearance, tone of voice, gestures, posture, and facial expressions

**4.** Knowledge of teaching material

**5.** Utilization of a variety of teaching methods and resources

**6.** Realistic appraisal of teaching needed, ability of learner, ability of teacher

7. Acceptance of learner at his level of ability based on health, culture, intelligence, and education

8. Reinforcement of learning and acceptance of minor setbacks

Whenever teaching situations are formally planned, the nurse should remember that a variety of teaching tools are available to facilitate the process. These include books, pamphlets, visual aids such as posters or film strips, audiovisuals, speakers such as representatives of community agencies or societies, and planned learning programs. Whatever the teaching aids may be, the attitude and interest of the teacher will be a major factor in the learning process.

## Recording

Recording in the realm of nursing usually includes nurses' notes (Fig. 12-2) and the charting or notations of specific nursing activities on other records. These include, for example, medication sheets, intake and output (I&O) records, and treatment records. These types of forms differ with each health-care agency.

Nurses' notes usually serve as a record of medical and related therapies as well as nursing actions that respond to the problems identified in the nursing plan. In some agencies only nurses are allowed to record on the nurses' notes, while in others auxiliary nursing personnel—aides, orderlies—also may record on the nurses' notes. Most of these types of rules are particular to a given agency. The nurse will need to familiarize herself with the agency where she is affiliated in order to learn its policies.

The nurse's notes are written communications with specific purposes. They are always written in ink (usually blue or black) and are set up in such a manner that no empty spaces are to be left between the end of the note and the nurse's signature. The nurse's legal signature followed by her status, R.N., is to be affixed to the note. In the case of the student nurse, S.N. denotes status.

The major function of the nurse's notes is to provide the following information:

1. The therapeutic measures carried out by members of the health-care team—dressing changes done by the physician, physical therapy.

2. The therapeutic measures ordered by the physician and carried out by the nursing personnel—medications, range of motion exercises, enemas.

3. Independent nursing interventions identified by the nurse as problems through the nursing care plan—bath demonstrations for new mothers, turning and positioning of client.

4. Observations of client behavior or condition considered important to his general health—fatigue or anxiety noted after visiting hours, fear of impending surgery.

5. Specific responses noted regarding therapy or care—decreased anxiety following inhalation therapy, relief of pain following medication.

NURSING OBSERVATION & TREATMENT RECORD

| DATE | TIME | TREATMENTS, TEST, SPECIMENS | OBSERVATIONS |
|---|---|---|---|
| 1-18 | 11am | Gaviscon tabs ii | Hiccoughs causing strain |
| | | | on suture line. Small sips of |
| | | | water not effective. Relief |
| | | | noted with medication. |
| | | | R. Jones, S.N. |
| | | | |
| 1-18 | 2pm | | Client crying softly. Stated |
| | | | he did not want to live in |
| | | | his condition. Sat with client |
| | | | and talked. Seemed relieved, |
| | | | looking forward to visiting |
| | | | hours. R. Jones, S.N. |
| | | | |
| | | | |
| | | | |
| | | | |
| | | | |
| | | | |
| | | | |
| | | | |
| | | | |
| | | | |
| | | | |
| | | | |
| | | | |
| | | | |

**Figure 12-2.** *Nurse's notes: The nurse's observations are an important means of communication and serve as a legal record of the client's care.*

## Discharge Planning

From the moment the nurse comes into contact with the client, plans for discharge from her care and/or the care of the health agency are instituted. The basis for the nursing process is to intervene when health-care assistance is needed and to strive to assist the client in gaining optimal health.

Planning for the future may include referral to appropriate community agencies, family teaching and counselling, client teaching and assistance. The nurse must be aware of the available community resources, available family resources, and the ability of the client to reach maximum self-care activity. All health-team members must be involved in the discharge-planning if it is to be effective.

## EVALUATING

Separating the nursing process into four distinct steps for the purpose of definition and discussion is an artificial act done to provide a clear picture of the total process. In so doing, one risks giving the impression that one step follows another in clear and concise succession. As has been stated before, this is not the case. The nursing process is continuous and circular, and encompasses all nursing activities from the time the client enters the health care system until his discharge—including discharge-planning.

With this in mind, the phase or step labelled evaluation can be discussed. The nurse if continuously involved in evaluating nursing actions. The care plan, and implementation of the care plan, serve as a framework for evaluating effectiveness of these actions.

The evaluation process, then, is continuous and dynamic. It considers the objectives of the care plan and develops evaluation criteria for:

1. **Measurable Effect** The nursing actions must be documented and should indicate whether the care given was effective or ineffective.

2. **Validation** This should include subjective feedback from the recipient(s) of the care, and objective feedback, such as observations, from members of the health team.

3. **Accountability** This involves being responsible for one's decisions and evaluating the outcome of the care based on questions regarding "how," "what," and "to whom" the actions were directed (Lewis, 1972).

The "how" is a measurement of the nurse's effectiveness against set criteria; in this case the planned nursing action would be the criterion. The "what" is less tangible, in that it must consider attitudes and subtle behaviors of the nurse in her care-giving activities. The "to whom" refers to accountability to client, family, group, doctor, nursing staff, agency administration, and community.

In all forms of evaluation the nurse will be participating in sharing information and learning new approaches to health care which will ultimately fulfill the main goal of the nursing process—assuring optimum health promotion.

Evaluation methods vary from agency to agency, but in general they involve an assessment of the effectiveness of the nursing actions. The following are examples of the types of tools useful in the evaluation process:

**1.** The process recording is a written account of the nurse-client interaction and an analysis of this interaction. The analysis includes communication patterns—verbal and nonverbal— and thoughts and feelings of the nurse.

**2.** Evaluation of nursing care in written form is a method of following the progression of the nursing process from *assessment* to *planning* to *implementing* to *evaluating*. The Problem-Oriented Medical Record method lends itself to this type of evaluation because of its internal structure.

**3.** The nursing audit is a method of evaluating effectiveness of care as it is reflected in the client's health-care record. There are three steps to this process: **(1)** development of criteria (the nursing care plan), **(2)** measurement of the care given, and **(3)** modifications or corrections and staff education. The audit may be done *retrospectively* by reviewing the chart after the client has been discharged from care, or *concurrently* as an ongoing process during care-giving functions. The latter is the ideal example of continuous evaluation.

Whatever the tool or method for evaluation, the student is cautioned to realize the importance of this step in the process. Assessment was said to be "the basis for all nursing care in the nursing process," without which care would be lacking a foundation and be haphazard at best. So the evaluation phase is the permit to continue building on the foundation. Because the evaluation phase requires skills in synthesis and analysis, it often does not receive enough attention in basic nursing courses. This may give the erroneous impression that is is not as important as the first three steps. Another issue in the evaluation phase is that it involves a potential threat to one's self-esteem. The nurse will need to separate her personal self from her professional self in order to effectively grow and learn from self- and peer-criticism of a constructive nature. This is not always an easy task, especially when clients and peers often have expectations of performance that may go beyond the capabilities of the beginning practitioner. This is an area where having a mentor (Ch. 1) can be a supportive experience.

## Problem-Oriented Medical Records

Problem-Oriented Medical Records (POMR or POR) is another method for documenting client care. It is in many ways a type of all-encompassing care plan. The development of the plan in this method involves the entire health team and is reflected in the record keeping. This plan is also problem-oriented, but the client's record becomes the tool on which all health team members

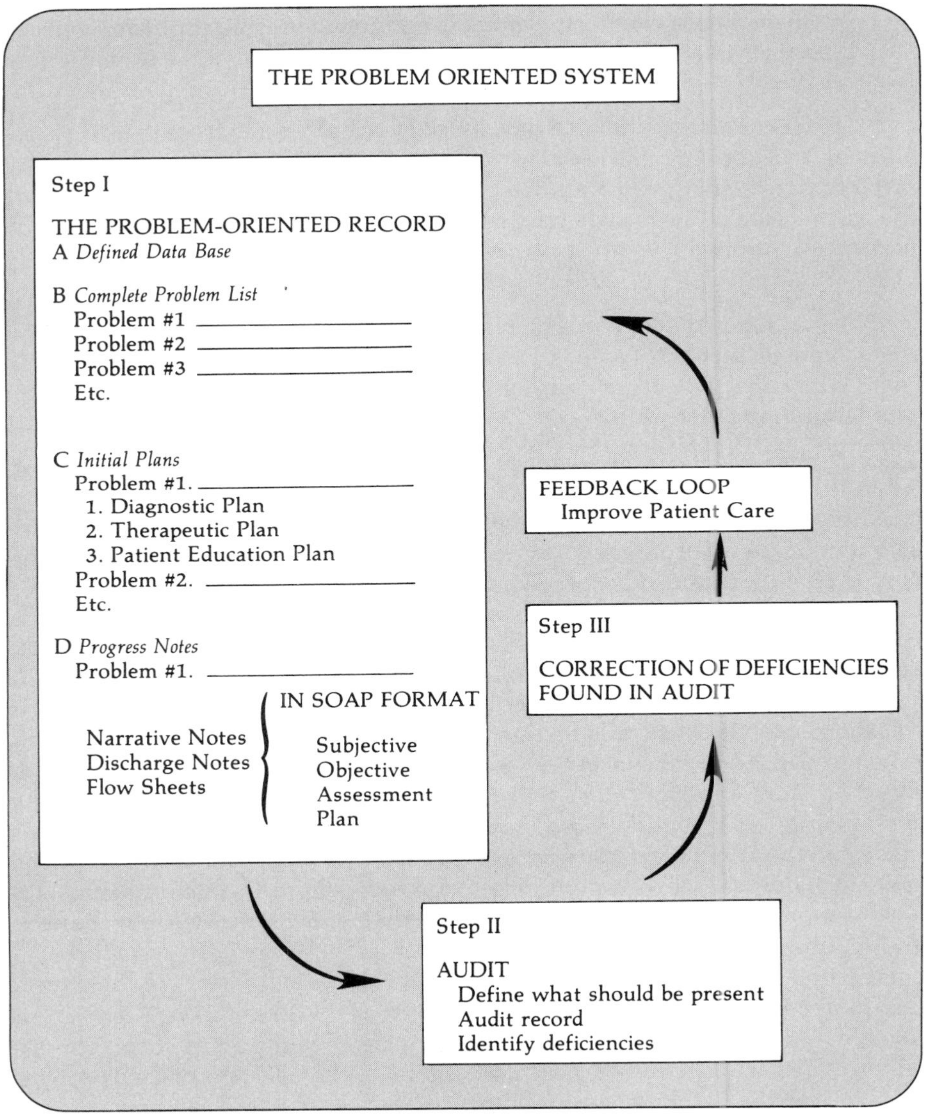

THE PROBLEM ORIENTED SYSTEM

Step I

THE PROBLEM-ORIENTED RECORD
A *Defined Data Base*

B *Complete Problem List*
Problem #1 _____
Problem #2 _____
Problem #3 _____
Etc.

C *Initial Plans*
Problem #1. _____
  1. Diagnostic Plan
  2. Therapeutic Plan
  3. Patient Education Plan
Problem #2. _____
Etc.

D *Progress Notes*
Problem #1. _____

IN SOAP FORMAT

Narrative Notes ⎫
Discharge Notes ⎬   Subjective
Flow Sheets     ⎭   Objective
                    Assessment
                    Plan

FEEDBACK LOOP
Improve Patient Care

Step III

CORRECTION OF DEFICIENCIES
FOUND IN AUDIT

Step II

AUDIT
  Define what should be present
  Audit record
  Identify deficiencies

Figure 12-3.   *The problem-oriented system. (Copyright 1973, American Journal of Nursing Company. Reproduced, by permission, from the* American Journal of Nursing, *73 [July, 1973], 1169–75.)*

correspond regarding meeting the needs of the client. The major components of the POMR are:

1.  Data base   The information necessary for developing the comprehensive care plan. Usually there is a standardized form or questionnaire that asks for the pertinent information. This is very similar to the nursing history form

and usually includes: chief complaint, description of present problem, medical, social, and psychological history, findings from the physical examination, laboratory and x-ray reports, and a nursing history.

**2. Problem List** This list is developed by the physician from the data base. Nursing and ancillary staff feed into the list. Each problem is listed in priority fashion, dated, and given a number. It then becomes an index for the rest of the client record, i.e., each treatment is numbered to correspond to the numbered problem it is meant to alleviate.

**3. Initial Plans and Orders** These are made to correspond to each problem on the problem list. The plan for each problem will be based on **(a)** the diagnostic measures, **(b)** the therapeutic measures, **(c)** the plan for client education. The doctor's order sheet is numbered to correspond with the problem numbers.

**4. Progress Notes** These notes are a record of the problems as identified. All health-team members record on these notes. The progress notes may refer to three distinct forms of record keeping: **(a)** The *narrative note*—these are also numbered according to problem number. They are dated, signed by the person writing the narrative and the title of the person noted (i.e., M.D., R.N., L.P.N., etc.). A specific format for these narrative notes is usually seen and is referred to as SOAP* or subjective and objective observations, assessments, and plan. Briefly the subjective observations refer to the problem as it is perceived and expressed by the client. The client's own words are to be used. If the client cannot speak this section is left blank. The objective observations refer to whatever the observer sees, hears, and/or feels. Tools such as thermometers and laboratory and *x-ray* findings may be included here. The assessments are the impressions, interpretations, and subsequent conclusions made by the observer from the observations. Finally, the plan states the specific action the observer intends to take in regard to this problem. **(b)** The *flowsheet*—these are graphic records that show specific interventions and/or observations in regard to a problem. These are also numbered to correspond to the specific problem. A temperature graph, or intake and output (I&O) sheet, are examples of flow sheets. **(c)** The *discharge summary* is usually the responsibility of the physician in charge of the client's care. The discharge plans are also numbered to correspond to the numbers of each problem on the problem list. In community health agencies where this form of client care plan is used, the nurse would probably be responsible for the discharge summary.

No matter what form of recording is used, certain factors are true of all record-keeping. Since the client's record is a legal document, it is to be kept in a manner lending itself to clarity, accuracy, brevity, and legibility. Erasures are never permitted. Each agency has its own policy for correcting mistakes, such

---

*A nursing adaptation of this format is SOAPIE. *I* stands for the implementation phase and *E* for the evaluation process.

as crossing out the mistake and writing "error" over the crossed out area. The charting should be accurate, truthful, concise, and complete. It is very important, also, that spelling be correct.

## SUMMARY

The last three phases of the nursing process are planning, implementing, and evaluating. The entire process has been presented in a theoretical manner. The student is encouraged to investigate the nursing process in more depth through further study and application.

The planning phase emphasizes goal-setting and the ability to set priorities. The implementing phase stresses the "doing" aspect of nursing. Evaluation leads to measuring the outcomes against the objectives and then making appropriate decisions regarding nursing care.

Included in the chapter in the appropriate sections were discussions of teaching-learning principles, recording, discharge planning, and problem-oriented medical records.

## LEARNING ACTIVITIES

Mr. P has been admitted to the hospital with a diagnosis of emphysema. He appears to be having an acute attack of shortness of breath and anxiety. Mr. & Mrs. P have smoked cigarettes all of their adult life. He is 47 years old and she is 45 years old. Mr. P is being forced to retire from his job early because of his Chronic Obstructive Pulmonary Disease (COPD). The doctor has advised Mr. & Mrs. P to stop smoking and to stay indoors when the pollution level is in the dangerous range.

You, the nurse, have taken a nursing history and found that:

Mr. P has an enlarged chest due to labored breathing; he has signs of oxygen deprivation as seen in the clubbing of his fingers; and his appetite is poor and he is very thin.

Mr. P is very anxious, perspires, and there is a quiver in his voice when he talks. This is Mr. P's third hospitalization and each time the symptoms are more severe.

Based on this information (and your imagination):

1. Formulate a nursing diagnosis.
2. Make a nursing care plan.
3. Discuss implementation of the plan including teaching, recording, and discharge planning.
4. Evaluate your actions.

## REFERENCES AND SUGGESTED READINGS

Barber, J.M.; Stokes, L.G.; and Billings, D.M., 1977. *Adult and child care: a client approach to nursing.* St. Louis: C. V. Mosby.

Blount, M., et al. Documenting with problem-oriented record system. *American Journal of Nursing,* September, 1978, pp. 1539–1542.

Lewis, E. P. Accountability: how, for what, and to whom? *Nursing Outlook,* 20 (1972), 315.

Little, D. E. and Carrevali, D. L., 1969. *Nursing care planning.* Philadelphia: J.B. Lippincott.

Marriner, A., 1975. *The nursing process: a scientific approach to nursing care.* St. Louis: C. V. Mosby.

Murray, R.B. and Zenter, J.P., 1979 *Nursing concepts for health promotion.* 2nd ed. Englewood Cliffs, N.J.: Prentice-Hall.

*The nursing process in practice.* Contemporary Nursing Series, New York: The American Journal of Nursing Company, 1974.

Orem, D.E., 1971. *Nursing: concepts of practice.* New York: McGraw-Hill.

Roy, C., 1976. *Introduction to nursing: an adaptation model.* Englewood Cliffs, N.J.: Prentice-Hall.

Sloboda, S. B. Understanding patient behavior. *Nursing 77,* September, 1977, pp. 74–77.

Yura, H. and Walsh, M.B., 1978. *The nursing process: assessing, planning, implementing, evaluating.* New York: Appleton-Century-Crofts.

# 4
# Basic Procedures in Nursing Care

Hygiene
Skin
Respiration/Circulation
Nutrition
Elimination: Bowel and Bladder
Fluid and Electrolytes
Medication Preparation and Administration
Activity, Rest, and Sleep
Body Temperature
The Sensory System and Pain

Part 4 describes the basic procedures which are essential to the delivery of nursing care of clients. Foundational concepts for these procedures are identified. Nutrition and its preventive implications are discussed. The preparation and administration of medications, a key nursing function in assisting the client's medical management, is described.

# 13

# Hygiene

Introduction
Factors Affecting Personal Hygiene
The Professional Nurse Assisting with Personal Hygiene
Summary
Learning Activities
References and Suggested Readings

## Behavioral Objectives

Upon completion of this chapter, the student will be able to:

1. Discuss factors affecting personal hygiene.
2. Assess a client's need for assistance in personal hygiene.
3. Plan, implement, and evaluate nursing interventions for hygiene.

## Key Terms

| | | |
|---|---|---|
| anemia | mitered corner | sacrum |
| anticoagulant | myocardial infarction | scrotum |
| canthus | pathogen | sordes |
| effleurage | perineum | stump |
| foreskin | periodontal disease | sutures |
| glans | petrissage | tapotement |
| hygiene: personal | podiatrist | urinary meatus |
| labia minora | prepuce | vaginal orifice |
| | pubic area | |

## Introduction

Personal hygiene may be defined as those practices of bathing, skin care, and grooming that enhance one's physical comfort and attractiveness. Nursing has long been associated with helping the client meet his needs for personal hygiene. Hygienic practices vary with the individual. Yet when personal hygiene needs have been met, each client is generally more comfortable than he was before.

In this chapter, we will discuss variations in hygienic practices. We will also discuss reasons why the professional nurse should assist her client with hygiene rather than delegate this responsibility to an auxiliary worker. Nursing measures that assist a person in meeting his hygiene needs are presented.

## FACTORS AFFECTING PERSONAL HYGIENE

Social and cultural factors influence hygienic practices. Knowledge about the importance of good personal hygiene also affects one's hygienic habits, as does one's attitude and feelings about oneself.

### Social Influences

Family hygiene practices learned in childhood probably affect the person's own practices later in life. In some families, daily showering is expected of every member; in others the Saturday night bath is the rule. One person showers at bedtime because it helps him to sleep and another showers first thing in the morning because it helps him to wake up. Many people must brush their teeth before they eat and others are quite content to wait and brush after they have eaten.

Peer group hygiene practices are important, especially to the adolescent. If all of a particular teenager's friends shampoo daily, so will she. The use of deodorant may also depend upon peer practices—to be natural is important to many people, and this might exclude the use of deodorants.

### Cultural Influences

Culture also dictates personal hygiene habits. For example, in the United States a woman usually shaves her legs and her axillae. This is not a common practice in many other countries.

Another factor affecting personal hygiene is the availability of water in some areas. For example, a couple drove from the city to their house in the country to spend a week's vacation. Upon arrival they discovered that the outside pump was not working. There was a mountain spring five miles away which delivered water safe for drinking. Since only one of the persons was physically capable of carrying water, only 4½ gallons of water was obtained. This amount of water lasted for three days for drinking, cooking, dish washing, and personal hygiene. The personal hygiene practices were altered considerably from those normally practiced.

### Knowledge

Knowing that disease-causing organisms are present on the skin may increase one's practice of hand-washing and bathing. Knowing that pathogens are present in the products of elimination (urine and feces) may increase the care one takes in cleansing after toilet use. Other information that may affect hygienic practices is knowing what is fact and what is fiction. For example, some people believe incorrectly that going to bed with wet hair can cause pneumonia or that too much bathing can cause colds.

## Self-esteem

How a person feels about himself may also affect personal hygiene habits. One person may feel he is at his best only if he showers and shampoos daily while another will be comfortable showering and shampooing less frequently. In general, most people feel better about themselves and the world around them when they feel clean, though their definition of cleanliness may vary. It is important for the nurse to take these factors into account as she assists the client with his hygienic practices.

## Implications for Nursing

Certain limitations placed on the client may dictate necessary adaptations in meeting hygiene needs. Often a decrease in attention to personal cleanliness and neatness is a sign of depression or emotional troubles. The person who is confined to bed is dependent upon others to bring him the equipment he needs for personal hygiene. Adaptations in personal hygiene are also required when a client has a physical disability—the use of only one hand, for example.

## THE PROFESSIONAL NURSE ASSISTING WITH PERSONAL HYGIENE

Why should the professional nurse assist the client with bathing when there are auxiliary workers who are capable of assisting him? One reason is that while the nurse assists the client or bathes him completely when he cannot do it himself, she indicates her interest in him. She probably spends more time with the person she bathes than with any other client. For this reason, and because the beginning nurse is known to be more comfortable around a client when she is "doing" something, bath time is a good time to establish a positive client-nurse relationship.

Also, during the bath, a health assessment can be easily and comfortably performed. The skin, hair, nails, and teeth are easily examined. As one senior nursing student related, "I like to give baths because it is easier for me to look at elbows and heels which I have a tendency to forget when I am caring for a bed-ridden person."

In addition, the client's energy level can be determined at this time. For example, how much bathing can the person with anemia perform before he is short of breath?   How is his respiratory rate altered during activity? This is an example of a physiological assessment that can be made during the bath. The client's psychological attitude toward his health can also be determined. Does he talk or is he silent? The client who is being bathed realizes the nurse is spending a set period of time with him; if she doesn't seem to be in a hurry, he is more apt to talk. Is the person with an amputation reluctant to wash his stump? If so, this might indicate that he is denying the loss of an extremity, or it might indicate fear that washing the stump will disrupt the sutures.

Another reason for the professional nurse to assist with bathing is that this time can be used for teaching the client—not just about personal hygiene, but about any aspect of his care. For example, the person who needs to exercise a paralyzed arm can be taught how to do this during the bath. The woman who does not know how to perform breast self-examination can also be taught at this time. While the nurse is bathing a diabetic's feet she has an excellent opportunity to teach the importance of good foot care.

The nurse plans with her client ways to meet his personal care needs. How much help with hygiene does he need? It is a good practice to ask the client how much help he thinks he will need. His need for assistance is also based upon any imposed physical restrictions. For example, the person who has a myocardial infarction (heart attack) is permitted only limited exertion no matter how well he feels.

Client energy needs to be conserved after surgery. Anesthesia causes fatigue. The person's energy should be conserved for woundhealing, ambulation, deep breathing, coughing, etc. For these reasons the nurse bathes the person after surgery.

The nurse and client together decide on the need for bathing. For example, the elderly person may not be bathed completely daily because soap and water are drying to the skin. His face, hands, axillae, perineum, and back are washed. The person who is very ill, as well as the person who finds a complete bath tiring, does not need a complete bath daily. In addition, many other people, both sick and well, do not feel the need for a complete bath daily. Their wishes should be respected.

## Giving a Bed Bath

The purposes of the bed bath are to cleanse the skin and to provide comfort. The person who has not previously had a bath in bed may need some suggestions on how to bathe himself. Some persons who are physically able but confined to bed can wash all of the body except the back. Sometimes the client needs to be taught the exercise value involved in bathing himself. The nurse and her client determine how much help he needs with bathing.

Sometimes it is difficult for a young man to permit a female nurse to bathe him or for a woman to permit a male nurse to bathe her. Whatever may be the nurse's personal beliefs in this respect, it is essential that the client's wishes be respected.

In addition to providing all the necessary equipment for bathing, the room must be arranged for convenience and privacy. The top bedding is removed and replaced with a bath blanket. Usually the equipment is placed on the over-bed table and clean clothing and grooming aids are placed within easy reach. It is important to know whether the male client wishes to shave before or after he bathes and if he uses a safety razor. Hotter water is needed for a shave than for a bath and the water must be changed after the shave.

When the person is not able to bathe himself, the following procedure is suggested. It is assumed that the client can have his bed raised and lowered and that routine hygienic care is needed.

## Special Considerations: Bath Procedure

First, the nurse washes her own hands before beginning the bath procedure. Generally, the bath water should be quite warm to the touch because it cools rapidly. Common sense is a good determinant of water temperature, since

---

### Performance Checklist

### Bathing a Person in Bed

1. Provide privacy.
2. Obtain articles needed for bathing and bedmaking.
3. Arrange articles for efficiency and convenience.
4. Offer the client the bedpan or urinal.
5. Remove the top bedding and fold that to be reused. Place linen not to be reused in a laundry hamper or plastic bag.
6. Place a bath blanket on the client.
7. Elevate the head of the bed to about 45 degrees during oral hygiene.
8. Then lower the head of the bed and remove all but one pillow.
9. Help the client to remove his clothing.
10. Arrange the washcloth like a mitt (no loose ends dangling).
11. Wash the person's face, ears, and neck. Many persons do not use soap on their faces. Check this with the client. Wipe the eye area from the inner canthus out. Use a different portion of the cloth for each eye.
12. Wash and dry the arms; soak the hands in the basin and dry.
13. Wash and dry the axillae and the chest.
14. Wash and dry the abdomen.
15. Drape the bath blanket around the upper thigh; lift the client's leg at the ankle and heel and place the foot in the basin of water. Wash, rinse, and dry the foot. Then wash the upper leg and thigh; rinse and dry.
16. Repeat for other leg.
17. Change the water. (You may have had to change it before this if it had become too soapy or too cool.)
18. Have the client turn on his side away from you, while lying close to the edge of the bed nearest to you.
19. Place the towel on the bed along the person's back and wash and dry neck, shoulders, back, buttocks, and upper thighs.
20. Back is usually rubbed at this time.
21. Have the client turn onto his back.
22. Wash the perineal area if the person cannot do this himself.
23. Remove and clean equipment.
24. Comb the client's hair if he cannot do this himself.

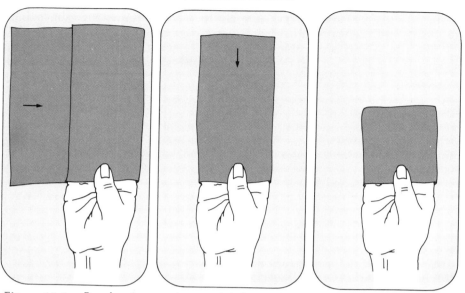

**Figure 13-1.** *Procedure for wrapping a washcloth around the hand to form a bath mitt.*

bath thermometers frequently are not available. It is easy to get too much soap in the bath water, so the water should be changed when necessary to prevent leaving soap on the skin, which could cause irritation.

Not all agencies have linen hampers and laundry bags for the disposal of used linens, but linens should never be placed on the floor. There is a danger of spreading pathogens from the floor and from the soiled linens. It is also inefficient to have to pick the linens up again when they could have been disposed of initially. The sequence for bathing the body parts can be altered somewhat according to client's wishes; however, the procedure on page 207 works well.

## Oral Hygiene

Many health-care workers are aware of the importance and benefits of good oral hygiene and dental care. Dental experts agree that the adult set of teeth should last a lifetime; however, by middle age many Americans have lost their teeth and many others have periodontal (gum) disease.

The objective of oral hygiene is to keep the mouth moist and the teeth free of food particles. Brushing the teeth after eating, using dental floss, and having plaque removed by a dentist several times a year all contribute to good oral hygiene. A healthy mouth and teeth also depend on good general health. When food and fluid intake are adequate, the mouth and gums are more easily maintained in a healthy state than when the oral intake is inadequate.

If the client cannot brush his own teeth, the nurse does it for him. The nurse should also teach mothers to brush their children's teeth until children can do it themselves. There is some controversy over the proper method for toothbrushing; however, the following method is one which successfully removes food particles and stimulates the gums. After a dentifrice has been put on the brush, use a rotary motion beginning at the front of the mouth and working towards the back teeth. The upper teeth are brushed downward from the gums and the lower teeth upward from the gums. The biting surface of the teeth and the tongue should also be brushed. The use of dental floss will ensure adequate cleaning between the teeth, and rinsing will remove the food particles. There is no known value in mouthwash over plain water for rinsing. Personal preference should determine which will be used.

When a person has no teeth, oral hygiene consists of rinsing the mouth of food particles. When oral intake is inadequate, the person's mouth may develop a bad taste and the tongue and gums collect debris and become covered with crusts (sordes). Sordes are accumulations of microorganisms, food, and epithelial tissue. To prevent the formation of sordes, the mouth must be kept moist and free from food particles.

When the client cannot perform his own mouth care, nursing judgment determines how often care is necessary to keep the mouth clean and moist. For example, persons who breathe through the mouth and those receiving oxygen require mouth care often (probably every two to three hours). If the person is unconscious, his mouth must be kept open with a mouth gag (gauze wrapped around a tongue blade and fastened with adhesive tape). A soft bristled toothbrush is effective for giving mouth care even if the person has no teeth. Gauze squares or applicator sticks are helpful in removing dried materials from all parts of the mouth. Gauze wrapped around the nurse's index and middle fingers also work well in cleansing the mouth, though care is needed to protect the fingers from being bitten. Various commercial products are available for mouth care. Glycerine and lemon swabs are pleasant-tasting and soothing when applied to the tongue and lips after the mouth has been cleaned. A female client's lipstick also serves as efficient emollient.

Fluid must be placed in the mouth of the unconscious person with great care to prevent aspiration. The toothbrush or gauze must be moist, but not wet enough to allow fluid to accumulate in the mouth. All the mouth surfaces, the teeth, and the tongue are cleansed. The nurse must be gentle when cleansing the mucous membranes of the mouth; they are fragile and easily injured. The tongue is not so easily injured. A suction apparatus is helpful for removing accumulated fluids from the mouth of the unconscious person.

When a person wears dentures, he usually prefers to remove and clean them himself. However, the nurse must remove, clean, and replace the dentures of the person who needs such assistance. Warm water and a brush will adequately clean the dentures. Some people, however, use a soaking solution to clean their dentures. Because dentures are slippery and may break if they are dropped, they should be placed in an emesis basin while the nurse is cleaning them. If the dentures are not to be replaced in the person's mouth, they are stored in a safe place. Most agencies provide plastic-covered denture containers. The client usually will inform the nurse whether to store the dentures dry or in solution. Usually the person with dentures should wear them. Prolonged disuse causes changes in the shape of the face and fit may become a problem. And of course, eating becomes a problem without teeth. Dentures should be removed before some surgical procedures. This depends upon the type of anesthesia to be used, so the nurse should check the agency policy. Removal of dentures is also important when the person cannot hold them firmly in his mouth, for then they can become an obstacle to breathing.

The nurse's responsibility in caring for the mouth of the seriously ill person is well recognized. Many persons also believe it is one of the most neglected aspects of personal care.

## Back Rub

The purposes of a back rub are to provide comfort and relaxation for the client and to stimulate the back muscles and peripheral circulation. A back rub can help a person rest or sleep because it soothes.

Either lotion or alcohol is used for a back rub. While alcohol has a refreshing effect and dries and hardens the skin, it should not be used when a person's skin is already dry. Lotion, therefore, is generally used for rubbing the backs of persons who are bedridden.

The nurse positions the bed to a comfortable working height and helps the client lie on his abdomen or on his side near the edge of the bed. Lotion is poured onto the nurse's hands where it is warmed and then, using long, firm strokes, it is rubbed into the back. A circular motion is used over the shoulder

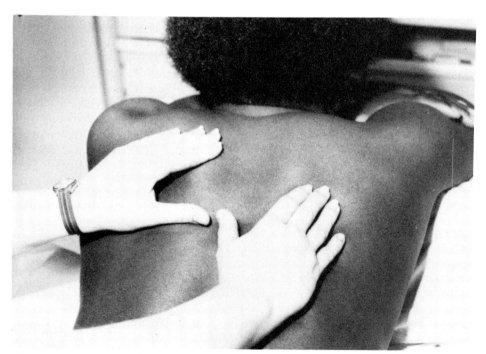

Figure 13-2. *A back rub provides comfort and relaxation. It increases the circulation and helps the client rest or sleep.* (Photo by Frank R. Engler, Jr.)

blades and the sacrum. The nurse starts the back rub at the client's sacrum and moves her hands up the center of the back to the shoulders. Here she uses circular motions to help increase the circulation to the bony prominences. Then the nurse brings her hands down the sides of the client's back to his hips and sacrum where the circular motions are repeated. This process is repeated until the client is refreshed and the lotion is absorbed.

Effleurage, petrissage, and tapotement are three strokes sometimes used in back massage. Effleurage is the smooth, long stroke described above in which the hands are moved firmly up the spine and lightly down the sides. In petrissage, large pinches of skin and muscle are taken along the sides of the vertebral column and then the entire back. In tapotement, the nurse uses the edge of the hand in a gentle hacking motion over the surface of the back. Effleurage alone is effective in providing a relaxing back rub.

## Perineal Care: Male and Female

When the client is unable to perform his own perineal care, the nurse must provide it. The nurse will frequently be required to give perineal care to a client of the opposite sex.

Male Perineal Care   The penis is washed first with a wash cloth and warm soapy water. If the client is uncircumcised, the foreskin is retracted, the glans and prepuce washed and dried, and the foreskin pulled forward. Next, the outside of the foreskin and the penis are washed. The scrotum is then lifted upward and forward and washed, rinsed, and dried. Then the person is turned on his side and after separating the buttocks, the skin from the scrotum to the anus is washed and dried.

Female Perineal Care   Personal hygiene plays an important part in the prevention of urinary tract infections, especially in females. The short female urethra and the proximity of the anus and the external genitalia to the urinary system permit bacteria to be transmitted easily from the perineum to the bladder. The female perineum is always washed from front to back (from the pubic area towards the anus). The outer perineum and the area between the thighs should be washed, rinsed, and dried first. Then, with another part of the wash cloth, the labia minora are washed. The urinary meatus and the vaginal orifice are washed last. Then the client is assisted to lie on her side and, after separating the buttocks, the anal area and the posterior perineum are cleansed in the same manner.

Women should be reminded to pay particular attention to perineal hygiene when they shower. Bubble bath, perfumed soaps, feminine hygiene sprays, and hexachlorophene should be used with caution since they may be irritating. Other ways to prevent urinary tract infections include wearing cotton underpants that have been carefully rinsed, removing damp swimsuits promptly, and giving prompt attention to vaginal discharges (Anderson, 1977).

## Shaving

The male client who has an electric razor can be shaved quite easily. The following procedure is suggested when shaving is done with a safety razor.

---

### Performance Checklist
### Shaving with a Safety Razor

1. Using a hot, wet wash cloth, wet the beard.
2. Place shaving cream on the face.
3. Dip the razor in hot water.
4. Using short strokes and tightening the skin when needed, draw the razor over the skin in the direction in which the hair is growing. The upper lip and chin usually require the most skillful attention.
5. Rinse the face and apply lotion if desired by the client.
6. Clean and replace equipment.

---

Clients on certain medications, anticoagulants for example, should be encouraged to use an electric shaver to minimize the danger of bleeding excessively if cut while shaving.

## Hair Care

The client's hair needs to be kept neat and clean. This may be important in maintaining his comfort and self-esteem. Many people can take care of their hair without assistance. However, an acutely ill person needs help in keeping the hair neat and free from tangles and matting. Brushing and combing are all that is required for short hair. Long hair may, with the client's permission, be kept in order by braiding it.

Persons who are in a health-care agency for a prolonged time period may need a shampoo. The ambulatory person's hair can be washed in the usual way in the shower or tub. The bedridden person who can be placed on a stretcher can be taken to a sink for the shampoo. If the person must remain in bed for the shampoo, the procedure will depend upon the equipment available. Two important points to remember are that the bed needs to be protected and the water used for the shampoo must be able to drain off the hair if the shampoo and rinse are to be effective. Basic supplies include pitchers of warm water, a rubber sheet formed into a trough and a bucket to collect the water run-off. Following the shampoo, the hair should be thoroughly dried and arranged as requested by the client.

For the client who has thick, curly or wiry hair, the nurse should use a large-toothed comb and a firm-bristled brush. After shampooing, the hair should be combed thoroughly before drying to eliminate tangles. Dry hair may need hair oil or conditioner.

## Nail Care

Fingernails should be filed or cut to an oval shape. Care should be taken to prevent injury to the skin at the cuticles and the corners of the nails.

Toenails should be trimmed straight across in a manner that avoids cutting the lateral corners. Nail clippers work better than scissors. Filing with an emery board completes the nail care. If the client has thick and brittle nails, the nurse should soak the feet before attempting to cut the nails. This makes the trimming easier. If the client has a circulatory problem (e.g. diabetes) and his nails are very thick and difficult to cut, it may be necessary to call a podiatrist.

## Assisting with a Tub Bath or Shower

The client who is not physically weak may need no assistance with either showering or taking a tub bath. The nurse should instruct the client on certain safety precautions, however. These include keeping the door unlocked in case help is needed, using a shower stool or chair, using the hand rails on entering and leaving the tub, and emptying the tub before stepping out of it. Rubber strips or mats are usually placed on the bottom of the tub to keep the person from slipping. Call bells are available in bathrooms and clients should be reminded to use them when necessary.

## Making an Unoccupied Bed

The client's hospital bed is made much the same way as his bed at home. After he has been bathed, if the client is permitted to get out of bed, he is helped to a chair while his bed is made. The top bedding has already been removed and any linens to be reused have been folded and placed conveniently on the back of a chair. The following procedure can be used when making an empty bed:

**Special Considerations**
The linens must be smooth and wrinkle-free for the client's comfort. Shaking and patting the linens into place can waste the nurse's energy and spread microorganisms through the air. Linens are folded "away from the nurse" so that organisms that may be on the bedding are not spread to the nurse's uniform. Linens that fall on the floor should be discarded for the same reason.

## Making an Occupied Bed

Making the occupied bed is similar to making the empty bed except that the client's safety and comfort must also be considered. Most of the time, the head of the bed can be lowered and the pillow kept under the client's head. If the client's condition does not permit lowering the head of the bed, it is somewhat more difficult to make a neat and comfortable bed. Because the nurse needs to use good body mechanics when she works, the mechanical bed should be raised so that the level of the bed is at a comfortable working height. After the bed has been made, it is lowered to the lowest level possible for safety and

## Performance Checklist
## Making an Unoccupied Bed

1.   Remove and place in a laundry bag the linens from the bottom of the bed.
2.   If contour sheets are used, place the sheet folded in half lengthwise on the side of the bed where you are working and cover half the mattress with it. If flat sheets are used, the bottom of the sheet is placed flush with the bottom of the mattress, the excess sheeting is tucked under the top of the mattress, the corner mitered, and the sheet tucked under the mattress.
*3.   Place the rubber sheet folded in half on the middle portion of the bed and tuck in the side closest to you.
*4.   Cover with a cotton draw sheet.
5.   Place the flat top sheet that is folded in half lengthwise even with the top of the mattress.
6.   Tuck the bottom of the sheet under the foot of the mattress and miter the corner.
7.   Place a blanket over the top sheet about six inches lower than the edge of sheet. Tuck the bottom of the blanket under the mattress and miter the corner.
8.   Place the bedspread even with the top of the mattress.
9.   Tuck in and miter the bottom corner of the bedspread.
10.   Go to the other side of the bed, pull the bottom sheet taut, and either put the contour sheet corners on the mattress or miter the top of the flat sheet and tuck sheet under mattress.
*11.   Pull the rubber sheet taut and tuck it under the mattress.
*12.   Pull the cotton draw sheet taut and tuck it under the mattress.
13.   Pull the top sheet taut, miter the bottom corner and tuck sheet under the mattress.
14.   Do the same for the blanket and spread.
15.   At the top of the bed, fold the spread over the blanket. Fold the sheet back over this fold so that the blanket is encased by the sheet and the spread.
16.   Fanfold the covers down to the foot of the bed.
17.   Cover the pillow by grasping the pillowslip at the middle of the closed end. Then flip the open part of the pillowslip back and insert the pillow into the cover.

*Steps preceded by an asterisk may be omitted if extra protection is not required.

convenience if the client is able to get in and out of bed by himself. About the only times the mechanical beds are left in the high position are when the client has left the unit on a stretcher and will be returned the same way, when orthopedic equipment may make it impossible to have the bed in the low position, and when the bed is awaiting occupancy.

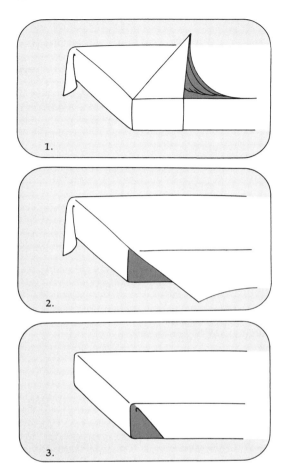

**Figure 13-3.** *Mitering a corner: (1) Pick up the side edge of the sheet and lay it on the bed so that a 90-degree angle is formed (2) and (3) Hold the sheet with one hand to maintain the sharp corner and tuck the rest of the sheet under the mattress.*

The top bedding should be removed and whatever is to be reused folded and placed on the back of a chair before the client is bathed. Since the occupied bed is usually made after the bath, the client will be covered with a bath blanket. The client should move to the far side of the bed so that the foundation can be made more easily. All the bottom linen on the side where the nurse is standing is loosened. The linen is then folded as close as possible against the client's back at the center of the bed. Clean bottom sheet, rubber draw sheet, and cotton draw sheet are then placed on the near side of the bed and tucked in as was done for the empty bed. The sheets are folded as close to the client's back as possible. Then the nurse raises the side rail on her side and has the client roll over the folded linens. From the other side of the bed, the nurse removes and discards the used linen and pulls the sheets tightly before she tucks them under the mattress.

The client is moved to the center of the bed and the top linens are placed on the bed as they were for the unoccupied bed. The bath blanket is removed after the top sheet is in place. Some plan is needed to allow space for the client to move his feet. One method is to make a toe pleat in the top covers. A two inch fold is made in the sheet and blanket either parallel or longitudinally to the foot of the bed. The linen is then tucked in. Another method is for the nurse to pick up and loosen linens over the client's feet.

After the bed is made the unit must be straightened up. All the used equipment is cleaned and put away if it is to be reused. The used linen is put in the laundry chute. Equipment the client will need is placed where he can reach it and, most important, his signal bell is attached to the linens in such a way that he always has the call bell within reach. Before leaving the unit, it is a good idea for the nurse to look around and be sure that the room is neat and that things are where the client can reach them.

## Use of Elastic Stockings

Many hospitalized persons wear elastic stockings in an attempt to prevent circulatory problems. Surgical patients especially wear them. When the person bathes himself or is bathed by the nurse, the elastic stockings are first removed. Unless the client knows this he may push them down while he washes his legs rather than remove them. This interferes with circulation because the bunched-up stocking acts like a garter. The stockings must be removed at least once a day so that the skin can be examined, and an appropriate time is during the bath. After the bath, the stockings are put on much as one puts on nylons. It is important to elevate the legs for a few minutes first to help increase venous flow; then, with the legs elevated on a pillow the nurse pulls on the client's stockings. Wrinkles must be removed. When the stockings are soiled they are washed and reused.

## Evening Care

Evening care usually includes oral hygiene, washing the face and hands, a back rub, and either changing the sheets or tightening them. The person is either offered the bedpan or urinal, or helped to the bathroom. The head of the bed is placed in a position comfortable for sleep. An extra blanket is provided if necessary. The call bell is placed within easy reach. Any other items the person thinks he will need during the night are also placed where they can be reached. Lights are adjusted.

## SUMMARY

The nurse assists the client with hygiene needs as required. While assisting with hygienic needs, the nurse should keep in mind the factors influencing personal hygiene and should respect her client's wishes in this regard. The nurse uses the time spent bathing the client to assess the skin, to determine energy limits, to teach the client certain hygienic practices and to establish a positive nurse-client relationship. She should know how to give hygienic care to clients of the opposite sex. The nurse assesses her client's need for daily bathing and remembers that the elderly person with dry skin may not need a daily bath.

## LEARNING ACTIVITIES

1. You are having clinical experience in an agency where the professional nurses think the aides and practical nurses should help the clients with personal hygiene. They ask you to explain why you believe this task belongs to the professional nurse.
2. Explain why personal hygiene practices may differ from one client to another.
3. Demonstrate to a family member how to clean the mouth of a helpless person.
4. Why is lotion preferred for back rubs?
5. How do you assess when a client's toenails need the attention of a podiatrist?

## REFERENCES AND SUGGESTED READINGS

Davis, E. D. Give a bath? *American Journal of Nursing*, November, 1970, pp. 2366–2367.

DeWalt, E. M. Effect of timed hygienic measures on oral mucosa in a group of elderly subjects. *Nursing Research*, March–April 1975, pp. 104–108.

Giles, S. F. Hair: the nursing process and the black patient. *Nursing Forum*, Vol. 11, No. 1 (1972), 70–88.

Michelsen, D. Giving a great back rub. *American Journal of Nursing*, July, 1978, pp. 1197-1199.

Reitz, M. and Pope, W. Mouth care. *American Journal of Nursing*, October, 1973, pp. 1728–1730.

# 14

# Skin

Introduction
Structure and Function of the Skin, Hair, and Nails
Wounds: Classification and Description
Physiology of Wound Healing
Nursing Interventions for Persons with Skin Problems
Decubitus Ulcers
Summary
Learning Activities
References and Suggested Readings

## Behavioral Objectives

Upon completion of this chapter, the student will be able to:

1. Describe the structure and function of the skin and its appendages.
2. Assess a client's skin, hair, and nails by inspection and palpation.
3. Implement nursing measures to prevent skin problems.
4. Plan, implement, and evaluate nursing interventions for persons with skin problems.

## Key Terms

| | | |
|---|---|---|
| abrasion | ecchymosis | necrosis |
| alopecia | eccrine glands | pallor |
| apocrine glands | edema | palpation |
| aseptic technique | epidermis | pathogens |
| clean wound | episiotomy | petechiae |
| cyanosis | erythema | puncture wound |
| contaminated wound | excoriation | purpura |
| contusion | exudate | sebaceous glands |
| compress | hematoma | shearing force |
| debridement | hemorrhage | shock |
| decubitus ulcer | hyperemia | subcutis |
| dehydration | inspection | suture |
| dermis | intentional wound | traumatic wound |
| diaphoresis | jaundice | turgor |
| dorsal | karaya | ulcer |
| dressings | laceration | wound |
| | melanin | |

# Introduction

The skin is the largest organ of the body. An intact skin prevents the entrance of microorganisms and other foreign bodies as well as ultraviolet irradiation. Nursing measures attempt to keep the skin from injury and to promote healing when skin injuries occur. Minor wounds are cared for so that infection is prevented. Surgical incisions are also kept clean and dry to prevent infection. Nursing measures are used to prevent and treat decubitus ulcers, which occur when a person is unable to change his body position independently and pressure results in breakdown of the skin surfaces.

Physical examination of the skin is readily accomplished without any specialized tools. Inspection and palpation are used to assess the health of the skin. A discussion of the physical assessment of the skin, hair, and nails will follow a brief review of the structure and function of the skin and its appendages.

## STRUCTURE AND FUNCTION OF THE SKIN, HAIR, AND NAILS

Briefly summarized, the skin consists of three layers: the epidermis, dermis, and subcutaneous fatty layer (subcutis). The epidermis includes keratinocytes, which make up the outermost layer (the stratum corneum) that continually flakes off. The barrier function of the skin prevents microorganisms and other foreign bodies and ultraviolet rays from entering the body. It also prevents the loss of water and electrolytes. Melanocytes yield melanin, which protects the body from ultraviolet irradiation. The epidermal appendages extend into the dermis. They include the hair and nails, the sebaceous, apocrine, and eccrine glands. The function of the sebaceous glands is to secrete sebum which lubricates. The eccrine sweat glands regulate body temperature by evaporation and excrete waste products. The apocrine glands are modified sweat glands; they respond to emotional stimuli. Hair has no known purpose other than ornamentation (Prior and Silberstein, 1973). The nails protect the fingers and toes.

The dermis holds the epidermis in place and contains peripheral blood vessels and the nervous system of the skin. The various skin sensations are received through these nerves, a function that protects the body from physical trauma. The dermis is the largest readily available storage area for water and electrolytes (Prior and Silberstein, 1973).

The subcutaneous fatty layer lies beneath the dermis and is the principal storage area for body fat. It is also an important temperature insulator.

## Assessment of the Skin, Hair, and Nails

Nurses have always assessed the skin, hair, and nails of their clients. They have looked at the skin (inspection) and they have felt it (palpation). Nurses

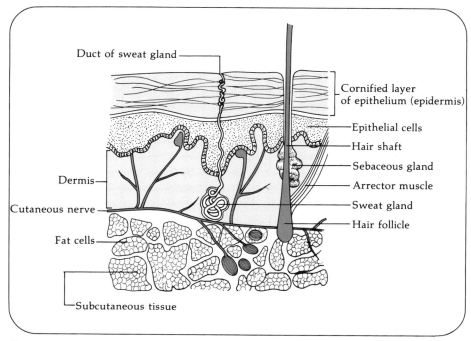

**Figure 14-1.** *Structure of the skin.*

are responsible for maintaining the good condition of the skin in clients of all ages. This necessitates a knowledge of the functions of skin and of its changes in the aging process.

Skin   Without any specialized tools, the skin can readily be assessed by inspection and palpation. Color, moisture, temperature, texture and mobility/turgor are factors to be assessed.

Inspection is defined as visual examination for detection of features or qualities discernible to the eye. Palpation is examination by feeling with the fingers or hand. Inspection is the most important part of the examination of the skin and it requires good lighting, adequate exposure of the skin, and good color sensitivity on the part of the examiner.

*Color*   Skin color not only varies considerably from person to person, but from one part of the body to another and from time to time in the same part of the body depending upon position and environmental factors. For example, the color of the palms differs from the color of the lower outer arms. The color and vasculature changes can be noted when the hand is raised and when it is lowered. The color of hands and feet differ when they are warm and when they are cold. A person may have normally pale skin or the pallor may be an indication of anemia. The best basis for assessing the individual's skin color is to ask him if his present skin color is normal for him.

The following skin colors may be detected when the skin is examined:

1. Tanning or freckles caused by diffuse melanin hyperpigmentation.

2. Erythema (redness) as seen in sunburn or fever, due to increased oxygenated blood flow in the dermis.

3. Cyanosis (a bluish, dusky color), which is due to deoxygenated blood hemoglobin.

4. Localized red or purple vascular changes, which might be hemorrhages into the skin (petechiae and ecchymosis).

5. Pallor caused by decreased hemoglobin, as in shock or anemia.

6. Jaundice (yellowish hue of skin and sclera) caused by increase in tissue bilirubin.

7. Yellowing of the skin (but not the sclera) caused by excessive ingestion of foods containing carotenoids (e.g., carrots).

**Accurate assessment** of skin color is based on knowledge and experience. Roach (1977) discusses the assessment of color changes in dark-skinned persons. As with light-skinned persons, changes are relative to normal skin color. She includes the following important points in the assessment of dark skin. Edema of the skin reduces the intensity of skin color and the skin appears lighter. Therefore, awareness of the presence or absence of edema is essential, as it masks pallor, erythema, and jaundice. Some dark-skinned persons normally have bluish lips and bluish pigmentation of the gums. They may also have brown freckle-like pigmentation of the gums, mouth, and nail beds. Color changes are best observed in those areas where pigmentation from melanin, melanoid, and carotene are not strong. These places include the sclera, conjunctiva, nail beds, lips, buccal mucosa, tongue, palms, and soles (unless heavily calloused, when they will have a yellowish cast).

Inspection and palpation are used together. Generally palpation is used to confirm and amplify findings observed by inspection. Temperature, moisture, texture, elasticity, and presence of edema are detected by palpation.

*Temperature and moisture* The dorsal surface of the fingers is more sensitive to temperature differences than the palmar surface. To check temperature, the examiner rests the back of curved fingers on the skin area to be tested, then moves the fingers to another part of the skin for comparison. Skin temperature depends upon the amount of blood circulating in the dermis. For example, there is local increase in blood flow and warmth in an area of inflammation, and general body warmth in a skin which is sunburned. If the skin of the person with fever is warm and moist, sweating is probably reducing the body temperature. The cold, clammy skin of the person in shock is caused by the generally reduced blood flow to the skin.

*Texture and thickness* Normally the skin is soft and smooth. But of course this varies with the area of the body examined. Some areas of the body are rougher, thicker, and drier than others. The skin of the soles of the feet, palms of the hands, elbows, abdomen, anterior thighs, and eyelids all have different textures and thicknesses. Age and sex also make a difference in texture and thickness. A baby's skin is generally soft, smooth, and thin while an elderly person's skin is often dry, rough, and thin. A man's skin has a texture and thickness different from a woman's.

*Elasticity* (*mobility/turgor*)   When a bit of skin on the inner forearm is gently picked up and released, the elasticity is demonstrated. If it quickly goes back into place, the skin has good elasticity and turgor. The skin of elderly or dehydrated persons exhibits loss of elasticity when this test is applied. The skin is loose and wrinkled and slow to go back into place when it is picked up (see Fig. 14–2).

*Edema*   Excessive body water is seen in soft, swollen tissues. Some people's ankles swell a bit at the end of a long day. When the thumb is pressed against the swollen area, pitting edema is exhibited if a pit (indentation) remains.

**Hair**   The condition of the hair is assessed by examining its texture, luster, distribution, amount. Normally, the hair is evenly distributed over the scalp, adult axillae and pubic area, and other body parts. In the older person, the hair grows more slowly than it did in earlier years. It also gets thinner, and sometimes baldness (alopecia) develops. Greying can be another sign of aging, although it may occur prematurely.

Healthy hair is shiny. Dry, brittle hair may be a sign of illness or the result of chemicals used to change the hair's color or consistency.

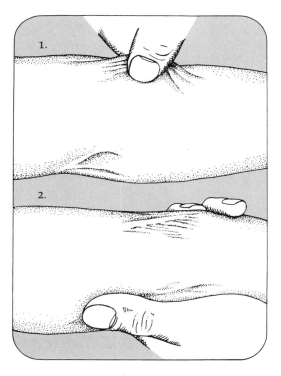

**Figure 14-2.**   *Assessing skin turgor: (1) Pick up some skin on the inner forearm and release it. (2) Skin is slow to go back into place. This demonstrates poor skin turgor.*

Nails   The nails are assessed for color, shape, angle, mobility, and lesions. Normally the nail beds are pink and the nails convex. Many of the changes seen in the nails reflect damage that occurred months earlier. The older person's nails grow more slowly than the young person's and they often become thickened and ridged. By comparison, the newborn's nails are very thin and pliable.

## WOUNDS: CLASSIFICATION AND DESCRIPTION

A wound is defined as an interruption in the continuity of any surface, either internal or external, that is caused by physical trauma. Wounds are classified according to the presence or absence of microganisms, presence or absence of a break in the surface covering, and the cause of the wound.

Presence or Absence of Microorganisms   A clean wound does not contain pathogens. (A surgical incision is an example of a clean wound.) Contaminated and infected wounds contain pathogenic microorganisms. Accidental wounds are considered contaminated. If the pathogens in a contaminated wound are of sufficient number and virulence, the wound becomes infected.

Presence or Absence of a Break in the Surface Covering   A *closed* wound has no break in the skin or mucous membrane. *Open* wounds involve destruction of the continuity of the skin or mucous membrane.

Causes   An *accidental* or *traumatic* wound is one that occurs by accident. An *intentional* wound is produced for a specific purpose (e.g., surgical incision).

Wounds are described as *incised, contused, abrasions, lacerated,* and *puncture* according to the manner in which they occurred.

A. **Incised wound**   a clean cut made with a sharp instrument—similar to those made during surgery.
B. **Contused wound**   made by blunt force with considerable soft-tissue injury, accompanied by hemorrhaging and swelling, but the skin remains unbroken (e.g., a bruise).
C. **Abrasion**   a wound that results from scraping off the outer skin layer (e.g., a skinned knee).
D. **Laceration**   a wound with jagged irregular edges produced by the tearing of body tissues (e.g., those caused by falls against a rough surface, glass, etc.).
E. **Puncture**   a small opening made in the skin by a pointed object (a nail, pencil, etc.).

Nurses will frequently care for persons who have incised wounds made during surgery. It is important to assess skin needs and the special skin care of these persons before they go to surgery.

## Preoperative Skin Care

In order for the client to be as free as possible from microorganisms before he goes to surgery, he should shampoo and shower. In addition, the skin is surgically prepared at the proposed incision site. Hair is removed because of the possibility that microorganisms on the hairs will cause infection at the site of the surgical incision. After the skin is shaved (the area shaved varies according to the type of surgery, surgeon, and the agency) the skin is cleansed with soap and water alone, or sometimes with antiseptics because of their effect on microorganisms. In many hospitals, a member of the operating room staff performs the preoperative skin preparation, but often the nurse may be required to do so.

## PHYSIOLOGY OF WOUND HEALING

### Inflammatory Response

Normally, when the body is injured, inflammation occurs. The inflammatory response is a defense that attempts to limit tissue damage, remove injured cells, and repair damaged tissues. It occurs in three stages: vascular, exudative, and reparative.

Vascular Stage   Following trauma, there is an immediate and brief blood vessel constriction in the injured area. Then the vessels dilate. The increased blood supply to the area causes redness and warmth (hyperemia). Plasma, blood cells, and antibodies move into the interstitial spaces because of increased capillary permeability and changes in the filtration pressure of the blood. Leukocytes surround the foreign bodies and the damaged cells, and the phagocytic process is begun.

Exudative Stage   Fluid exudate is formed of the fluid and cells from the blood, damaged tissue cells, and any foreign bodies. The amount and type of exudate vary with the kind and extent of the injury. Localized pain and swelling result from the collection of exudate in the interstitial spaces.

Reparative Stage   Damaged tissue cells are replaced with new cells or scar tissue. This stage is often called wound healing. The three phases of wound healing are the *lag phase*, *fibroblastic stage*, and *contraction*. The lag phase comes first; blood, serum, and red blood cells form a fibrin network in the wound. The wound is held together by this network (scab). If the damaged tissue is healed by cell replacement, the healing is called regeneration.

In the fibroplasia phase, fibroblasts grow along and in the fibrin network. The fibrin network is gradually absorbed. Granulation tissue, formed from fibroblasts and accompanying small blood vessels, fills in the injured area. The wound then appears pink, soft, and tender. Epithelial cells begin to grow from the edges of the wound. Connective tissue cells then fill in the area and form the scar, which is considerably stronger than the granulation tissue. This type of healing is called *replacement healing.*

In the contracting phase, the small blood vessels in the new tissue disappear and the scar shrinks. This phase may last indefinitely. It is desirable for healing to occur with a minimum of scarring because of the inelasticity of scar tissue. Because of its limited blood supply, scar tissue is also prone to infection and can create future difficulty in healing.

## Types of Healing

**Healing by First Intention**  Tissues return to normal with minimal inflammation and scarring. Incised wounds with well-approximated edges (suturing or use of butterfly strips) and no infection may heal by first intention. Few accidental wounds heal in this manner.

**Healing by Second Intention**  Extensive granulation tissue fills in a wound which either was infected or had wound edges not well approximated. Healing is usually prolonged.

**Healing by Third Intention**  This occurs when secondary wound closure is necessary for drainage, debridement, or wound disruption. After the secondary wound closure, healing occurs by secondary intention.

## Factors Affecting Wound Healing

Factors affecting the body's response to injury include the person's age, general health, and the extent of the injury. The very young and the very old heal less readily than persons of other ages. An adequate blood supply is essential for healing. If arteriosclerosis is present, then the blood flow to the wound is impeded. People with anemia have difficulty in healing (Van Ort and Gerber, 1976). Edema slows wound healing because it interferes with cell nutrition. Poor wound healing also occurs in those who are obese and in people with debilitating conditions, such as cancer. Certain medications adversely affect the healing process—for example, steroids with their anti-inflammatory characteristics, because inflammation is part of the wound healing process, and anticoagulants, which may cause hemorrhaging. Tissue healing is promoted when adequate rest and relief from stress are provided. The diet should include a high protein intake, increased vitamin C, and adequate fluids.

## Complications of Wound Healing

Two common complications of wound healing, infection and hemorrhage, will be discussed here. Additional wound complications are addressed in advanced nursing texts. The infected wound is red, swollen, warm to the touch, and painful. There may also be a purulent (pus) discharge. The person's temperature and pulse may be elevated. Hemorrhage in the process of wound healing may be caused by the rupture of a weakened blood vessel, the disruption of sutures, or a problem in the clotting mechanism of the blood. The presence of bright red blood on the dressing of a healing wound is indicative of possible hemorrhage. Medical opinion should be sought immediately and the wound observed every 15 minutes to determine whether or not the bleeding is increasing. If bleeding becomes excessive the person may go into shock.

Concealed bleeding may occur in the wound under the skin. This hemorrhage may stop spontaneously with a resultant clot formation in the wound (hematoma). A small clot may be absorbed without treatment; a large hematoma will need to be removed or healing will be delayed. The doctor will evacuate the hematoma and, usually, pack the wound. Healing will occur by granulation.

Those factors discussed earlier that affect wound healing are also factors in the person's ability to resist infection. In addition, the nature of the wound has an effect on the incidence of infection. Extensive wounds and those containing foreign bodies frequently become infected. Improper technique during dressing change can also lead to infection. An important nursing responsibility is vigilance in seeing that everyone carries out proper aseptic technique in dressing changes.

The following organisms frequently cause wound infection: Staphylococcus aureus, Escherichia coli, Proteus vulgaris, Aerobacter aerogenes, and Pseudomonas aeruginosa. These organisms are found in the nose, throat, skin, and intestinal tract. Equipment used in dressing wounds may also harbor pathogenic organisms. Some nurses put their bandage scissors in their pockets without disinfecting them. This practice can be responsible for the spread of organisms from one person to another. A study that examines the cultures of organisms from bandage scissors might yield results that would alert nurses to the danger of not disinfecting scissors.

Because the skin and mucous membranes harbor microorganisms, one way to lessen the dangers of infection in the client's environment is to help the client keep his hands clean and to remind him not to touch or scratch the skin around the wound.

## NURSING INTERVENTIONS FOR PERSONS WITH SKIN PROBLEMS

### Care of Wounds: Without Dressings and With Dressings

An open wound that has sealed itself and can be protected from injury and irritation does not need to be covered with a dressing. Many small lacerations and abrasions as well as surgical incisions can be left uncovered. Some of the principles involved in the decision to leave a wound uncovered are:

1.  Healing tissue may be damaged by the irritation and friction caused by a dressing.
2.  Microorganisms thrive in the dark, warm, moist area under a dressing.
3.  Organisms normally found on the skin can be rubbed into the wound by a dressing.

4. A dressing tightly applied may interfere with healing by decreasing the blood supply.
5. Some wounds are in a site that is difficult to dress (e.g., episiotomy).

On the other hand, a dressing on a wound often serves several purposes. When properly used, a dressing helps prevent microorganisms from entering a wound, helps absorb drainage, and helps restrict movement that may interfere with healing. In addition, a pressure dressing is used to stop hemorrhaging. Sometimes a dressing is used to cover a wound that the client might find upsetting to see.

## Putting on Sterile Gloves

A nurse must wear sterile gloves on many occasions: in the specialized areas of the operating and delivery rooms; when performing certain basic nursing skills, such as changing sterile dressings, or when inserting urinary catheters, for example.

**Special Considerations**
Gloves are packaged so that they can be put on without contaminating them. When they are packaged separately, the glove for the left hand, palm side up, is on the left side of the package and the right glove on the right. When the gloves are packaged with other sterile equipment, they are placed on the top so that they can be put on before the other materials are handled. A cuff 2 to 4 inches wide is folded down over each glove. The following is a method for putting on gloves without touching the outside.

---

### Performance Checklist
### Putting on Sterile Gloves

1. Select the correct sized gloves (small, medium, large).
2. Open the package, touching only the edges.
3. Open the right side of the folder without touching the glove.
4. Touching only the folded cuff, pick up the right glove with the left hand.
5. Insert your hand into the glove.
6. Pick up the left glove under the cuff.
7. Put on the left glove, touching the outside of glove only with the right hand.
8. Turn up cuffs by flipping them against skin.
9. Adjust gloves as you would any others.

---

## Changing a Sterile Dressing

Dressings (also called compresses, four by fours, and flats) are packaged two or three to a sterile paper pack or as part of a more complete package containing sponges, fluffs, and abdominal pads for use when the wound is large and draining. The package containing the material the nurse expects to use should be selected. It is inefficient and expensive to open a large pack when a small one would be sufficient.

The surgeon usually changes the initial dressing on a postoperative wound. If drainage soaks through the dressing, the nurse can "reinforce" it until it can be changed. Reinforcing means to add sterile dressings to the top of already existing dressings.

Often the client will not desire to see his wound, and this wish should be respected. The first few postoperative dressings are done by hospital personnel and there is little need for the client to be involved. Later, but well before discharge, the client or a family member should be taught how to change the dressing and told where to obtain supplies.

It is essential that the nurse not display shock, disgust, or some other disturbing emotion to the client when she changes the dressing. She should tell the client that she will not talk while changing the dressing and that she will move quickly because of the presence of microorganisms in the air and in her respiratory tract. In some agencies, nurses are required to wear masks while changing a dressing. Any questions the client has may be answered after the dressing is changed. Clients frequently ask how long the incision is, how it is held together, and whether or not there will be a scar. It is safe, generally, to tell a client that surgical incisions usually heal with minimal scarring.

### Special Considerations

Privacy should be provided before the dressing change is begun. The curtains around the bed may be pulled, or the door in a private room closed. The client should be helped to a comfortable position. If indicated, pain medication can be given before the dressing change. Good lighting and a satisfactory work area (such as an overbed table) are important.

The following supplies are needed for a dressing change: a sterile forceps or sterile gloves for removing the soiled dressing without contaminating the wound or the hands; materials for cleansing the wound and surrounding tissue; a second sterile forceps or pair of gloves for applying the clean dressing; dressings and material for securing them; and a receptacle for the safe disposal of used dressings and instruments.

The directions on page 229 are given for changing a dressing when there is drainage; if there is no drainage, these directions can be easily adapted.

## Securing the Dressing

Adhesive tape is used most frequently for attaching dressings. Nonallergenic tape is available for those persons allergic to tape. Special adhesive straps (Montgomery straps) are used when frequent dressing changes are needed. Binders are also used to hold some dressings in place.

## Protecting the Skin Around a Draining Wound

The skin around a draining wound is kept clean and dry by applying a protective substance (e.g., karaya) on the skin to keep drainage from coming in

---

### Performance Checklist

### Changing a Sterile Dressing

1. Obtain equipment. Be sure dressings are sterile by checking the sterilization date on the package, and examine for dampness or tears.
2. Wash hands.
3. Put on mask if required by agency policy.
4. Place overbed table in a convenient position.
5. Place a waterproof disposable bag for holding contaminated articles within reach, but away from the sterile field.
6. Drape the client to expose the wound area.
7. Open instrument and dressing packages and use inside of wrappers as sterile field.
8. Loosen tape on dressing by pulling straight back toward wound to lessen discomfort. Solvent such as acetone may be necessary to make tape removal easier.
9. Remove dressing by using forceps or sterile gloves. If dressing sticks, moisten area with sterile saline, water, or hydrogen peroxide.
10. Assess the amount and type of drainage.
11. Discard dressing and forceps or gloves in the waste bag without touching the outside of the bag so that safe disposal is made easier.
12. Put on new sterile gloves or use another sterile forceps.
13. To decrease the chances of infecting the wound, using antiseptic cleansing solution and sponges, cleanse the wound as follows:
    a. use a fresh sponge for each stroke.
    b. starting with the top of the wound, move down and out gradually.
    c. discard sponges in waste bag.
    d. dry the area well with sterile material.
14. Assess condition of wound.
15. Place sterile dressings over the wound (once placed, they are not to be moved). Add absorbent dressings as needed.
16. Remove sterile gloves. Only outermost dressing may be touched with the bare hands.
17. Secure the dressing with tape.
18. Answer any questions the client may have and provide physical comfort as needed.
19. Remove and discard the waste bag and its contents in such a manner that no one else will touch contaminated material.
20. Wash hands.
21. Chart the dressing change: include type and amount of drainage, appearance of the wound, and any special procedure for dressing change that might help the person doing the next dressing.

---

contact with the skin. The protective substance is usually removed once a day, the underlying skin cleansed, and the protective substance reapplied. Care is used to keep friction to a minimum during the procedure so that epithelial cells are not damaged.

## DECUBITUS ULCERS

Decubitus ulcers (decubiti) are a type of pressure sore. Frequently these ulcers are called bedsores, but this is incorrect. Pressure sores can develop in persons not confined to bed. The cause of decubitus ulcers is excessive or prolonged pressure, causing decreased or absent blood flow. Cellular death (necrosis) results from this interference in cell nourishment and removal of cellular wastes. Decubitus ulcers describe an area in which the skin is destroyed and, progressively, the underlying tissues are destroyed. Both the amount and duration of pressure are important. While the skin can withstand high pressure for a short time without breaking down, it frequently breaks down because of low to moderate pressure over a prolonged period.

Development of pressure sores is also related to shearing force. For example, when the head of the bed is raised 30 degrees or higher, the person slides down toward the foot. Tissues attached to bony structures, such as the sacrum and the heels, move with the person; however, because of the friction between the skin and the bed linens, the skin tends to stay in a fixed position. This pushing force causes obstruction of subcutaneous blood flow because of the sliding of one tissue layer over another; and eventually, deep ulcers can form.

### Prevention of Decubitus Ulcers

It is easier to prevent the formation of pressure sores than it is to treat them. Carbary (1974) states that "superb nursing care is most important in prevention and treatment of bedsores." Even when vigorous nursing measures are implemented to prevent pressure sores, some persons will develop decubiti.

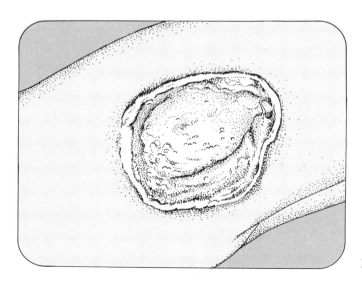

Figure 14-3.   *Decubitis ulcer.*

Especially susceptible are those people who cannot change their own body position (for whatever reason), those who are overweight or underweight, older people with dry wrinkled skin, people whose skin cannot be kept clean and dry, people with fever or with edema, and people suffering from the problems of poor nutrition.

Prevention of decubiti includes daily assessment of the skin of susceptible persons, elimination of sources of pressure, keeping the skin clean, dry, and well lubricated, and maintaining good nutrition.

Initially, pressure causes ischemia (decreased blood supply to an area) and the area looks pale. We can demonstrate this when we press a fingernail against the finger and note the blanching that results. This reaction is similar to the body's first response to pressure, signaling the onset of a pressure sore. It is most easily visible on a client's heels. In other susceptible body areas, redness is the first visible indication of pressure. We see this when we cross our legs for five minutes. When we uncross them, we find large, red, circular pressure areas and increased warmth. The redness and warmth (hyperemia) are caused by the rush of blood to the area after the pressure is removed. This normal reaction quickly supplies cell nutrients and oxygen and removes cellular wastes.

If the pressure on an area continues, the skin turns dusky and does not blanch under pressure. However, if the skin can be kept intact, infection can be prevented. Any break in the skin increases the chance that pressure sores will develop.

The nurse should look particularly for color changes in the pressure sites formed by the bony prominences. The less the muscle and subcutaneous padding over a bony prominence, the more susceptible the area is to pressure. If the client can hold a mirror, he should be taught to inspect his own skin.

The pressure points for a person in four common positions are:

a. **Supine Position**   sacrum, heels, elbows, scapula, back of head.
b. **Side-lying Position**   ankle, greater trochanter, medial and lateral condyles, ribs, acromion process, cheek, and ear.
c. **Prone Position**   toes, knees, iliac crests, breasts, male genitalia, acromion processes, cheek, and ear.
d. **Sitting**   ischial tuberosities.

There are many ways to eliminate pressure. The normally mobile person changes his own position when discomfort tells him there is too much pressure on an area. When a person cannot feel pressure (e.g., if he is paralyzed), the nurse is responsible for hourly turning to prevent skin breakdown. The person is turned from back to abdomen and to each side in regular order unless a certain position is contraindicated.

If the immobile person can be moved from the bed to a tilt table or a chair, pressure is redistributed. However, even when a person is sitting in a chair, position change is necessary. The nurse must encourage the person who has no feeling in his buttocks to raise himself up every 30 minutes by placing his weight on his arms. Artificial sheepskin or foam protect pressure points, especially in the sacral area, elbows, and heels. Sheepskins help absorb moisture and, therefore, are valuable in keeping the skin dry as well as in relieving pressure and friction between the skin and the bed sheets. Some people, however, find sheepskin uncomfortably warm and decline to use it. The value of the sheepskin is decreased when health-care workers have to place an incontinence pad on top of it.

Overbed cradles keep the bed clothes off the feet and thereby prevent pressure. An alternating pressure mattress is another way to prevent these problems. The electrically operated pneumatic mattress has air strips that alternately inflate and deflate at three to five minute intervals. Therefore, no one area of the body is exposed to pressure for more than a few minutes at a time. Additional ways to relieve pressure include: keeping the bed linens free from wrinkles and foreign objects such as crumbs, pins, and needles; keeping equipment, such as intravenous tubing or boards, nasal catheters, or nasogastric tubes from exerting pressure on the skin; using a pull sheet to lessen friction when moving a helpless person up in bed; providing an overhead trapeze for those people who can move themselves; keeping the bed as flat as possible to lessen shearing force; avoiding the use of a too firm mattress; and eliminating plastic or rubber sheets on the bed because they add to skin irritation.

It is important to keep the skin clean, dry, and well lubricated, although good skin care alone will not prevent the development of pressure sores (Bliss and McLaren, 1967). Any break in the skin will predispose subcutaneous tissue to infection; therefore, it is essential to inhibit the growth of microorganisms by keeping the skin clean and dry. When the person is debilitated, infection spreads rapidly. Wrinkled, dry skin may crack or peel and allow bacteria to enter. Therefore, the person who has dry skin must be well lubricated. The skin folds of an overweight person, who may perspire excessively, must be kept clean and dry. When a person is incontinent of urine or feces, cleaning the skin immediately and changing the bed linen helps prevent excoriation of the skin and a decrease of skin turgor due to the contact with moisture. If there is a draining wound and the skin cannot be completely protected from secretions, a protective skin barrier (karaya, zinc oxide, petrolatum) can be used to prevent excessive irritation. Massaging with lotion helps to relieve skin dryness, to reduce friction, and to improve circulation. Alcohol should not be used because of its drying nature.

Because protein is necesary to maintain tissue integrity, the protein intake is increased. Fluids are encouraged to maintain skin turgor and prevent infection. Vitamin C is given to decrease capillary fragility and hasten healing.

## Treatment of Decubitus Ulcers

Despite the implementation of nursing measures to prevent decubiti, some people still develop them. The preventive measures described are also used therapeutically in addition to other procedures. No one method has proven successful in treating decubiti. However, some of the methods in current use are:

**Water Mattresses**    These distribute pressure evenly over the body surface. They are used on the principle that when pressure is increased on an enclosed liquid, it is distributed uniformly and undiminished to all parts of the liquid.

**Flotation Pads**    These usually contain silicone gel and are designed to imitate fatty tissue. They are used especially for persons who sit in chairs for long time periods.

**Adhesive-Backed Foam Rubber**    This is used to distribute the pressure equally. An appropriate-sized hole is cut in the foam to allow air to reach the skin.

Local therapeutic measures in decubiti care include:

1. Oxygen is applied at 15 liters for five minutes.
2. Ultraviolet irradiation.
3. Exposure to the air several times daily.
4. Exposure to an electric light bulb.
5. Packing the wound with granulated sugar.
6. Cleansing with mild soap and water, sterile water, saline, or peroxide.
7. Topical enzymatic or proteolytic digestive agents (e.g., Elase, Varidase).
8. Gelfoam, which forms a lattice-work for fibroblastic activity.
9. Gelusil or Maalox applied directly and allowed to dry.
10. Vitamin E.
11. Cortisone.
12. Topical antibiotics.

The ulcer site is often cultured. If indicated by the results of the culture, oral antibiotics are prescribed. When the ulcer cannot be debrided by use of topical agents, surgical intervention is required.

Evaluation of nursing intervention in decubiti care is essential. Many persons cite the need for more scientific evaluation of the effectiveness of the therapeutic agents used in decubiti care. No one method has been found to be the best prevention or treatment. Van Ort and Gerber (1976), using a small (14), predominantly female sample, tested the hypothesis that "there would be a significant increase in the rate of healing for those who received topical insulin therapy as evidenced by a decrease in the diameter of the ulcer." Ten units of U-40 insulin were dropped into the wound twice a day and the wound was then exposed to the air. Treatment continued for 15 days. The hypothesis was supported: photographs indicated that the diameters of the ulcers decreased. Evaluation of similar interventions in prevention and treatment of decubitus ulcers is necessary.

## SUMMARY

Nurses have always assessed the skin, hair, and nails of their clients. They have also been held accountable for maintaining the integrity of their client's skin. Whether the client was a healthy newborn or an immobilized older person, the nurse was responsible for preventing skin breakdown. Today, the nurse continues to be responsible for the assessment of the skin, hair, and nails of all her clients—both well and ill. She knows the physiology of wound healing and the factors that hasten or delay healing. She can change a sterile dressing and teach others how. In addition, while the nurse focuses on prevention of decubitus ulcers, she is able to use various methods to treat them. Evaluation of the success of the treatment is an important aspect of nursing intervention.

## LEARNING ACTIVITIES

1. Compare the skin of an infant with that of a healthy 85-year-old.
2. List four functions of the skin.
3. Describe how to assess pallor in a dark-skinned person.
4. Describe three factors which determine the skin's resistance to injury.
5. Classify wounds according to their cause.
6. List two complications of wound healing.
7. Make a plan to be used in teaching a family member to change a dressing on a draining abdominal wound.
8. Compare two methods used in prevention of decubiti.
9. Compare two methods used in the treatment of decubiti.
10. Identify one area in decubiti care that you would like to research.

## REFERENCES AND SUGGESTED READINGS

Bliss, M. R. and McLaren, R.   Preventing pressure sores in geriatric patients. *Nursing Mirror*, 123 (February 3, 1967), 405.

Carbary, L. J.   Bedsores: a real challenge. *Nursing Care,* November, 1974. pp. 22–25.

Derbes, Vincent J.   Rashes: recognition and management. *Nursing 73,* March, 1973, pp. 44–49.

Gruis, Marcia L. and Innes, Barbara.   Assessment: essential to prevent pressure sores. *American Journal of Nursing*, November, 1976, pp. 1762–1764.

Henderson, John, 1973.   *Emergency medical guide.* New York: McGraw-Hill.

Luckmann, Joan and Sorensen, Karen, 1974.   *Medical-surgical nursing.* Philadelphia: W. B. Saunders.

Prior, John and Silberstein, Jack, 1973.   *Physical diagnosis.* St. Louis: C. B. Mosby.

Roach, Lora B.   Color changes in dark skin. *Nursing 77,* January 1977, pp. 48–51.

Van Ort, Suzanne R. and Gerber, Rose M.   Topical application of insulin in the treatment of decubitus ulcers. *Nursing Research,* January-February 1976, pp. 9–12.

# 15

# Respiration/Circulation

Introduction
Structure and Function of Respiratory/Circulatory Systems
Prevention of Respiratory/Circulatory Problems
Assessment of Respiratory/Circulatory Functioning
Assisting Clients to Achieve Adequate Ventilation/Circulation
Summary
Learning Activities
References and Suggested Readings

## Behavioral Objectives

Upon completion of this chapter, the student will be able to:

1. Identify the structures of the respiratory/circulatory systems and briefly describe their functions.
2. Plan and implement measures for the prevention of respiratory/circulatory problems.
3. Assess the respiratory/circulatory systems of a client in health and in illness.
4. Plan and implement, after practice, nursing measures to assist clients with a variety of respiratory/circulatory problems and evaluate the results.

## Key Terms

ABG (arterial blood gases)
accessory muscles of inspiration
alveoli
apical-radial pulse
apnea
arrhythmia
biopsy
blood pH
bradycardia
bradypnea
breath sounds
bronchi
bronchioles
bronchitis
bronchoscopy
cannula

cardiac catheterization
carotid sinuses
catheter
chemoreceptors
chest p – t (percussion and vibration)
Cheyne-Stokes
cholesterol
costal breathing
CPR (cardiopulmonary resuscitation)
cyanosis
diastolic pressure
diffusion
dyspnea
electrocardiogram
external respiration

fluoroscopy
glomerulonephritis
heart structures
Heimlich maneuver
hematocrit
hemoglobin
Hering-Breuer reflex
hypoxia
internal respiration
intradermal
IPPB
isolette
Kussmaul respirations
kyphosis
larynx
mucus

nebulizer
orthopnea
otitis
palpatory estimate
patent
peripheral pulses
pharynx
pleura
postural drainage
precordial thump

Pulmonary Function Tests
pulse deficit
pulse pressure
râles
respiration
respiratory center
rheumatic fever
scoliosis
sinusitis
sphygmomanometer
streptococcal infection

systolic pressure
tachycardia
tachypnea
tidal volume
trachea
tracheostomy
triglycerides
venules
wheezes
xiphoid

## Introduction

Nurses learn early that maintaining a patent (open) airway is the priority for life. The body cannot live without oxygen and since oxygen cannot be stored, a constant supply is required. Atmospheric air provides all the oxygen that is required in health and, if the passages from the nose to the alveoli are open, there is no problem in ventilation. Because blood transports the gases to and from the cells, the circulatory system must be functional if life is to be maintained. This chapter discusses briefly the structure and function of the respiratory and circulatory systems. It focuses on nursing assessment of the respiratory/circulatory systems and presents nursing measures for prevention of problems. Hypertension screening, detection of strep throat, and pollution prevention are discussed. Selected common diagnostic measures are included. Nursing measures to assist a client with respiratory/circulatory problems are stressed. Interventions range from care of the common cold to cardiopulmonary resuscitation. All interactions are evaluated.

## STRUCTURE AND FUNCTION OF RESPIRATORY/CIRCULATORY SYSTEMS

### Respiration

Oxygen is essential for life and necessary for the process of respiration. Normally, all the oxygen required is provided by atmospheric air which, at sea level, provides 20.95 percent oxygen and 0.04 percent carbon dioxide. An unobstructed airway is required for the passage of oxygen from the atmosphere to the alveoli, and carbon dioxide from the alveoli to the air. Respiration includes two processes, external and internal respiration. External respiration refers to the absorption of oxygen and the removal of carbon dioxide from the body as a whole. Internal respiration refers to the gaseous exchanges between the cells and their fluid medium. Successful gas exchange depends on efficient functioning of both the respiratory and circulatory systems.

**Mechanics of Respiration**   Respiration consists of two phases: inspiration and expiration (inhalation and exhalation). Breathing is accomplished by movements of muscles of the chest wall (the intercostals) and the diaphragm. In addition, in forced breathing, abdominal and neck muscles may be brought into use. During inspiration, the diaphragm descends as it contracts, and the rib cage is lifted up and out. During expiration, the diaphragm ascends as it relaxes, and the rib cage is drawn down and in. Relaxation of the abdominal muscles allows greater diaphragmatic contraction. While most people use both costal (rib) and diaphragmatic breathing, some use more of one type than the other. Costal breathing is more shallow than diaphragmatic breathing.

**Anatomical Structures**   All the anatomical structures involved in respiration must be intact and capable of moving air in and out with ease if gas exchange is to occur. Air passes through the nasal passages, pharynx, larynx, trachea, bronchi, and bronchioles to the alveoli, and then returns. The air is humidified, warmed, and cleansed as it passes through the respiratory tract which is lined with mucous membrane, part of which contains cilia and excretes mucus to trap organisms and other foreign matter. The lungs are cone-shaped organs containing the alveoli, bronchi, and bronchioles. The

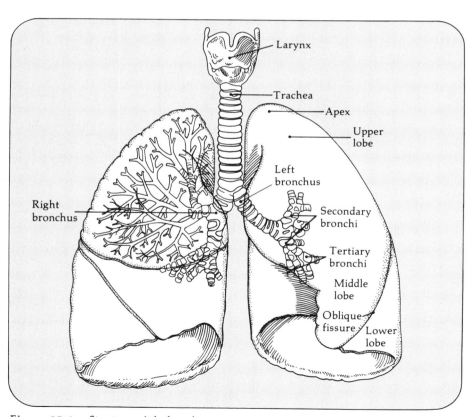

**Figure 15-1.**   *Structures of the bronchorespiratory tree.*

alveoli are tiny sacs, each composed of a thin elastic tissue wall containing a network of capillaries and a thin layer of epithelial cells through which molecules of gas can diffuse. The left lung is made up of two lobes; the right lung of three. The lungs are surrounded by a potential space called the pleura. The inner lining of the pleura is the visceral pleura and the outer lining the parietal pleura. The space between these linings maintains a pressure that is more negative than the pressure within the lungs. Because of this constant negative pressure the elastic lungs remain expanded.

When oxygen enters the alveoli, it passes into the blood as a result of diffusion. Oxygen passes from the area of higher pressure (inspired air) to the area of lower pressure (oxygen in the venous blood). Diffusion also accounts for the passage of carbon dioxide from the blood to the alveoli.

Respiratory Control   The respiratory process is controlled principally by the respiratory center in the medulla. Changes in respiration are initiated by impulses from specialized receptors. For example, impulses from stretch receptors located principally in the visceral pleura surrounding the lungs initiate the Hering-Breuer reflex: at a specific point during inspiration these receptors carry impulses to the respiratory center; then inspiration is quickly inhibited and the expiratory phase of respiration is triggered. During expiration the reverse occurs. Chemoreceptors located in the respiratory center, aorta, and carotid sinuses respond to changes in the chemical composition of the blood and other body fluids. The respiratory rate is stimulated by a lower concentration of oxygen, a higher concentration of carbon dioxide, a lowered blood pH, and an elevated body temperature. Changes in arterial blood pressure affect pressoreceptors in the aorta and carotid sinuses, which transmit impulses to the respiratory center in the medulla. A sudden rise in blood pressure will cause a decrease in respirations. Exercise acts to stimulate respirations as the proprioceptors located in muscles and tendons of movable joints are stimulated.

Other factors influencing respirations include anxiety, pain, fear, and anger, which usually increase the respirations.

## Circulation

The transportation of oxygen to the cells and carbon dioxide from the cells depends upon an adequate circulatory system: the heart, blood vessels, and blood must be functioning properly. The heart must contract, blood vessels must be intact, and the quantity and quality of blood must be adequate.

The heart has four chambers: the right atrium, right ventricle, left atrium, and left ventricle. It is enclosed in a protective sac called the pericardium. The superior and inferior vena cava return unoxygenated blood to the right atrium. The right atrium is separated from the right ventricle by the tricuspid valve. The pulmonary artery, the only artery in the body carrying unoxygenated blood, originates in the wall of the right ventricle. Right and left branches of this artery lead to the right and left lungs.

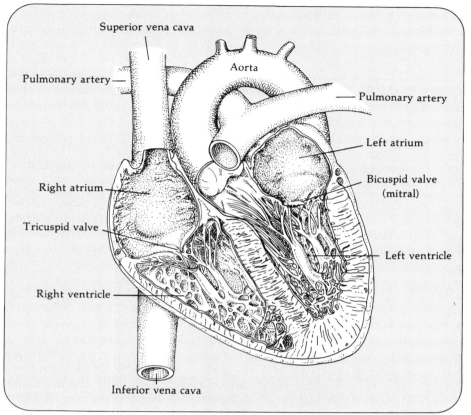

**Figure 15-2.** *Structures of the heart.*

In the lungs, carbon dioxide is exchanged for oxygen at the alveolar-capillary membrane. Minute branches of the pulmonary arteries (pulmonary capillaries) lie immediately adjacent to the alveoli; oxygen readily diffuses into the capillary and carbon dioxide diffuses outward into the alveoli. This phase of gas exchange depends upon adequate gas pressures, the presence of hemoglobin, and appropriate capillary membrane structure. After diffusion at the alveolar level is complete, oxygenated blood returns by the pulmonary vein to the left atrium. The mitral valve separates the left atrium and ventricle. The aortic valve separates the left ventricle from the aorta, which delivers oxygenated blood to peripheral arteries and arterioles, and these deliver oxygen to the cells. Carbon dioxide is removed from the cell by venules that empty into veins and eventually return to the pulmonary artery.

A problem at any point in the respiratory/circulatory system can affect the intake and use of air. For this reason, prevention of respiratory and circulatory problems is vital.

# PREVENTION OF RESPIRATORY/CIRCULATORY PROBLEMS

Prevention and early treatment of respiratory infections, maintaining a balance between activity and rest, and appropriate nutrition are important factors in maintaining a healthy respiratory and circulatory system throughout the life cycle.

## Upper Respiratory Infections (Common Colds)

About twice a year, most people are affected by an upper respiratory infection. Sneezes, coughs, scratchy throat, and drippy nose are encountered. At present there is no vaccine for the prevention of a common cold, because any one of 200 different viruses might be the cause. There is some hope that, in the future, a drug may be developed to cure colds, but there is no cure now. However, there are some ways to decrease one's chances of catching a cold:

1. Avoid overheated places. Some people believe that warm, dry air makes the mucous membranes more susceptible to infection. Air can be made more humid by placing water in containers around the warm, dry room (for example, plants growing in water) or by using humidifiers.
2. Avoid unnecessary stress. Some researchers believe that stress alters the body's hormonal balance and thereby increases susceptibility to infection.
3. Avoid smoking. Smokers have more colds than nonsmokers; their colds last longer and are more serious.
4. Wash the hands frequently. One researcher believes that most colds are not spread by airborne virus particles or by kissing, but by physical contact with the mucous membranes of the nose. Shaking hands may cause colds because people harbor large colonies of viruses on their hands from smothering coughs, sneezes, and blowing their noses. They deposit these viruses on everything they touch. Since these viruses survive for several hours, healthy people can pick them up when they touch tables, telephones, and other smooth surfaces that have been contaminated. When a healthy person rubs his eyes or his nose after he's touched a contaminated surface, chances are he'll catch a cold.

Treatment Colds usually do not last more than a week or two. There are ways to speed recovery and to increase comfort: Rest is important in fighting any infection. Fluids—especially hot fluids—are beneficial. Aspirin relieves pain and inflammation. The use of Vitamin C in cold prevention and treatment is highly controversial.

It is important to watch for signs of secondary infection (fever, earache, bronchitis, etc.). Some of these complications can be treated with antibiotics.

## Detection of Strep Throat

The diagnosis of streptococcal infection is important because of the serious complications it can cause, such as sinusitis (inflammation of the sinuses), otitis (inflammation of the ear), acute glomerulonephritis (inflammation of the glomeruli of the kidney), and acute rheumatic fever with cardiac damage. When a person has a sore throat, a culture should be taken to identify the causative organism so that treatment can be instituted. Early detection and treatment can help prevent the serious complications listed above.

## Hypertensive Screening

Having the blood pressure checked is a painless, simple technique that aids in preventing heart disease and stroke by early identification and referral for treatment. Community health fairs are one means of screening large numbers of apparently healthy individuals for hypertension. Nursing students often find cases as they measure blood pressure and recommend further serial blood pressure readings for those people with a systolic pressure above 150 mm Hg and a diastolic above 95 mm Hg. Serial readings are required, because blood pressure is influenced by various environmental factors (e.g. time of day, position, activity, and anxiety). At present, there is some indication that the position of the arm while blood pressure is being taken affects the reading, but, further research is needed to determine whether or not position of the arm does, in fact, make a difference.

## Pollution Prevention

The hazards of air pollution and smoking are well documented. Nurses are urged to become actively involved in alerting their clients to ways to protect themselves from pollution whether from smoking or from other atmospheric pollutants. In Chapter 9, The Environment, we discuss pollution and its prevention.

## ASSESSMENT OF RESPIRATORY/CIRCULATORY FUNCTIONING

## Respirations

Normal respirations are quiet and effortless. A respiration consists of an inspiration and an expiration. In the adult, an inspiration lasts about 2 seconds and an expiration about 3 seconds. Normal respirations have an even rhythm and the chest and abdomen work as a unit. When the lungs expand during inspiration, the pressure within them decreases and air moves in. (As the volume of the area within which a gas is present increases, the pressure of the gas decreases. When the volume of the area decreases, the pressure of the gas increases.) Therefore, when the lungs are filled with air, the rise in pressure forces the air to be exhaled. With each respiration we use 300 to 500 ml of air. This is called *tidal volume*.

Adults breathe approximately 16 to 20 times per minute. In the newborn, the respiratory rate is 30 to 80; in early childhood 20 to 40; during late childhood, 15 to 25. The adult respiratory rate is reached at about 15 years of age (Bates, 1974).

Special Considerations

The rate, rhythm, and depth of respirations are assessed. Depth of respirations is seen as the chest expands and then returns to its normal position after exhalation. Normally, chest expansion is deep and even.

Respirations are usually counted after the pulse has been counted. The nurse should be careful to count the respirations when the client is not aware of it, so that he will not consciously control his breathing. It is easiest to count a child's respirations when he is asleep.

---

Performance Checklist
Assessment of Respirations

1. After taking the pulse, with fingers still on the radial artery, observe the respirations by watching the rise and fall of the chest, shoulder, or abdomen.
2. Using a watch with a second hand, count for a full minute each inspiration and expiration as one respiration.
3. After gaining experience and skill, count the respirations for 30 seconds and multiply by 2 if the person has no abnormalities in rate, rhythm, or depth. If he does, regardless of your experience and skill, count for one full minute.
4. Record respiratory rate, depth, and rhythm.

---

## Respiratory Abnormalities

When respirations are labored, the accessory muscles of inspiration (sternocleidomastoid, upper trapezius, and intercostals) contract vigorously. During expiration, the abdominals may contract forcefully. Abnormalities in respiration may be indicated by a rapid rate (tachypnea) or a slow rate (bradypnea). Kussmaul respirations are defined as gasping for air while the respirations are deep and rapid. These respirations are seen when a person has excessive amounts of carbon dioxide (for example, in metabolic acidosis). Dyspnea is defined as occurring any time a person believes he is having difficulty breathing. Orthopnea occurs when the upright position is necessary for comfortable breathing. Cheyne-Stokes respirations occur in cycles. First the breathing is very deep, then it gradually decreases in depth, and finally respirations cease for a brief period (apnea). This respiratory pattern is related to heart failure.

## Skin Color

The color of the skin and mucous membranes is examined when the respiratory system is assessed. Cyanosis is a bluish tinge to the skin and mucous membranes, frequently associated with insufficient oxygen. It may appear as a general duskiness of the entire body or it may be observed as a bluish tinge to the lips or the area around them (circumoral pallor) or blueness in the earlobes and in the nail beds. Cyanosis is not considered a very reliable indicator of respiratory status because it is influenced by hemoglobin level, blood flow to the tissues, blood volume, and normal skin color. Generally, cyanosis is considered a late sign of oxygen deficiency; over 5 g percent of hemoglobin must be without oxygen for cyanosis to be exhibited.

The nurse needs considerable skill to detect cyanosis in dark-skinned persons. It is more easily detected in these clients in the buccal mucosa and conjunctiva than in other parts of the body.

## Pulse

When the heart contracts, it forces blood into the arteries and the arterial walls expand. This arterial expansion creates the pulse. The pulse can be felt most easily at points where the artery is close to the skin and is located over a bone. The major arterial pulses are the radial, temporal, carotid, facial, femoral, popliteal, brachial, posterior tibial, and dorsalis pedis.

Rate   Pulse rate, rhythm, and volume are assessed. A considerable variation in normal pulse rate may exist. In the adult, 60 to 100 beats per minute is generally considered normal (Bates, 1974), though the American Heart Association lists the normal range as 50 to 100. Athletes frequently have normal pulses of 40 to 50. The client's current pulse should be compared with his normal pulse—not with someone else's.

Factors affecting pulse rate include body temperature, emotions, exercise, medications, age, body size, sex, pain, and disease. When the pulse rate exceeds 100 it is called tachycardia; when it is less than 50 it is described as bradycardia.

Rhythm   Normally the intervals between the heartbeats are equal and the rhythm of the pulse is regular. An irregular rhythm is called an arrhythmia.

Volume   In health, the amount of blood pumped with each heartbeat is constant and the force of the pulse is constant. The pulse is described as bounding when it is difficult to compress the pulse wave with mild pressure of the fingertips. If this pressure very easily stops the feel of the pulse, the pulse is described as feeble, weak, or thready. A thready pulse is usually rapid. Neither a thready nor a bounding pulse is normal.

## Measuring the Radial Pulse

Because the radial pulse is easily accessible, it is the one most frequently measured. With the person lying or sitting, the arm supported, and the palm of the hand down, the nurse places the first three fingers along the radial artery (on the thumb side of the wrist) and gently compresses it against the radius. The thumb rests on the back of the client's wrist. Using a watch with a second hand, the nurse counts the pulsations for one full minute, assessing the volume and rhythm of the pulse, at the same time.

When the nurse has acquired skill in assessment and when the person's pulse is normal she may count for 30 seconds and multiply by two to measure the pulse. However, when the pulse is considered abnormal, it is always necessary to count it for a full minute.

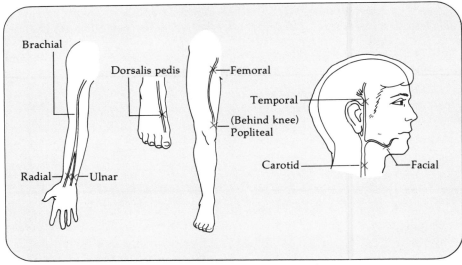

**Figure 15-3.** *Frequently used sites for determining peripheral pulse.*

## Apical, Apical-Radial Pulse

When it is difficult to measure a peripheral pulse, the apical pulse is taken by listening with a stethoscope placed slightly below the level of the nipple to the left of the sternum over the apex of the heart. Apical pulses are also taken to assure accuracy when certain cardiac drugs are administered.

Occasionally an apical-radial pulse is taken to determine whether or not there is a pulse deficit (the difference between the apical pulse and the radial pulse). The procedure differs from measurement of the radial pulse in the following ways:

1.  Two persons are required: one to listen to the apical pulse at the same time the other person is counting the radial pulse.
2.  With a watch placed so that each person can see it, one person calls the signal to begin and stop the count.
3.  If a difference exists between the apical beat and the radial, a pulse deficit exists and is so recorded.

## Blood Pressure

Blood pressure is the force of the blood flowing through the arteries. It is the force present when the heart contracts and the blood vessels offer resistance. The greatest pressure on the arterial walls occurs when the heart pushes blood into the aorta. The maximal pressure in the arteries as the left ventricle contracts is called systolic pressure. The minimal pressure exerted against the arterial walls when the left ventricle and arteries are at rest is called diastolic pressure. The difference between the systolic and diastolic pressure is called the pulse pressure.

Blood pressure is measured in millimeters of mercury (mm Hg) and recorded, for example, as 120/80 where 120 is systolic and 80 is diastolic

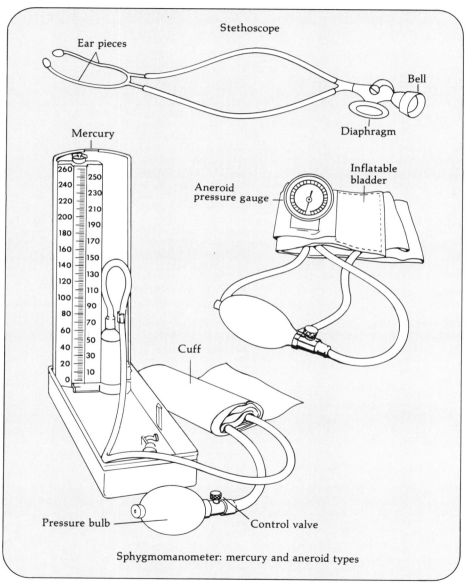

Figure 15-4.   *Equipment used in measuring blood pressure.*

pressure (normal for young adults). At birth a normal newborn has a systolic pressure of approximately 20 to 60 mm Hg. Blood pressure increases gradually until, at about age 20, adult pressure is reached. In old age, a small steady rise in blood pressure is normal because of decreased elasticity in the arteries. Position affects blood pressure. In the supine position the pressure is usually lower than when the person sits or stands although the difference may be insignificant.

Arterial blood pressure is measured by using a stethoscope, sphygmomanometer (the instrument, either mercury or aneroid type [spring]) that indicates the level of the pressure, and a blood pressure cuff. In the mercury manometer, a vertical cylindrical gauge measures the pressure on a mercury column. The spring sphygmomanometer consists of an aneroid gauge and the pressure is indicated on a dial.

The blood pressure cuff consists of a cuff—a flat rubber bladder covered with cloth—a hand bulb, and connecting tubing which are attached to the sphygmomanometer. The cuff is wrapped around the upper arm and inflated to the point at which the blood flow through the artery is temporarily occluded. Then, when pressure from the cuff is released, the stethoscope is used to detect the systolic and diastolic pressures.

## Special Considerations

The size of the cuff used depends upon the size of the extremity. The American Heart Association suggests that the cuff be 20 percent wider than the diameter of the limb on which it is to be used. For an adult of average weight, a 4½ to 5½-inch cuff is usually adequate. Of course, for children smaller cuffs are used and for persons with large arms or for leg pressures larger cuffs are used.

When the pressure in the cuff is released, Korotkoff sounds are heard. The first Korotkoff sound, a clear tapping sound when blood first flows through the compressed artery, is identified as the systolic pressure. Sounds continue until cuff pressure begins to equalize with pressure in the artery at rest. Muffling of sounds occurs at this time and the American Heart Association suggests this point be recorded as diastolic pressure. Other authorities regard the cessation (not muffling) of sound as the true diastolic pressure. Nurses must determine which measure their agency uses for diastolic pressure and proceed accordingly. It is sometimes wise to record both diastolic pressures (e.g., 120/80/74).

The same technique can be used to take an infant or child's pressure. Specific techniques for use when the blood pressure is difficult to obtain in children are outlined in pediatric texts.

If the blood pressure cannot be measured on an arm, the thigh pressure can be taken by using a wide cuff. The client lies on his abdomen; the nurse places the inflatable bag over the back of the thigh and positions the stethoscope over the popliteal artery (the back of the knee). Systolic pressure is a little higher in the thigh than the arm; diastolic pressure is about the same.

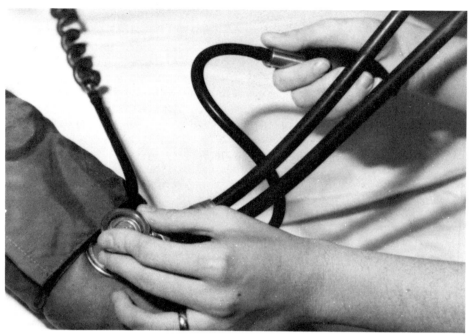

**Figure 15-5.** *The blood pressure cuff must be the proper size and correctly applied if an accurate reading is to be obtained. (Photo by Frank R. Engler, Jr.)*

If it is necessary to check a blood pressure reading by taking the pressure a second time, a lapse of at least 15 seconds should be allowed before reinflating the cuff. This will permit venous congestion, which alters the reading, to subside.

If the client requires frequent blood pressure measurements, the cuff is kept in place, with care taken to ensure that it is completely deflated when not in use.

Blood pressure may also be measured by palpation using the same technique as for auscultation except that, rather than using a stethoscope, the fingers are placed on the radial pulse and the first pulsation felt as the pressure is released is recorded as the systolic pressure (palpatory estimate). Determining diastolic pressure by this method is difficult (change in character of pulse) and not considered accurate.

It is also possible for arterial blood pressure to be measured by placing a catheter within the artery. This method is the most accurate, but also dangerous and used only when accurate pressure measurement is vital.

Electronic instruments are available for measuring blood pressure and their use removes the variable of observer hearing acuity as a factor in accurate readings.

Performance Checklist
Blood Pressure Measurement

1. Wash hands.
2. Explain procedure.
3. Gather all equipment.
4. Position client comfortably with forearm in supine position.
5. Attach blood pressure cuff appropriately:
   a. check width of cuff
   b. position bladder over brachial artery
   c. place cuff ½-inch above elbow
   d. check snugness of cuff
   e. if using aneroid sphygmomanometer, position within 3 feet and view gauge from directly in front
   f. if using a mercury manometer, position within 3 feet, with gauge vertical, read from level of meniscus
6. Clean ear pieces and stethoscope diaphragm.
7. Palpate brachial artery and place diaphragm over it.
8. Close valve on pump; inflate cuff to 30 mm above normal systolic reading.
   a. ask client or check chart for normal systolic pressure
   b. or make palpatory estimate
9. Place stethoscope; release pressure at constant rate of 2 to 3 mm/beat.
10. Remember the first beat heard is systolic and last (or muffled) sound is diastolic.
11. Open valve until all air is removed.
12. Wait 15 seconds before repeating reading, if second reading is necessary.
13. Remove equipment.
14. Record systolic and diastolic pressures.
15. Clean stethoscope and return equipment to storage.

## Physical Assessment Skills

Physical assessment of the respiratory and circulatory systems is based on a thorough understanding of the anatomy and physiology of these systems. In addition to the assessment skills already described, the beginning student will find a few other assessment skills valuable. Auscultation of the lungs is useful in determining air flow. A stethoscope is used to detect the movement of air in and out of the lungs while the client breathes through his mouth somewhat more deeply than normal. The lung sounds on one side of the body are compared with the sounds on the other side. The quality and intensity of breath sounds, which are decreased or absent when air flow is decreased, are listened for. Vesicular, bronchovesicular, and bronchial sounds should be identified. Vesicular breath sounds are soft sounds of low pitch, with inspiration greater than expiration heard throughout most of the chest. Bronchovesicular sounds are of medium pitch and sound with equal inspira-

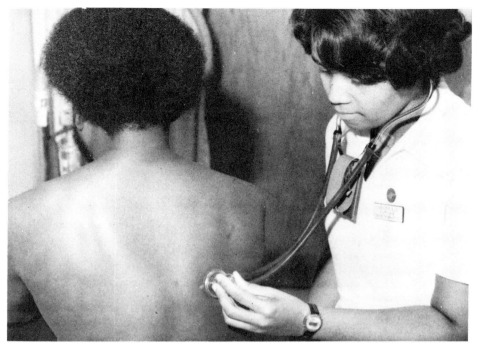

**Figure 15-6.** *Auscultation of the lungs is useful in determining air flow. (Photo by Frank R. Engler, Jr.)*

tion and expiration. They are detected near the main stem bronchi below the clavicles and between the scapula, especially on the right. Bronchial breath sounds are loud and high pitched, with the expiratory phase longer than the inspiratory phase. They are heard over the trachea.

Adventitious or abnormal sounds—for example, wheezing and rales—are usually heard in conjunction with normal breath sounds. Wheezing is a musical, high-pitched sound heard on expiration as air passes through a narrowed lumen. Persons with asthma or chronic bronchitis produce wheezing respirations. Râles are bubbly breath sounds heard on inspiration near the base of the lung. They usually indicate fluid in the respiratory tract.

Gait and posture are also assessed because of their influence on the respiratory system. Kyphosis (a rounded thoracic convexity) and scoliosis (a lateral spinal curvature) interfere with respirations.

Evaluation of the venous pressure is an important part of the physical assessment. The venous pressure can be assessed by inspection of the venous pulses. Any pulsations or distention of the internal or external jugular neck veins while the client is upright should be recorded. This inability of the veins to drain into the right side of the heart could indicate congestive heart failure.

The rhythm of the heartbeat is identified by auscultation. When the apical heart rate is assessed its regularity or irregularity is noted. If the rate is irregular, it is important to try to identify a pattern. Do the early beats appear in a regular rhythm? Does the irregularity vary with inspirations? Is there no identifiable pattern to the arrhythmia?

Physical assessment of the respiratory and circulatory systems provides baseline information that can be used to increase the client's ability to maintain his health.

## Respiratory Assessment Guide

The following guide is intended to assist the student determine relevant information about the client's respiratory-circulatory systems. These are questions the student might ask the client:

1. How many pillows do you use for sleeping?
2. Have you ever had a chest x-ray? If so, why?
3. Do you have any trouble breathing?
   If you do, what brings on your breathing difficulties
   (air pollution, pollen, other allergens)?
   Is your breathing difficulty related to the time of day?
   How long have you had this trouble?
4. If you have trouble breathing, what do you do to ease your breathing?
   Do you take any medications (including over the counter medications)?
5. Do you smoke? If so, how much? Does anyone in your house smoke?
6. Do you have a cough? Sputum? Chest pain? If so, describe.
7. Is there a family history of respiratory problems?

After these questions have been answered:

1. Check your client's respirations, pulse, and blood pressure.
2. Check his color for cyanosis.

## Selected Respiratory/Circulatory Diagnostic Tests

In addition to their value in early detection of health problems, diagnostic tests provide baseline data for future comparisons. The nurse should always encourage her clients to seek early diagnosis. An understanding of the commonly used diagnostic measures is necessary if the nurse is expected to help her clients understand the purpose and procedures of the test.

Much has been written about the anxiety associated with diagnostic tests. Understanding that this emotion is frequently associated with the unknown helps the nurse to seek and use appropriate techniques to lessen the client's anxiety. Knowing what is expected of him during the procedure is important to the client. And if the client knows when the results will be available, he will be better able to deal with the situation. For example, if the client knows that it takes 48 hours before a skin test can be read, he will not expect the results before they are available. Often the nurse is influential in relaying to the physician the client's concern about test results. Unnecessary delays in telling the client the results can then be avoided.

Here we will discuss only a few of the commonly used diagnostic measures from the wide variety available.

**Chest X-Ray**  X-ray examination of the chest is considered a most important diagnostic aid. Infectious processes (e.g., tuberculosis), space-occupying lesions, and the size and shape of the lungs and heart are demonstrated. Preparation consists of removing any neck jewelry and clothes from above the waist. The client must carefully follow the technician's directions regarding breathing. Fluoroscopy permits observation of the movements of the chest, heart, and lungs.

**Skin Tests**  Skin testing is frequently part of the diagnostic procedure when tuberculosis or other lung infection is suspected. A small amount of dilute antigen is injected intradermally (between the layers of the skin) and the person is observed at a specified time for a skin reaction at the site of the injection. A reaction indicates presence of antibodies resulting from previous contact with the antigen.

**Cultures** are taken to identify a specific organism. To take a throat culture the nurse uses the following procedure:

---

Performance Checklist
Throat Culture

1. Obtain a flashlight, tongue depressor, culture tubes (prepared commerically or in the agency laboratory), and applicator sticks.
2. Illuminate the throat.
3. Remove a sterile applicator from its container.
4. Have the client say "ah" as you depress his tongue with the tongue blade (to lessen the gag reflex).
5. Swab one tonsillar site with the sterile applicator using one downward stroke. Place applicator in culture tube.
6. Using the second applicator, swab the other tonsillar site and then place applicator in culture tube. Follow any additional directions on commercial packages.
7. Make the client comfortable.
8. Discard tongue blade.
9. Label tubes, send to laboratory, and record procedure.

---

**Nasal Culture**  Using one applicator stick for each nostril, the nurse swabs the mucous membrane deep in the nasal passage, places the applicators in the culture tube, labels, sends to laboratory, and records.

**Sputum Specimen**  A sputum specimen may be examined in the laboratory for cells, pus, bacteria, or blood. Specimens obtained early in the morning or following respiratory therapy are the most effective in securing material actually coughed up from the lungs. Saliva and nasal mucus do not constitute a sputum specimen. The amount of sputum required for most tests is about a teaspoonful. Special sputum containers are supplied and the client expectorates directly into the container. The container is always covered when not in use.

It may be necessary to use a catheter to obtain a specimen from a person who cannot cough. Gastric washings, in which a stomach tube is inserted into the empty stomach, can also be used to obtain a specimen of swallowed sputum.

**Blood Tests**   Because blood is the medium for oxygen transport, specific blood components may be examined to determine efficiency.

*Hematocrit* determines the quantity of cells in the blood. In the laboratory, blood is centrifuged until the cells are packed in the bottom of the tube. Normal hematocrit is 41 to 48 percent.

*Hemoglobin* is measured to determine the oxygen-carrying capability of the blood. Normal hemoglobin is 14 to 16 g/100 ml of blood.

*White blood cells* are counted to indicate presence or absence of infection, which could interfere with oxygen transport. An elevated white count (normal: 5,000 to 10,000/cu mm) could indicate infection.

*Cholesterol* and *triglyceride* levels are taken to diagnose potential or actual coronary artery disease. Normal levels for cholesterol are 250 mg or below; for triglyceride, below 160 mg/100 ml.

*Arterial blood gases* are drawn from the femoral or brachial arteries to determine the partial pressure of oxygen and carbon dioxide in the blood ($PO_2$; $PCO_2$). A glass heparinized syringe is used for blood withdrawal. The syringe is immediately packed in ice and taken to the laboratory. Normal blood gases are: $PO_2$ 80 to 100 mm Hg; $PCO_2$ 35 to 45 mm Hg. External pressure is applied to the puncture site for at least one minute to prevent bleeding and ecchymosis.

**Bronchoscopy**   In bronchoscopy a lighted instrument (bronchoscope) is passed through the anesthetized pharynx so that the bronchial tree can be visualized. The client fasts for 6 to 8 hours before the examination and following the examination until the gag reflex has returned. In addition to visualization of the bronchi, washings or biopsy (removal of tissue for microscopic examination) may be performed. The client must be watched closely for any signs of respiratory difficulty following this procedure, because hoarseness, bleeding, or swelling of the larynx may occur. Bleeding or swelling of the larynx constitute a medical emergency because the airway will become obstructed unless corrective measures are taken.

**Pulmonary Function Tests**   Many different tests of pulmonary function may be performed. The most common is vital capacity which uses a spirometer to measure the inspiratory capacity and expiratory reserve of the lungs. Normally a person who inhales deeply and exhales forcefully moves a volume of 4,000 to 5,000 ml of air.

Maximal breathing capacity measures the maximum amount of air a person can breathe in and out per minute. This is considered a good measure of a person's ventilatory ability. The normal rate for a female is 100 1/min.; for a male: 125 to 150 1/min.

**Electrocardiography** The electrocardiograph is a machine that records the heart's electrical potential—the spread of the cardiac impulse through the conduction system of the heart. Heart rate, position, and arrhythmias are recorded. Leads from the machine are attached to body sites (arms, leg, and various points on the chest). A paste or other conducting material is placed under each lead. A record of the cardiac activity is produced on a narrow strip of paper. There is no pain or discomfort associated with the procedure; however, the client may feel a slight "pull" as the suction cup is placed on different parts of the chest wall.

**Cardiac Catheterization** A catheter is passed through the saphenous vein to the right side of the heart and blood samples are taken to determine the amount of oxygen in the blood within the heart. X-rays are taken to record structural defects. The client is awake throughout the procedure. A local anesthetic is injected at the site of the catheter insertion. The procedure is not without risk and the client is made aware of this prior to the procedure. Following the procedure, the catheter insertion site must be checked for signs of bleeding and the extremities examined for color, temperature, and presence of pulses. The heart rate must be monitored regularly to detect signs of hemorrhage or cardiac irregularities.

## ASSISTING CLIENTS TO ACHIEVE ADEQUATE VENTILATION/CIRCULATION

Preventing respiratory and circulatory problems is a priority in nursing. However, once a deficit occurs in respiratory/circulatory function, nursing goals consist of assisting the client to conserve energy, achieve adequate ventilation and circulation, and prevent further deterioration. If appropriate nursing interventions are to occur, the nurse needs knowledge and skill in the therapies which provide air (oxygen).

### Cardiopulmonary Resuscitation

When cardiac or respiratory arrest occurs, a well-trained layperson can perform basic life-support measures until advanced life support is available. Basic life support is the emergency first aid procedure which begins with the recognition of cardiac and respiratory arrest and the application of cardiopulmonary resuscitation to support life until further aid is available. Today, grade-school children are being taught resuscitation procedures. It is hoped that soon at least one member of every family will be trained in cardiopulmonary resuscitation (CPR). Health professionals are expected to be proficient in this technique.

**Figure 15-7.** *Cardiopulmonary resuscitation: (1) Open airway. (2) For mouth-to-mouth resuscitation, pinch victim's nostrils. (3) Rescuer makes a seal with his lips over the victim's mouth. (4) If cardiac massage is necessary, rescuer locates landmarks on the sternum. (5) Rescuer places hands properly and keeps elbows straight while compressing the heart. (6) Location and technique for delivering precordial thump. (Reproduced with permission of the* American Journal of Nursing, *75 [Feb. 1975].)*

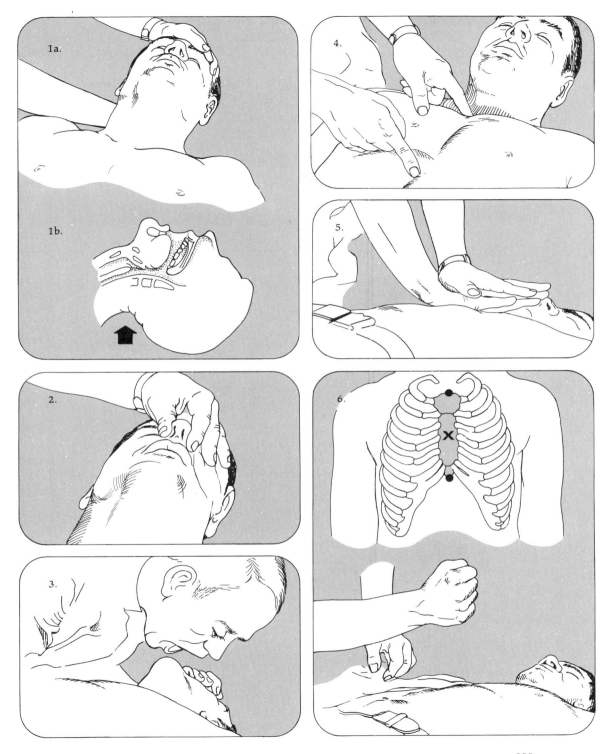

Body tissues respond in varying ways to oxygen deficiency, but authorities agree that irreparable brain damage occurs when the brain has been without oxygen for as little as 4 minutes. In persons with hemoglobin below normal and with circulatory deficits, brain damage occurs even sooner.

The American Heart Association, in cooperation with the National Academy of Sciences—National Research Council, has issued guidelines and standards for basic life support (1974). Reprints of the supplement from the *Journal of the American Medical Association* (1974) in which these guidelines appeared are available from local heart associations. Actions required for basic life support follow (adapted from Lingvarski, Argondizzo, and Boos, 1975).

When the rescuer does not actually observe the victim's collapse, the situation is called an *unwitnessed arrest* and the following steps are taken:

---

### Performance Checklist
### CPR Performed by One Rescuer

1. Establish unresponsiveness by shaking shoulder and shouting "Are you OK?"
2. Open airway: person on his back, tilt his head back as far as possible by placing one hand beneath neck and lifting it; use other hand to press forehead back. Establish breathlessness by placing ear over victim's mouth.
3. If breathing is absent, give four ventilations (quickly)
   a. keeping the head tilted back as far as possible, pinch nostrils closed with thumb and finger of hand used to press forehead down
   b. open his mouth wide
   c. take a deep breath
   d. make an airtight seal over the victim's mouth
   e. exhale forcefully into victim's mouth
   f. remove mouth and allow victim to exhale passively
4. Establish pulselessness by palpating the carotid pulse.
5. If a pulse is absent, perform external cardiac compressions in addition to ventilations (ratio of 15 compressions to 2 ventilations within 5 seconds of each other).
   a. place victim supine on floor (or on a board, if in bed)
   b. locate the lower half of the sternum by feeling the tip of the sternum (xiphoid process)
   c. apply long axis of the heel of one hand over lower half of the sternum 1 to 1½ inches above the tip of the sternum, toward the victim's head.
   d. keep fingers off chest wall.
   e. place second hand on top of first one, bringing your shoulders directly over victim's sternum
   f. keeping arms straight and elbows locked, apply firm, heavy pressure to depress the sternum vertically 1½ to 2 inches
   g. compressions must be regular, smooth, and uninterrupted. Compression rate for adult victim is 80 per minute
6. Check carotid pulse and breathing for return of pulse and respirations.

Reproduced with permission from the *American Journal of Nursing*, February, 1975, Vol. 75, No.2.

## Performance Checklist
### Witnessed Cardiac Arrest

1. Establish unresponsiveness.
2. Open airway.
3. Establish pulselessness by palpating carotid artery.
4. If pulse is absent, deliver one precordial thump:
   a. locate the midportion of the sternum, between the sternal notch and the xiphoid process
   b. deliver a sharp, quick, single blow over the midportion of the sternum with the bottom, fleshy portion of the fist; strike the blow from 8 to 12 inches over the chest
5. If breathing is absent, deliver four quick ventilations.
6. If pulse and breathing do not return immediately, begin cardiopulmonary resuscitation.

### Infant and Child Resuscitation

1. Establish unresponsiveness and breathlessness.
2. Open airway. Do not exaggerate the tilted position of the head, because forceful tilting may obstruct airway.
3. Cover mouth and nose of victim. Use less air than in resuscitating adults. Inflate lungs 20 to 24 times per minute.
4. Establish pulselessness.
5. If pulseless, one hand can be placed under child's back as firm support, while other hand compresses the chest.
   a. apply compression to mid-sternum of infants or children: for small child, use heel of one hand to depress sternum ¾ to 1½ inches; for infant, use tips of index and middle fingers to depress sternum ½ to ¾ inch
   b. ratio of compressions to ventilations is 5/1. Compress chest 80 to 100 times per minute; deliver one quick breath after every five compressions.

### Airway Obstruction

1. If airway obstruction is suspected, roll victim on his side, place a knee under his shoulder, and force his mouth open with crossed-finger technique.
2. Run index and middle fingers along base of cheek toward base of tongue, deep into victim's throat.
3. With a sweeping motion, move fingers across back of throat and remove any foreign matter.
4. If airway is still obstructed, roll victim on side so that he faces you.
5. Deliver one or two sharp blows with heel of hand between victim's shoulder blades.
6. If still unsuccessful, repeat mouth to mouth resuscitation, blows to back, and probing of upper airway with fingers.
7. If the victim is a small child, pick him up quickly, turn him over your arm, and deliver blows with flat of palm between shoulder blades.

Reproduced with permission from the *American Journal of Nursing*, February, 1975, Vol. 75, No.2.

## Special Considerations: Two Rescuers

One rescuer performs ventilation and the other cardiac compression. The ratio of compressions to ventilations is 5:1. Ventilations are performed, without pause, between the fifth and the next compression.

## Heimlich Maneuver

People can be protected from choking by being reminded of the importance of chewing food adequately before swallowing, not eating too fast, and not laughing and talking with food in their mouths. Children can be protected by keeping small objects that they might put in their mouths out of reach and not giving them food that they are unable to chew. In one instance, a two-year-old was admitted to the emergency room after he had fallen down a couple of steps while he was being fed peanuts by an older sibling. When he fell, his airway was obstructed by the unchewed peanut and by the time he reached the hospital he was in respiratory arrest. He was successfully treated for airway obstruction and given oxygen. The following day he was well enough to be up and about. The Heimlich maneuver, if performed immediately, would probably have saved him and his family a lot of distress.

Food-choking can be easily recognized. The victim cannot speak or breathe; he becomes pale, then deeply cyanotic, and collapses. Dr. Heimlich (1975) has suggested a universal signal that the victim can use and a rescuer can

---

### Performance Checklist

#### Heimlich Maneuver with Rescuer Standing

1. Stand behind the victim and wrap your arms around his waist.
2. Grasp your fist with your other hand and place the thumb side of your fist against the victim's abdomen, slightly above the navel and below the rib cage.
3. Press your fist into the victim's abdomen with a *quick upward thrust*. Repeat several times if necessary.
4. When the victim is sitting, the rescuer stands behind the victim's chair and performs the maneuver in the same manner.

#### Heimlich Maneuver with Rescuer Kneeling

If the victim has collapsed or the rescuer cannot lift him, the following procedure is used:

1. Victim is lying on his back.
2. Facing victim, kneel astride his hips.
3. With one of your hands on top of the other, place the heel of your bottom hand on the abdomen slightly above the navel and below the rib cage.
4. Press into the victim's abdomen with a *quick upward thrust*. Repeat several times if necessary.
5. Should victim vomit, quickly place him on his side and wipe out his mouth to prevent aspiration.

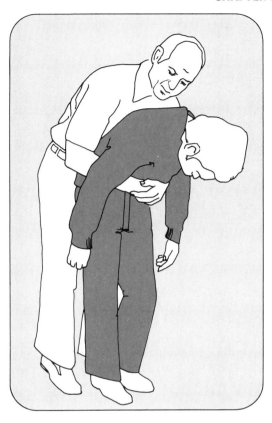

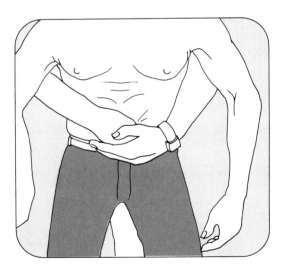

**Figure 15-8.** *Heimlich maneuver: With the victim standing, the rescuer grasps his own fist with his other hand and presses the fist (thumbside against abdomen) into the victim's abdomen with a quick upward thrust.*

recognize to indicate that choking has occurred. He recommends that the victim grasp his neck between thumb and index finger of one hand to indicate he is choking on food.

**Special Considerations:**
The principle on which the Heimlich maneuver is based is as follows: food-choking probably occurs during inspiration, which causes the food bolus to be sucked against the laryngeal orifice. Therefore, at the time of the accident the lungs are expanded. Even during normal expiration, however, some tidal air (500 ml) and the entire expiratory reserve volume (1,900 ml) are present in the lungs. Pressing one's fist upward into the epigastrium elevates the diaphragm. Sudden elevation compresses the lungs and increases the pressure within the tracheobronchial tree. This pressure is forced out through the trachea and will eject the food (or other small object) that is occluding the airway (Heimlich, 1975).

## Coughing, Deep Breathing, Turning, Positioning

Proper respiratory functioning in health is effortless. However, when there is a problem related to respiration (such as pain following surgery, limited lung expansion, or cough with expectoration), the client is helped by instruction. Pre-operative instruction regarding the need for proper positioning, turning, coughing, and deep breathing improves the postoperative course. In addition, a person with a productive cough is taught proper ways to cough and dispose of secretions to help prevent the spread of pathogenic organisms.

Coughing is a protective reflex for expelling foreign material from the respiratory tract. The cough reflex may be stimulated, for example, by dryness, pressure, cold, smoke, or excessive laughing or talking. During coughing, about 2 liters of air are inhaled: the epiglottis closes and the vocal cords shut tight. Then suddenly there is a forceful expiration and the epiglottis and vocal cords open wide and the air is forced out under great pressure. Foreign matter from the trachea and bronchi is carried with it. If the client has a cough that produces secretions, instruct him to use tissues (not cloth handkerchiefs), dispose of them promptly, and wash his hands to help prevent the spread of organisms released with the cough.

Following surgery, persons frequently breathe guardedly. They have pain if they take a deep breath or they fear they will disrupt the stitches if they cough. If shallow breathing and limited coughing are permitted, lung expansion will be less than optimal and secretions will be retained and the oxygen-carbon dioxide exchange will be inadequate.

While there is no universal agreement on the best technique for deep breathing and coughing, the following method is appropriate:

**Deep Breathing** The client inhales slowly and evenly (he should feel a "pull" between the ribs) and expands the chest as far as possible. He holds his breath at least 3 seconds, then exhales normally. He should breathe according to these directions at least 4 to 5 times every hour.

Coughing  The client assumes a sitting position. He inhales deeply and then coughs forcefully. The surgical incision should be supported during coughing by the client's hands, the nurse's hands, a pillow, or a folded bed sheet placed over the area of the incision. The nurse should stand behind the client while she supports the incision. The client should cough in this manner 4 to 5 times an hour.

Turning and Positioning  Good body alignment, as described in the chapter on activity, rest, and sleep (Chapter 20), encourages proper breathing—movement of the diaphragm and expansion of the chest—whether the client is lying, sitting, or standing. Changing position in bed regularly (at least once every hour) promotes proper respiration. Until the client is able to move independently, he should be assisted in changing position. Early ambulation (walking soon after surgery) contributes to increased respiratory efficiency.

## Humidification

Increasing the concentration of moisture in the air is a common treatment for respiratory problems. High humidity provides extra moisture to the mucous membrane lining the respiratory tract. This moisture helps soothe irritation, dilute thick secretions, and loosen the crusts that form on the mucous membranes as the result of infection. With humidification, the secretions can be more easily coughed up and expectorated. Increasing fluid intake is another way to help thin mucus.

High humidity environments are created by using tents (Isolettes, croup tents), special rooms, and popularly, a steam kettle or home humidifier. Appliances that provide either hot or cold humidity are available. Humidity may be delivered continuously or at scheduled intervals throughout the day and night (e.g., for ½ hour q 4 h).

When the client is receiving some form of humidification the following aspects of assistance are important:

1.  Explain the purpose and procedure for humidification.
2.  If hot steam inhalations are used, protect the client from burns.
3.  Drugs may be added to the water of the steam inhalator.
4.  If the entire room is being humidified, keep the door closed and the apparatus placed so that the client can easily inhale the humidified air.
5.  Protect the client from drafts and change the linens when they become damp (especially when the person is in a tent).

6. Provide a container for expectorated mucus and encourage the client to cough and expectorate.
7. Monitor body temperature regularly, because increased humidity can produce an increase in body temperature.

## Intermittent Positive Pressure Breathing (IPPB)

IPPB is a mechanical means of providing, under positive pressure, gases (air or oxygen) or drugs intermittently by inhalation. It is frequently used to aid respiratory ventilation after surgery; it is also used to relieve those confined to bed for prolonged periods, and to administer aerosal therapy. It is a method of helping persons expectorate respiratory secretions. A portable machine (a Bird or a Bennett respirator, for example) provides a specific amount of gas and medication under increased pressure. With IPPB, positive pressure forces deeper inspiration. Expiration is normal. The amount of pressure used is prescribed according to the client's needs. Each treatment lasts from 15 to 20 minutes (or until all medication has been inhaled) and is administered 2 to 4 times daily.

In many agencies, respiratory therapists administer IPPB therapy. However, the nurse will want to know how the equipment in her agency works.

## Nebulizers

Aerosol inhalation or nebulization is a method whereby a nonvolatile drug is inhaled into the respiratory tract. Oxygen or compressed air, as it passes over the drug in solution, picks up small particles and forms a spray. The client breathes deeply to inhale the small drug particles deep into the respiratory tract. Many aerosal treatments are given by IPPB, but other equipment such as ultrasonic and hand nebulizers are also used. The size of the drug particles inhaled depends upon the source of nebulization: particles formed by a hand nebulizer are larger than those formed by either the ultrasonic or IPPB nebulizers.

Clients frequently use hand nebulizers and it is necessary for the nurse to know the action of the drug, its side effects, and the amount and frequency of the treatment. When a client is initially given a hand nebulizer, this information is given to him.

## Postural Drainage

The purpose of postural drainage is to facilitate the drainage of secretions from the respiratory tract. The body position the client assumes for postural drainage depends upon the area of the lung to be drained. Gravity assists in moving the mucus; therefore if the lower lobes are to be drained, the person lies with his chest lower than his hips. He may lie prone across the bed with his waist at the edge of the bed, upper part of the body supported by arms resting on the floor. Tissues and a container for the sputum are placed where they can be reached easily.

Other positions are assumed when different areas of the lung require draining. Length of time per treatment (usually 10 to 15 minutes) and frequency (usually 3 to 4 times a day) are prescribed. Drainage is scheduled so that it does not follow a meal.

## Chest Percussion and Vibration

Chest percussion and vibration over the affected area of the lung are additional methods used to loosen mucus so that it can be expectorated more easily. In percussion, the closed hand strikes the area over the lung. In vibration, the open hand is used in firm, strong circular movements.

In many agencies, the physical or respiratory therapist is responsible for performing postural drainage, percussion, and vibration, and for instructing the family members who may need to perform these techniques in the home. The nurse learns these techniques best by asking the therapist to demonstrate them and/or by reading specialized texts on respiratory treatments.

## Oxygen Therapy

When a person has an inadequate supply of oxygen (hypoxia), oxygen therapy must be instituted. Respiratory and cardiac problems frequently decrease the supply of oxygen to the cells. Persons who have difficulty breathing (dyspnea) are restless and apprehensive. Oxygen therapy relieves these symptoms and decreases the work load of the heart.

The percentage of oxygen in the atmosphere is approximately 21 percent. Oxygen is colorless, odorless, and tasteless. It is a gas that supports combustion; therefore, special precautions must be taken by client, staff, and visitors to prevent fire or explosion during treatments. "No Smoking" signs must be prominently displayed and the rule enforced. Wool and synthetic fabrics must be avoided because they develop static electricity. See that electrical equipment is carefully inspected. Faulty wiring might create a spark. Portable oxygen tanks must be properly secured to prevent them from falling.

In most intensive care centers oxygen is piped into client units and dispensed directly through wall outlets. The flow of oxygen is measured in liters per minute. The rate of administration depends upon the condition of the client and the equipment used. Oxygen is stored under pressure ranging from approximately 50 lbs/square-inch to 2,000 lbs/square-inch. Flowmeters are attached to the wall outlet or the portable tank. The flowmeter opens the outlet and a valve permits regulation of the oxygen flow.

Oxygen is delivered to the respiratory tract artificially and under pressure. To prevent excessive drying of the mucous membranes, the oxygen is humidified by passage through water (or another solution), regardless of the method of administration.

Oxygen is usually administered by nasal cannula, catheter, or face mask. Tents are used infrequently except for supplying high humidity to children and this method, therefore, will not be discussed.

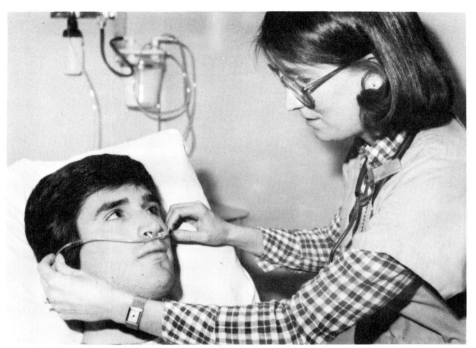

**Figure 15-9.**  *Oxygen is often delivered by use of a nasal cannula. The prongs fit into the nostrils and an adjustable elastic band placed around the head holds them in place.  (Photo by Frank R. Engler, Jr.)*

Nasal Cannula   Oxygen is administered directly into the client's nostrils by means of the nasal cannula. The cannula is a plastic disposable device consisting of two prongs for insertion into the nostrils, an elastic strap that fits around the head, and a tube connected to the oxygen supply. This method is simple to use, efficient, and comfortable.

---

### Performance Checklist
### Nasal Cannula

1. Attach cannula tubing to the oxygen supply and humidifier at prescribed rate (usually 2 to 4 l/min). Test by feeling the oxygen flow through the cannula prongs.
2. Place cannula prongs in nostrils. Secure fastenings for comfort.
3. Check oxygen flow regularly.
4. Remove and clean cannula at least every 8 hours.
5. Instruct client to breathe through his nose.
6. Cleanse nostrils of secretions as necessary.

**Nasal Catheter** A nasal catheter is used somewhat less frequently than a cannula because it is not as comfortable, although it delivers oxygen at a relatively high concentration.

---

### Performance Checklist
### Nasal Catheter

1. Attach catheter tubing to oxygen supply and humidifier and adjust to prescribed flow rate (usually 4 to 7 l/min). Test by placing tip of catheter in cup of water and observing for bubbling.
2. Lubricate catheter with water soluble lubricant to lessen irritation by reducing friction. Size of adult catheter is usually 10 to 12 French.
3. Measure and mark distance from nostril to earlobe. Insert catheter up to this mark through nostril along floor of the nose. If resistance is met, remove catheter and place in other nostril.
4. Check level of catheter tip by using tongue blade and flashlight. The tip should be visible slightly to the side of the uvula. Adjust catheter if necessary. (If catheter is inserted too far, it may cause gagging or stomach distention; if not inserted far enough, oxygen will escape.)
5. Secure catheter at temple with adhesive tape. (See illustration).
6. Monitor rate of oxygen flow regularly.
7. Remove and clean or replace catheter at least every 8 hours. Alternate nostril whenever possible.
8. Cleanse nostrils of secretions as necessary.

---

**Face Mask** Masks are effective when high concentrations of oxygen (40 to 95 percent) are required. Various types are available—some cover both the nose and mouth. Clients frequently object to the mask and considerable psychological support is needed if they are to keep the mask in place.

The mask is different from the catheter and cannula in that the oxygen is humidified by the air that is exhaled into the mask; therefore, it is not necessary to have oxygen pass through water before it is inhaled.

---

### Performance Checklist
### Face Mask

1. Initially, turn the oxygen flow rate high (10 to 15 l/min) so that the client feels the oxygen and is less anxious.
2. If the mask covers both nose and mouth (and most of them do), place the mask so that the narrow part covers the nose and the wider part the mouth.
3. If the mask does not fit the face tightly, pad it with gauze to obtain a close fit.
4. Adjust strap comfortably around the client's head.
5. Monitor oxygen flow rate frequently and adjust as required.
6. Clean or replace face mask at least every 8 hours.

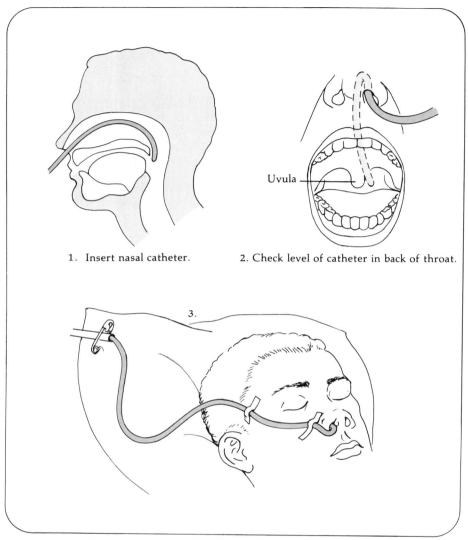

1. Insert nasal catheter.

2. Check level of catheter in back of throat.

Uvula

3.

**Figure 15-10.** *Insertion of nasal catheter: (1) and (2) After the catheter is inserted, its proper location (on the level with the uvula) is checked. (3) The catheter is taped to the side of the face to minimize pressure and discomfort.*

## Additional Nursing Measures for Those Receiving Oxygen

Physical comfort, emotional support, and safety precautions are important while the client is receiving oxygen. He may be restless, apprehensive, and so dyspneic that he welcomes the administration of oxygen. He may, at the same time, feel that his condition must be very serious or he would not be given oxygen. A straightforward explanation to the client and his family should provide effective reassurance. They should be told of the effect of oxygen on the workload of the heart; they should be told, too, that oxygen is frequently prescribed.

Physical comfort includes attention to the skin and mucous membranes of the face. If the client's skin is irritated by the tape, nonallergenic tape must be used and care taken to tape a different area whenever the catheter is changed. When a mask is used, the face must be washed, dried, and powdered. Frequent mouth care (e.g., every 3 hours) is essential for comfort during oxygen therapy.

For safety, "No Smoking" signs must be placed conspicuously and this rule must be vigilantly enforced.

## Insertion of Airway

When a person is unconscious and there is danger that his airway will become occluded, a plastic disposable airway may be inserted into the mouth. It is shaped to follow the contour of the mouth and upper respiratory tract. When this device is placed properly, it keeps the tongue from dropping back and occluding the airway. Persons in the postoperative recovery room, for example, frequently have an airway in place until they regain consciousness.

To insert an airway, a tongue blade is used to hold the tongue flat. Then the disposable airway is introduced upside down. As the tip of the airway reaches the palate, the airway is turned right side up. It will slip smoothly into the correct position.

## Tracheostomy Care

A tracheostomy is a surgically produced opening in the trachea. A tube is placed in the tracheal opening and the person breathes air or oxygen through it. Suctioning through the tracheostomy removes secretions that cannot be coughed up. With the advent of polyvinyl chloride endotracheal tubes, tracheostomies are no longer as frequently performed.

Tracheostomy tubes are made of different materials—usually silver or plastic. Some polyvinyl chloride tubes contain an inflatable cuff that serves to occlude the area of the trachea around the tube. Generally, the tracheostomy set consists of an inner and outer cannula. The outer cannula is tied with cotton tapes around the neck. The inner cannula locks in place into the outer cannula. Frequent suctioning through the inner cannula is required (depending upon the amount of secretions present).

The suctioning procedure is usually a nursing function, although clients with long-term tracheostomies are taught to suction themselves. The procedure for suctioning is similar to that for pharyngeal suctioning.

The suctioning procedure must be sterile. A catheter no larger than half the diameter of the tracheostomy tube is used. Suctioning lasts no more than 4 to 5 seconds (the time required to withdraw the catheter without pausing), because oxygen as well as mucus is being aspirated while the catheter remains in the tracheostomy tube.

At stated intervals, (usually every 4 to 8 hours), the inner cannula is unlocked, removed, and cleaned. Commercially prepared cleansing sets are available. The cleansing agents may differ from one agency to another; however, water and hydrogen peroxide 3 percent are appropriate cleansing agents. Containers for the solution, gloves, a wire brush, tapes, and dressings are usually included in the packs. The inner cannula is placed in peroxide, which helps loosen the mucus that has gathered in it. It is then cleaned on the inside with the brush and rinsed in the water (sterile), dried, and replaced. Parts of one set are not interchangeable with those from another. This cleansing process is a sterile procedure and the inner cannula remains clean (but not sterile).

Tracheostomy dressings are placed around the skin opening (stoma) to prevent irritation from the mucus that is coughed up. The dressings are changed as needed. The compress is usually 4 × 3 inches, cut halfway through the middle with the split edges reinforced to prevent fraying. The dressing is inserted from the bottom so that the open part fits around either side of the tube and the uncut part is at the bottom, where it can collect the mucus and protect the skin.

The tapes also are replaced as needed. A beginning student or inexperienced nurse should ask a second person to help: one person holds the tube securely in place, while the other changes the tapes and ties them with a square knot at the side of the neck. Tying at the side is safer and more comfortable for the client. There is no uncomfortable knot at the back of the neck, and the tracheostomy tapes cannot be easily mistaken for ties on the gown and loosened inadvertently.

Whenever a tracheostomy tube is in use another tracheostomy set must be in the room in clear view (either attached to the wall or the bedside table) so that the tube can be replaced immediately if it is accidently coughed out. A sterile hemostat must also be kept in clear view at the bedside to be used to hold the trachea open in a similar emergency.

Because the air inspired through the tracheostomy is not warmed and humidified by passage through the nose and pharynx, a humidifying apparatus is placed over the tracheal opening. Either oxygen or air is given through this apparatus. Frequent mouth care is important for a person with a tracheostomy. Emotional support is vital, because the client cannot talk until he is taught how to occlude the opening in the tube when he wants to speak. Many people prefer to communicate initially by writing because they have trouble, or fear that they will have trouble doing without oxygen when the tube is occluded.

More detailed information on nursing responsibilities when the client has a tracheostomy can be found in medical-surgical textbooks, as well as in the suggested readings at the end of the chapter.

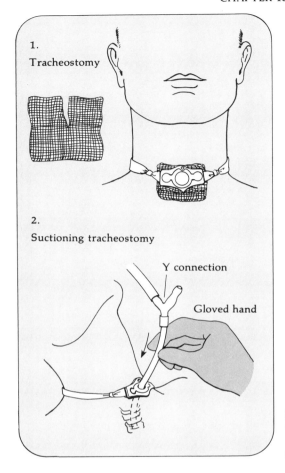

1.

Tracheostomy

2.

Suctioning tracheostomy

Y connection

Gloved hand

**Figure 15-11.**   *Tracheostomy: (1) Tube in place with dressing properly placed. (2) Technique for inserting catheter in tube for suctioning.*

## Pharyngeal Suctioning

The purpose of pharyngeal suctioning is to help a client clear his airway by removing secretions and foreign matter from nose, mouth, and pharynx. For suctioning, a sterile catheter is inserted into the nose or mouth.

**Special Considerations**
The catheter should be inserted without force. If an obstruction is encountered in one nostril, the catheter is inserted into the other. If blood appears in the material suctioned, the amount of suction is reduced and/or a smaller catheter is used. If the client vomits, his head must be turned to the side and the catheter withdrawn. As vomiting subsides, the suctioning is resumed. The client is placed in lateral, prone or semiprone positions to encourage drainage of secretions.

## Performance Checklist
### Pharyngeal Suctioning

1. When appropriate, explain what you are going to do and why.
2. Encourage the client to cough while you are suctioning.
3. Pour water or saline into a disposable cup.
4. Attach a sterile rubber or plastic catheter with a narrow lumen, a "whistle" tip, and several openings on the sides to the tubing on the suction apparatus. If a "y" connector for controlling suction is not a part of the tube, attach a separate "y" connector.
5. Turn on suction and regulate pressure for the least amount required to remove secretions (usually low to moderate, 10 to 40 mm Hg).
6. Place a sterile glove on the hand used to manipulate the catheter.
7. Test suctioning apparatus by placing catheter tip in cup of water and placing *ungloved* finger over control vent ("y").
8. To suction through the nose:
   a. measure distance from tip of nose to lobe of ear
   b. dip catheter tip in solution to lubricate it
   c. gently insert catheter into nostril and advance it the distance measured
   d. close the "y" to initiate suction
   e. release suction and slowly rotate catheter while it is being withdrawn
   f. cleanse tube by drawing solution through it by closing "y"
   g. permit client to rest
   h. insert catheter into opposite nostril and suction as described above
   i. suction until all secretions are removed
   j. make the client comfortable
   k. dispose of catheter (or have it sterilized) and cup of solution
   l. set up equipment for future suctioning
   m. record results of suctioning (amount, color, consistency of mucus), and client's response to suctioning
9. To suction through the mouth:
   a. use same equipment as that for nasal procedure with addition of tongue blade if necessary
   b. aspirate mouth secretions
   c. pass catheter into esophagus
   d. suction as previously described
10. To suction through an airway:
    a. insert catheter through the lumen of the airway and proceed as described previously
    b. suction secretions from oral cavity
11. If necessary to suction nose, use fresh catheter.

## SUMMARY

In health we pay little attention to the body's need for air. Oxygen is inhaled and carbon dioxide is exhaled without obvious effort. However, when the air is filled with smoke or other pollutants, we begin to focus on the need for pure air. In addition, when there is a problem with the respiratory or circulatory system, we become painfully aware of the need for air.

A patent airway is essential for normal respiratory function. Maintaining an intact respiratory/circulatory system is a nursing priority. Attention to the effect of pollutants on breathing is as important for the nurse and her client as the need for deep breathing and coughing after surgery. The client is taught ways to prevent, detect, and treat upper respiratory infections so that their complications can be avoided. Especially in children, screening to detect strep throat is important for prevention of rheumatic fever. Hypertension detection helps prevent circulatory problems that interfere with gas transport. Screening for high blood pressure is one way nursing students can easily become involved in community activities.

Assessment of respiratory/circulatory functioning requires a background in anatomy and physiology. Measuring pulse, respirations, and blood pressure are valuable assessment techniques. Assessing air movement, venous pulsation, and cardiac arrhythmias provides additional information upon which nursing actions can be based.

When the client has a health problem, whether major or minor, the nurse can assist in achievement of adequate respiration and circulation. After practice, she is prepared to provide basic life support and to save the life of a choking victim. She can help maintain an open airway by giving coughing and breathing instructions and providing humidification of the environment. Suctioning, airway insertion, tracheostomy care, and oxygen administration are additional methods of assistance the student can practice and use after completion of this chapter.

## LEARNING ACTIVITIES

1.  Plan a program to instruct an adult who is in to have abdominal surgery in turning, positioning, coughing, and deep breathing.

2.  Describe the mechanics of respiration.

3.  Describe in two or three sentences how we are affected by air pollution.

4.  Assess the respiratory functioning of a healthy young adult.

5.  Describe râles and wheezing and, after practice, identify them on a client by use of a stethoscope.

6.  In a simulated setting, demonstrate a one-rescuer cardiopulmonary resuscitation on an adult.

## REFERENCES AND SUGGESTED READINGS

Acute respiratory insufficiency. *Nursing 77*, December, 1977, pp. 26–31.

Bates, Barbara, 1974. *A guide to physical examination.* Philadelphia: J. B. Lippincott.

Blood gas and acid-base concepts in respiratory care. *American Journal of Nursing,* June, 1976, pp. 963–992.

Burgess, Ann W., 1978.   *Nursing: levels of health intervention.*   Englewood Cliffs, N.J.: Prentice-Hall.

Bushnell, S., et al., 1973.   *Respiratory intensive care nursing.*   Boston: Little, Brown.

Diekelmann, Nancy, 1977.   *Primary health care of the well adult.*   New York: McGraw-Hill.

DuGas, Beverly, 1977.   *Introduction to patient care.*   Philadelphia: W. B. Saunders.

Foss, G.   Postural drainage. *American Journal of Nursing,* April, 1973, pp. 663–669.

Fuerst, Elinor; Wolff, LuVerne; and Weitzel, Marlene, 1974.   *Fundamentals of nursing.* 5th ed.   Philadelphia: J. B. Lippincott.

Guyton, Arthur, 1976.   *Textbook of medical physiology.* 5th ed.   Philadelphia: W. B. Saunders.

Heimlich, Henry.   A life-saving maneuver to prevent food-choking. *Journal of the American Medical Association,* 234 (October 27, 1975), 398–401.

Leitch, Cynthia and Tinker, Richard, 1978.   *Primary care.*   Philadelphia: F. A. Davis.

Lewis, LuVerne, 1976.   *Fundamental skills in patient care.*   Philadelphia: J. B. Lippincott.

Lingvarski, Peter; Argondizzo, Nina; and Boos, Patricia.   CPR: current practice revised. *American Journal of Nursing,* February, 1975, pp. 236–241.

Patient assessment: pulses. *American Journal of Nursing,* January, 1979, pp. 115–132.

Vraciu, J. K. and Vraciu, R. A.   Effectiveness of breathing exercises in preventing pulmonary complications following open heart surgery. *Physical Therapy, 57* (December, 1977), 1367–1371.

West, John B., 1974.   *Respiratory physiology—the essentials.*   Baltimore: Williams & Wilkins.

Wood, Lucile, 1975.   *Nursing skills for allied health services, Vol. 2.*   Philadelphia: W. B. Saunders.

# 16

# Nutrition

## Behavioral Objectives

Upon completion of this chapter, the student will be able to:

1. Identify factors affecting clients' nutrition.
2. Plan a balanced diet based on these factors for a person at any age.
3. Discuss the problem of waste and food additives in the promotion of good nutrition.
4. Plan, implement, and evaluate methods of assistance for a client with a nutrition-related health problem.

## Key Terms

| | | |
|---|---|---|
| absorption | excretion | metabolism |
| additives | fiber | minerals |
| adipocytes | fluoride | nausea |
| anorexia | gastrointestinal tract | nutrients |
| antioxidants | gastrostomy | nutrition |
| appetite | gavage | nutrition process |
| aspirate | glycogen | overnutrition |
| basic diets | hunger | proteins |
| calorie | hyperalimentation | RDA |
| carbohydrates | hypertonic | regularity |
| carcinogens | ingestion | satiety |
| Celsius | kosher | transportation |
| CHO | Kwashiorkor | undernutrition |
| cholesterol | lactation | USDA |
| digestion | malnutrition | vegetarian |
| edentulous | marasmus | vitamins |
| emesis | megavitamins | vomiting |

## Introduction

Currently, some milk cartons advise the public: "To be healthy, check with your doctor; check with your nurse. Ask your Heart Association for Helpful Heart Hints." Dr. Stare wrote in the preface to the *Manual on Nutrition,* of which he was co-author (Latham et al. 1970) that nutrition is a largely neglected field in health and medicine. A decade later, medical and nursing students are receiving more formal education in nutrition. Since health is so dependent upon nutrition, it is hoped that by presenting a few facts about nutrition in this chapter, nursing students will be encouraged to seek more information so that they can maintain their own health and assist others who seek their advice.

## FACTORS AFFECTING NUTRITION

Nutrition is the science of food. Nutrients are the chemical substances in food required by the body. The study of nutrition tells us what these substances do and how they interact. Culture, religion, psychological, and socio-economic factors as well as age, sex, and state of health all influence our food intake.

People often eat what they are accustomed to and can afford to buy. This statement describes the basis for the nutritional habits of many people in the United States today. The more adventuresome try new foods when the opportunity arises; others prefer the foods they have eaten since childhood. Cost of food is a factor in nutritional changes for some people, while others eat what they like regardless of the price and economize in other ways. If it is true that man eats what he is accustomed to, the importance of establishing good eating habits in early life is obvious.

### Culture

Any number of cultural influences on nutrition can be cited. Think of the feasting associated with Christmas and Hanukkah. Each year, many of us may diet periodically to overcome the effects of these feasts.

Traditional breakfast menus in this country differ markedly from the coffee and roll served in continental Europe. As delicacies, one person may prefer stuffed pig stomach and snails, while another person may prefer braised kidneys. Still others will choose steak when they are offered a treat. Wide individual preferences exist within our culture, and it is essential that we respect the food preferences of all clients—those whose cultural backgrounds are similar to ours as well as those whose cultural habits are different. It is difficult, if not impossible, to know the food habits of clients unless they are asked. The client or a family member can give the information needed so that the nurse can assist in meeting nutritional needs. Changes in food habits are more difficult for the ill person than for the healthy, so providing accustomed food whenever it is possible to do so is important.

Time for meals also differs. Three meals spread throughout the day is the usual pattern. Some people have their biggest meal of the day at noon and others have it in the evening. Those who prepare their own food after a day in the working world may have dinner at 8 out of necessity rather than choice.

## Religion

Religions often have nutritional requirements for their members. For example, Seventh Day Adventists do not eat meat; Muslims do not eat pork. On a few specified days of the year, Catholics fast and do not eat meat. Some Catholics never eat meat on Fridays, though the Church law no longer requires this. Orthodox Jews have strict requirements for food preparation and service. Foods that meet Jewish dietary regulations (called *kosher*) are becoming increasingly available in institutions where there is a demand for them.

When a person is ill, he is usually not bound by his religion to dietary constraints. However, some persons prefer to retain the restrictions, and the client's wishes are a primary concern of the nurse.

## Psychological Factors

Mealtime is often looked upon as a pleasant time for sharing the day's activities with other family members. Some hospitals attempt to increase the pleasure of meals by encouraging family members to stay with the client. Persons who are able to eat in a dining room are encouraged to do so when such a facility exists. Group eating is fostered more often for children than adults. The social aspect of eating—so important in many cultures—is emphasized in such instances.

In childhood, food is often used as a reward for good behavior or withheld as punishment. While these practices are no longer popular, adults who grew up under such circumstances may still see food in this light. The psychological meaning of food to each person is often even harder to identify than the religious or cultural implications.

## Socioeconomic Factors

While persons of moderate means may continue to eat as they choose even when prices rise, those on limited incomes are forced to eat less expensive foods. These tend to be starchy and easily lead to weight gain. When there is severe financial want, food is not available and malnutrition results.

A national nutrition survey showed that in the U.S. where half the families earned less than $3,000/year (in 1970), more than 16 percent had serious protein deficiencies—some well below the levels normally associated with malnutrition in underdeveloped countries (Lappé, 1975). The cost of the cheapest adequate diet recommended by the USDA rose well over twice as much as welfare benefits for poor workers between December 1970 and December 1973 (Lappé, 1975). The cost of the recommended diet already exceeds food stamp benefits.

## Hunger, Appetite, and Satiety

The individual consumption of food is affected by hunger, appetite, and satiety. *Hunger* is a complex of unpleasant sensations resulting from prolonged food deprivation. Hunger pains are felt when an empty stomach contracts. The feeling of emptiness or weakness, or headache, may also result from hunger. *Appetite* is a complex of sensations, in general pleasant, by which one is aware of the desire for food. It may be present in the absence of hunger, as when we smell fresh bread baking and so forth. *Satiety* describes a feeling of fullness and satisfaction.

## State of Health

Nutrition is an important factor in health, growth, strength, and endurance at every stage in life. Changes in required calories and specific nutrients are necessary at certain stages. An increase in calories and special attention to good nutrition are of special importance for the pregnant woman, the developing fetus, the growing child, and the adolescent. However, good nutrition is essential for the maintenance of health in all age groups.

Illness usually increases nutritional needs. For example, fever causes a higher metabolic rate with a greater caloric requirement. Wound healing requires an increase in calories, protein, vitamins, and minerals. Unfortunately, illness may adversely affect the appetite. Food is less appealing and fatigue may make eating difficult. An unpleasant taste in the mouth, a sore tongue and gums, and the absence of teeth are among the factors that affect appetite or the ability to chew. Nursing measures to improve the condition of the mouth and adaptations in the consistency of the diet help to meet nutritional requirements.

## NORMAL NUTRITIONAL NEEDS THROUGH THE LIFE CYCLE

Over 50 known nutrients are necessary for health. They are divided into 6 groups: proteins, fats, carbohydrates, minerals, vitamins, and water. Protein, carbohydrates, and fat provide calories. Both protein and carbohydrates provide 4 calories per gram, while fat provides 9 calories per gram. A calorie is the amount of heat required to raise the temperature of one gram of water one degree Celsius.

The body requires a diet made up of the essential nutrients obtained from a variety of foods. Requirements change throughout the life cycle and these will be indicated in the brief summary that follows.

## Protein

Proteins contain carbon, hydrogen, oxygen, nitrogen, and sulfur. They break down into amino acids, the basic structural unit incorporated into cells for growth and repair of muscles and other important tissues. The body can synthesize all but 8 of the 22 essential amino acids. These 8 must be ingested. A complete protein contains all 8 amino acids in proper proportions; if the protein does not contain all 8, it is called an incomplete protein. In general, animal proteins (meat, eggs, and dairy products) are complete; vegetable proteins usually are incomplete.

Foods high in protein are eggs, milk, fish, cheese, poultry, soybeans, and legumes. The Recommended Dietary Allowance (RDA) is 65 g/day or less. The need varies according to body size, age, and activity and whether pregnancy or lactation is present. But 65 grams is considered more than adequate. The average intake in America is 106 g/day. Any excess protein is converted to glucose to be burned as energy or stored as fat; the nitrogen is excreted.

Adequate protein intake is vital during the growth periods of infancy, childhood, adolescence, and pregnancy and lactation.

## Carbohydrates

Carbohydrates consist of sugars and starches and are energy foods; they can be broken down and used more quickly than fats and proteins. Grain products are the major source of carbohydrates, although all fruits and vegetables contain some. Refined simple sugars are an important source of energy but have no other nutritive value. If a person fills up on sugary foods, he usually doesn't eat enough of the other nutrients. Foods high in sugar lead to tooth decay, atherosclerosis, heart disease, and obesity. A limited amount of excess carbohydrates is converted to glycogen for storage in the liver but the rest is converted to fat and stored.

Starches (as found in rice, wheat, corn, and potatoes) are broken down into glucose. Carbohydrates form the majority of the calories required in most diets, because they are low in cost and readily available. Some carbohydrates are essential for fat metabolism.

Carbohydrates are especially needed for the energy requirements of adolescence and infancy. A full-term infant can digest a simple carbohydrate; following maturation of the gastrointestinal tract within the next few months, starches can be utilitzed.

## Fats

Fats serve as a concentrated energy source and as a medium for transport of fat-soluble vitamins. They add flavor and moisture to foods and have a satiety value. Large amounts of fat can quickly increase the caloric intake (9 calories/gram). Generally, no more than 25 percent of dietary calories should be obtained from fats.

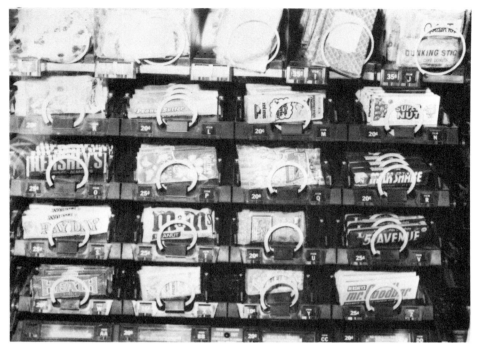

**Figure 16-1.** *Junk food. (Photo by Frank R. Engler, Jr.)*

Considerable attention is being paid to the saturation of fats. Animal fats are saturated fats and tend to raise the blood cholesterol level. Polyunsaturated fats are obtained from vegetables and tend to lower the cholesterol level, thus protecting against coronary artery disease.

## Minerals

Many minerals are required nutrients. Some are needed in large amounts and others only in traces. Calcium, iron, phosphorous, iodine, and fluoride are among those required. Iron and fluoride are essential in infancy and childhood because these are periods of rapid growth and increasing blood volume. A deficiency in fluoride at these times leaves the teeth relatively susceptible to caries. Calcium is required in large amounts during infancy, childhood, adolescence, and in pregnancy and lactation because it is necessary for bone growth. Women during pregnancy and lactation and growing children have an increased need for iodine. Iodine is obtained from certain foods, water, and iodized salt. Seafood is particularly rich in iodine. Iron deficiency is most common in young children and in women of child-bearing age. Calcium and phosphorous occur together in the body mainly in the bones. These minerals are needed in larger amounts during periods of growth.

## Vitamins

Vitamins are organic substances present in minute quantities in foods and are necessary for metabolism. Vitamins are sometimes classified as either fat- or water-soluble. The fat-soluble vitamins can be stored; the water-soluble cannot. Vitamins A, D, E, and K are fat-soluble. One medium-sized carrot contains all the Vitamin A needed daily. Few foods contain Vitamin D naturally. It is generally added to milk. Sunshine and enriched milk are major sources of Vitamin D, which is especially needed by children to prevent rickets (a bone weakness). Vitamin E is widely distributed in foods. The richest sources are vegetable oils. Vitamin K assists cells in forming prothrombin (a blood-clotting factor). It is plentiful in most foods.

The water-soluble vitamins are B and C. They cannot be stored and may be partially damaged by cooking. The B complex vitamins, of which there are 9, are necessary for the development of red blood cells, for tissue growth, and for digestion. They are found in meat, eggs, milk, green vegetables, and whole grains. The elderly are frequently deficient in these substances. Vitamin C is important for building and maintaining teeth, bones, muscles, gums, and connective tissue. It promotes wound healing. A common source is citrus fruits. A 6-ounce glass of orange or grapefruit juice will provide the daily needed amount.

## Water

Water forms nearly 70 percent of the body's weight. It furnishes no calories or vitamins. It may provide minerals (calcium or magnesium in hard water) and fluoride if this has been added. Six to seven 8-ounce glasses a day furnish enough water for an adult's metabolic requirements.

## Adults and Older Persons

In adulthood, caloric requirements decrease because growth needs are minimal and the metabolic rate decreases. A person who leads a sedentary life has an additional reason to decrease caloric intake—he still requires all the nutrients, but fewer calories.

The older person requires all the nutrients that other adults require; he too, needs fewer calories. Nutrients often lacking or deficient in the diet of the elderly include calcium, vitamin C, protein, iron, water, vitamin A, and the vitamin B complex. Some problems related to nutrition in the elderly include: difficulty in chewing because of dental disease or absence of teeth, with related digestive problems; difficulty and lack of motivation in getting and preparing food; lack of appetite due to an impaired sense of smell and taste. There is a 1% annual decrease in receptor neurons for smell throughout life (Noback and Demarest, 1975). What can the nurse do to help? Foods that can be easily chewed should be provided for these clients, as well as a dental consultation for tooth repair or replacement. Community services often include transportation to and from the grocery store. Food stamps, for those who qualify, may enable the elderly to purchase nutritious food. Easily prepared meals include TV dinners that can be heated in an electric skillet or an oven. Meals on Wheels provide nutritious meals at low cost to housebound persons. Many communities also offer lunch programs. For a small fee, eligible persons can obtain a hot, well-balanced meal.

## SELECTING AN ADEQUATE DIET

A diet consisting of a wide variety of foods usually includes all the necessary nutrients. Food guides are available that translate the RDA into patterns that meet the recommended levels (see Table 16-1). There are 4 food groups: milk, meat, breads and cereals, and vegetables and fruits. Each group contributes a number of nutrients, and when the recommended servings are eaten an adequate amount of nutrients are supplied. Additional servings from any group will increase the caloric intake when this is necessary.

## PROMOTION OF GOOD NUTRITION

Knowing what constitutes good nutrition includes a knowledge of waste, vegetarianism, fiber, cholesterol intake, and facts/fiction about foods, food additives, and the importance of diet in controlling hypertension.

### Waste

It has been estimated that, in the United States, 25 percent of all food bought is wasted (Hoffman, 1977). In a world where people are starving, reducing this waste is important. It could make more food available. The ways we waste food are legion. The hostess, for example, encourages her guests to eat more than they want because she doesn't want any leftovers. Food is wasted not only when it is thrown away but when it is consumed needlessly. Restaurants often serve larger portions than required. The food sent back to restaurant kitchens (or home in doggy bags) would feed a lot of hungry people. Restaurants are beginning to solve this problem by offering smaller portions for less money.

Persons who cook only for themselves have difficulty preventing waste because food processors and stores do not provide portions suitable for one serving. Leftovers are often forgotten or not wanted, though they can sometimes be frozen for future use.

In the United States, our diet is meat-centered and this is extremely wasteful in terms of food production. Approximately 78 percent of all grain harvested in the U.S. is fed to animals (Hoffman, 1977). Can adequate protein for health be obtained without eating meat? The answer is "yes" and in the following section we shall discuss ways to provide high quality protein while consuming less meat.

Table 16-1.    Daily Food Guide—the Basic Four Food Groups

| Food group | Main nutrients | Daily amounts [2] |
|---|---|---|
| **Milk** | | |
| Milk, cheese, ice cream, or other products made with whole or skimmed milk | Calcium Protein Riboflavin | Children under 9: 2 to 3 cups<br>Children 9 to 12: 3 or more cups<br>Teenagers: 4 or more cups<br>Adults: 2 or more cups<br>Pregnant women: 3 or more cups<br>Nursing mothers: 4 or more cups<br>(1 cup = 8 oz. fluid milk or designated milk equivalent[3]) |
| **Meats** | | |
| Beef, veal, lamb, pork, poultry, fish, eggs | Protein Iron Thiamine | 2 or more servings<br>Count as one serving:<br>2 to 3 oz. of lean, boneless, cooked meat, poultry, or fish |
| Alternates: dry beans, dry peas, nuts, peanut butter | Niacin Riboflavin | 2 eggs<br>1 cup cooked dry beans or peas<br>4 tablespoons peanut butter |
| **Vegetables and fruits** | | 4 or more servings<br>Count as 1 serving:<br>1/2 cup of vegetable or fruit, or a portion such as 1 medium apple, banana, orange, potato, or 1/2 a medium grapefruit, melon |
| | Vitamin A | Include:<br>A dark-green or deep-yellow vegetable or fruit rich in vitamin A, at least every other day |
| | Vitamin C (ascorbic acid) | A citrus fruit or other fruit or vegetable rich in vitamin C daily |
| | Smaller amounts of other vitamins and minerals | Other vegetables and fruits including potatoes |
| **Breads and cereals** | | 4 or more servings of whole grain, enriched or restored<br>Count as 1 serving: |
| | Thiamine Niacin Riboflavin Iron Protein | 1 slice of bread<br>1 ounce (1 cup) ready to eat cereal, flake or puff varieties<br>1/2 to 3/4 cup cooked cereal<br>1/2 to 3/4 cup cooked pastas (macaroni, spaghetti, noodles)<br>Crackers: 5 saltines, 2 squares graham crackers, etc. |

[1]From Williams, Sue Rodwell, 1977, *Nutrition and diet therapy*, 3rd ed., St. Louis: C. V. Mosby. By permission.
[2]Use additional amounts of these foods or added butter, margarine, oils, sugars, etc., as desired or needed.
[3]Milk equivalents: 1 ounce cheddar cheese, 3 servings cottage cheese, 1 cup fluid skimmed milk, 1 cup buttermilk, 1/4 cup dry skimmed milk powder, 1 cup ice milk, 1-2/3 cups ice cream, 1/2 cup evaporated milk.

Grains and legumes (beans, peas, and lentils) can be eaten together at the same meal. Eggs can be combined with salads or with cheeses in casseroles. Cereals can be supplemented with low-fat milk. A small amount of animal protein can, in this way, complement a plant protein.

## Vegetarianism

Nurses should be prepared to help vegetarians plan and obtain an adequate diet. Vegetarians are classified as those who avoid red meat only but eat poultry and fish; lacto-ovo-vegetarians avoid flesh foods but eat milk, cheese, and eggs; and strict vegetarians (vegans) avoid all foods of animal origin.

A nutritionally adequate diet is more difficult to achieve when food choices become more restrictive. Therefore, while a strict vegetarian diet can be nutritionally adequate, greater knowledge of food composition is required in order to choose foods containing the needed nutrients.

The basic principles for planning any nutritionally adequate diet are followed. Calorie intake must be adequate to attain and maintain ideal weight. Protein should supply all of the needed amino acids. In the vegetarian diet, this is achieved by complementing or supplementing one protein with another.

A vegetarian may have an adequate diet at home but the choices offered by a hospital menu may not provide the combination and variety of foods required unless special efforts are made.

## Fiber

The role of fiber in the diet is receiving increased attention. Since 1900, processed foods have caused dietary fiber to be decreased by 50 percent. There are several reasons why fiber is being added to the diet today. It has a role in weight loss; it is important in regularity; it can lower serum cholesterol by increasing cholesterol output; it is effective against chronic diarrhea because it absorbs water; and there is speculation that it decreases the incidence of cancer of the colon by rapidly removing the carcinogens from the intestinal tract.

Dietary fiber is that part of plant material that is not digested in the alimentary tract and is excreted in the feces. Fiber increases the rate at which food passes through the intestine and adds to the weight of the feces.

Whole grains, whole bran breakfast cereals, and many fresh fruits and vegetables all contain fiber. Eating bran and bran products easily increases total fiber intake, while large amounts of the other sources of fiber are required to increase the fiber intake substantially.

## Cholesterol Intake

There is ongoing controversy about the nature of the relationship between elevated cholesterol levels and cardiovascular disease. Widespread research efforts in this area are supported by the federal government and private funds. Dr. Wissler (Mallison, 1978) stated, at a symposium on cholesterol, that no one seriously claims that diet and cholesterol are not related. There is

## Table  16-2    Facts and Fiction

| | |
|---|---|
| Vitamin C in large amounts will prevent or cure colds. | Fiction. There is no conclusive evidence that a specific vitamin will prevent or cure a cold. |
| Vegetarians can't get enough complete protein. | Fiction. Complementary plant proteins can be used or they can be supplemented with small amounts of animal protein. |
| Increased fiber intake will lessen risk of colon cancer. | This is speculative. Rapid movement of carcinogens through the colon *may* play a part in preventing colon cancer. |
| Vitamin E is good for your sex life. | Fiction. Experimental rats totally deprived of Vitamin E became sterile. That's how the fallacy arose. |
| Megavitamins are good for you. | Fiction. There is no proof that they are helpful; indeed they may be harmful. |
| Athletes should eat steak before a game. | Fiction. It takes too long to break it down. Carbohydrate is better. |
| Fat babies become fat adults. | Maybe. They form more fat cells than others. They are also environmentally programmed to be fat. |

evidence from animal studies that advanced and complex atherosclerosis can be reversed by keeping the serum cholesterol at about 140 mg percent. The importance of a permanent change in the diet is stressed.

**Control of Hypertension**    Hypertension is another disease that can often be affected by diet. Dr. Christakis (Mallison, 1978) pointed out that each permanent 4-pound weight loss lowers diastolic pressure by one mm Hg. It is important for the public to be taught the importance of prudent diet, weight control, cessation of smoking, and blood pressure control in prevention of cardiac problems.

## Additives

Many substances added to our foods are safe, but we should not rely totally on foods high in additives. The Food and Drug Administration tries to regulate the use of these substances, and they are looking closely at old additives while making it much harder to introduce new ones. Coloring agents, artificial sweeteners, thickeners, antioxidants, and preservatives are among the additives. Many foods could not be preserved without additives and unfamiliar natural food colors might displease consumers. The nurse should keep abreast of current research in this area and be able to inform clients of the latest findings while respecting their individual attitudes toward food additives.

## ASSISTING A CLIENT WITH A PROBLEM RELATED TO NUTRITION

The nutrition process provides nutrients for essential body activities. Ingestion, digestion, absorption, transportation, metabolism, and excretion constitute the nutrition process. Ingestion is the taking in of food—usually through the mouth, although it can be taken directly into the stomach or blood stream. Digestion is the breaking down of foods into simpler substances. It begins in the mouth and is completed in the small intestine. Absorption occurs primarily in the small intestine as the end products of digestion are passed from the GI tract into the blood and the lymph system. Transportation is the delivery of nutrients to the body cells. It takes place, in general, in the circulatory system. Metabolism refers to the physical and chemical changes occurring within the cells. Nutrients are required for body function, maintenance, growth, and repair. Excretion is the means by which waste products are disposed of. Metabolic wastes are reabsorbed into the blood stream and excreted through the lungs as carbon dioxide and through the kidneys as urea. GI wastes are excreted through the anus as feces. A health problem at any stage of the process has an effect on nutritional status. For example, when a tooth is filled and you can't chew on it, digestion is affected as well as ingestion. Diarrhea affects absorption, as increased intestinal motility lessens the time available for absorption. Of course, more serious problems create greater difficulties.

Promoting good nutrition in the person who is well is sometimes difficult; it is much more difficult when the person is ill.

### Assessment Guide

Assessment of the client's nutritional state precedes any assistance offered by the nurse. The following nutrition assessment guide can be used to determine the client's perceptions of his nutritional habits and status:

1. How much do you weigh? How tall are you? Do you consider your weight correct for you?
2. Do you have any trouble with your mouth or teeth?
3. How does your diet compare with that included in the basic food groups? (Explain what they are, if necessary).
4. If not, what are you lacking? Any specific foods you don't eat?
5. Are you a vegetarian? Are you on a special diet?
6. Do you take diet supplements?
7. Do you smoke? If so, how much?
8. Does "junk food" make up any part of your diet? If so, how much?
9. Do you know the content of the foods you eat: sugar, salt, nitrates, other additives?

10. Do you prepare your own food? If so, do you know: the effects of frying food; the length of time for boiling vegetables; the effects of saturated fats vs. polyunsaturates?

11. Do you eat at home or in restaurants? Alone or with others?

12. How many meals a day do you eat? At what times?

13. How is your appetite?

In addition to a dietary history, physical findings help in assessing the nutritional status. Weight, height, and condition of mouth have been discussed. Condition of the hair and skin and the general energy level are also important factors.

## Malnutrition

Two types of nutritional problems will be included under the general classification of malnutrition: overnutrition and undernutrition. In overnutrition, we will consider obesity, and in undernutrition, the problem of calorie and protein deficits.

Overnutrition    Overnutrition, or obesity, an excess of adipose tissue, usually occurs when the intake of food and the expenditure of energy are not balanced. It is often considered a disease of an affluent society. Obesity is essentially an increase in adipose tissue of 20 percent above normal. Since this is difficult to determine, we usually consider a weight increase greater than 20 percent to signify obesity. The social and psychological effects of obesity are well-known. The ten-year-old who is told by the clerk to go to the "husky" department for jeans suffers, as does the  middle-aged woman who sews her own clothes rather than buy them at a half-size outlet. These inconveniences seldom match the physiological results of obesity. Cardiovascular disease, hypertension, gall bladder disease, diabetes, and joint problems are among the many problems linked to obesity.

Obesity is difficult to overcome, so its prevention is important. Good dietary patterns established in childhood are the basis for health—and the prevention of obesity. Mothers should not tell their children to eat all their food or "I'll know you don't like my cooking." Neither should they use food as a reward. A larger number of fat cells (adipocytes) formed during early growth makes later treatment more difficult. Studies indicate that when one parent is obese, 40 percent of the children are obese.

Obesity is a major nutritional disease which occurs at all socioeconomic levels and among persons of all races.

No specific diet makes people obese and, in general, no specific diet favors weight reduction. The best way to lose weight is to establish new behaviors related to foods, reduce caloric intake, and increase physical activity. If we take in more calories than we use, we will gain weight; if we burn more than we take in, we will lose weight.

Fad diets should be avoided. There is no evidence that extreme diets, especially those not including all nutrients, have any advantage over a balanced calorie-restricted diet.

New eating habits must be formed. It is important to cut down on fats, sauces, desserts, fried foods, etc., and on the overall amount of food consumed. A sample diet for weight reduction might include the following: 1200 cal/day: 45 to 50 g protein, 42 fat, and 100 to 150 carbohydrate. On this diet, a person of average height can expect to lose one pound a week. This is a good plan for those who have less than 30 pounds to lose. There is no risk and no expensive items are required. Because it takes a long time, new eating habits can be learned. There may be some discouragement, however, because of the long time required to lose a noticeable amount of weight.

Undernutrition    When children's diets are deficient in protein and calories, a wide range of malnutrition problems occur. Kwashiorkor and marasmus are the most severe. Mild to moderate calorie and protein deficiencies, however, are hardly less important in the long run, if the child's growth and development is to progress normally.

Monitoring growth and development in children is an important way to prevent malnutrition. Low weight and height for the child's age may be indications of undernutrition. If the nutritional state is not improved, permanent stunting of physical growth may occur. There is some indication that intellectual and psychological development are also affected.

*Kwashiorkor* is a disease of undernutrition where protein is the deficiency nutrient. In *marasmus* there is an overall deficit in both protein and calories. Kwashiorkor usually occurs in children 1 to 3 years of age. It has been reported in poverty areas of the United States, but it is common in countries where there is a short supply of protein. These children, who have been taken off the breast and fed a starchy diet, show growth failure, tissue wasting, edema, mental changes, skin and hair changes, diarrhea, and anemia. Their condition improves when they are fed dried skimmed milk, vegetable oil, and casein. Marasmus is more common in children under one year of age who lack food of any kind. These babies fail to grow, show tissue wasting, but have a good appetite, and appear bright-eyed and alert. They are anemic and have intermittent bouts of diarrhea. They respond to an adequate intake of calories and protein. It is important to ensure continuing adequate nourishment for these children by teaching the parents and making proper food available.

## Anorexia, Nausea, and Vomiting

Anorexia is a loss of appetite or lack of interest in food. There are many causes of anorexia: stress and illness are two that are seen frequently. In both these instances, nutrients are more necessary than ever. Special attempts must be made to increase the appetite and to provide foods containing the essential nutrients. If this fails, parenteral feeding methods are required. Determining the cause and removing it are essential in all instances of anorexia, nausea, and vomiting.

Nausea is the feeling that vomiting is going to occur. It may preceed vomiting but both nausea and vomiting can occur separately. Vomiting is the ejection of stomach contents through the mouth. There are many physical and psychological reasons for nausea and vomiting—some more serious than others. It is important ot assess the reason for the symptoms and find ways to treat the cause.

When a client says he is going to vomit, the nurse should respond quickly by providing a large container so that he doesn't have to be concerned about soiling his clothing or bedding. An emesis basin is usually not large enough; a bath basin is.

You can help the person who is nauseated or vomiting in the following ways:

1. Suggest he take deep breaths. This relaxes the muscles and may keep the nauseated person from vomiting.

2. Remove annoying sights or odors. If the appetite is poor, the sight of a disliked food can cause nausea or vomiting. A soiled dressing should be changed before mealtime.

3. Limit food and fluid intake until nausea and vomiting subside, and then offer ice chips or fluids in small amounts. Carbonated beverages are sometimes tolerated more readily than others.

4. Assist the client with oral hygiene after he vomits. Help him wash his face and hands and change any clothing that is soiled.

5. Measure (or estimate) amount of emesis (vomitus). Describe its appearance and record amount under "output."

6. Drugs may be required to control prolonged nausea and vomiting. Intravenous fluids will replace lost fluids.

7. Protect the person who is vomiting from aspiration. Have him in a sitting position, if possible. If not, place him in a prone or semiprone position. Side-lying will also permit vomitus to escape without danger of aspiration.

## Dental Caries

People with cavities (caries) or without teeth (edentulous) have difficulty eating a balanced diet. Dr. Shannon, director of an oral disease research laboratory in Houston, told conference members (*Washington Post*, January 7, 1979) that there are an estimated 1 billion unfilled cavities in the U.S. today. Most of the cavities are blamed on the everpresent disguised sugar in American foods. Many dental authorities believe it is the sticky, adherent carbohydrate food that stays in contact with the teeth and gums for a prolonged time that causes caries. If candies or other sweets are eaten after a meal, the teeth should be carefully flossed and then brushed.

Fluoridation of community water supplies is very important for cavity prevention. Fluorides can be added to infant vitamins and toothpaste, but water fluoridation is more efficient and effective.

Nurses are in a good position to teach dental hygiene to their clients. Many people who visit a dentist regularly are not aware of the importance of flossing for plaque removal (and caries prevention). Dentists have been in the past more concerned with restoration than with prevention of decay, but times are changing. As the public seeks ways to stay well, more preventive dentistry may be seen.

## Improving the Appetite

As suggested earlier, persons who are not feeling well may not have an appetite. Because they need even more nutrients than when they were well, it is important for the nurse to try to improve her clients' appetites in the following ways:

1. Provide a pleasant atmosphere and attractive food service.
2. Serve foods at the proper temperatures and properly seasoned (within dietary constraints). If hot foods get cold, reheat them.
3. Encourage physical activity.
4. Eliminate unpleasant sights, noises, and odors.
5. Alleviate physical discomfort.
6. Provide oral hygiene.
7. Help the client to a comfortable position for eating.

In many agencies, the dietary department is responsible for serving and removing trays; however, the nurse retains the overall responsibility for assisting her client to eat.

## Assisting a Client To Eat

**Special Considerations**
Some clients will be unable to feed themselves; others will need assistance. The client, should be encouraged to do as much for himself as possible. The nurse should always ask her client if he needs help, and use her good judgment.

Some clients need to have their meat cut, bread buttered, and cartons opened and then they can feed themselves. The tray should be placed appropriately in front of the client.

Feeding a client has sometimes been considered a skill not requiring a professional nurse's talents. But much valuable information about the client's physical and psychological status can be obtained during this time. It can also be a time for conversation and for showing interest. Hospitalized persons often look forward to their meals as a pleasant experience among others that are not so pleasant.

### Feeding Client
1. Place the tray so that you are in a comfortable working position.
2. Show (or tell) the person what he has to eat and ask him in what sequence

he wants you to feed him. If he can't tell you, feed him the way you would feed yourself.

3. If he wishes, let him feed himself finger foods. It is all right if he is slow, clumsy, and messy in feeding himself unless he objects to this. Respect his feelings.

4. Relax. People who are fed sometimes say that they don't want any more, when in fact they feel that they are taking too much of the nurse's time. If you act relaxed and unhurried the person you are feeding may be more willing to eat what is before him.

5. Record the foods and amounts eaten. It is helpful to know the person "ate all of regular diet except potatoes." It is not so helpful to know that he "ate well."

Family members or volunteers are valuable adjuncts to the nursing staff at mealtime when there are many people who need to be fed. They are often a positive influence on the client. Family members should be encouraged to bring food from home if the client is allowed a regular diet.

There are many devices available to assist people with a physical handicap to feed themselves. The purpose is to encourage independence. Guards to keep food on the plate, forks and spoons with modified handles, rocking knives, and special cups are among the devices available.

---

### Performance Checklist
### Assisting a Client To Eat

1. Prepare the room for pleasant eating.
2. Prepare the client:
   a. offer bedpan or urinal and remove after use
   b. wash client's hands
   c. give dentures or glasses as required
   d. provide medication for pain relief
3. Wash your hands.
4. Have client sit in chair if possible or in High Fowler's position. Turn him on side if there is no other alternative.
5. Check items on tray with menu. Serve immediately.
6. Provide napkin or towel for protection of clothing.
7. Feed client (see page 288).
8. Remove tray.
9. Provide comfort by removing crumbs, repositioning, washing face, etc.
10. Record foods eaten.

---

## Basic Diets and Teaching Diet Adaptations

Some of the basic diets for people who have problems related to nutrition are presented below. The person who is required to change his diet for either a short or long period of time needs an explanation of the reason behind it. Either he or a family member who is responsible for food service needs to be helped with any required changes. In addition to explaining the reasons why a diet change is required, it is necessary to take into account all the previously stated factors influencing nutrition. The new diet should fit, wherever possible, into the client's habitual diet. It is difficult to change the eating habits of a lifetime, so new procedure should be made as easy as possible. We must consider, too, how a change will affect the rest of the family. Will the diet cost more than the family usually spends for food? Does it have to be prepared separately? If so, will that put an added burden on the person who cooks? A diet change must be evaluated for its success. When client and family are anxious (as they frequently are during an illness), learning is difficult. The nurse may have to arrange a home visit to review the teaching as well as to evaluate it.

**Table   16-3.     Types of Diets**

| | |
|---|---|
| *Clear liquid* | Contains, essentially, simple carbohydrates which are easily ingested and leave the stomach in a few hours. It is never a nutritionally adequate diet, although it can be used for short periods, as before x-ray examinations and surgery, or postoperatively. It is also valuable when there is nausea, vomiting, or diarrhea. |
| *Full liquid* | Any food that is liquid at body temperature, e.g. ice cream. This can be an adequate diet if composed of regular foods blended and liquified. It is used when the client has difficulty swallowing or in a progression to soft diet. |
| *Soft* | Diet is composed of foods that are easy to chew and digest. Fiber content is reduced. It is used as one progresses from liquid to regular diet and can be adequate if carefully selected. |
| *Bland* | Made up of nonirritating foods. It is usually given persons with gastrointestinal problems. It can be nutritionally adequate. |
| *High Protein* | Includes more protein than a regular, well-balanced diet and may include concentrated protein supplements. It is used when tissue healing or regeneration is desired and when added calories are important. |
| *Restricted Protein* | Diet is high in fat and carbohydrates and low in protein. It is used when kidney or liver disease is present. |
| *Low Cholesterol* | A nutritionally adequate diet, used in the prevention or treatment of atherosclerosis. Polyunsaturated fats are eaten instead of saturated fats. |
| *Low Sodium* | Requires careful selection of food to limit sodium intake to prescribed level. Foods are quite tasteless. Selection is important because many additives common in prepared foods contain sodium. This diet is used when the person is retaining fluids. |

The assistance of a nutritionist is invaluable when a diet must be planned. Many sample menus are available to help nurses plan and teach new routines.

## Gavage

Gavage feeding is prescribed when the client can digest the food if it is placed in his stomach but he cannot ingest or swallow it with ease. Tube feeding (gavage) is the insertion of a liquid diet into a tube which has been passed into the stomach by way of the nose or mouth. It can provide food either intermittently or continuously.

### Special Considerations

The tube may be removed and reinserted for intermittent feedings, or it can be left in place. Infants are gavage fed if they need to conserve energy, and adults with swallowing difficulties may be tube fed.

The tube is inserted by nurse or doctor (depending upon agency policy) according to the directions in the chapter on elimination. For long-term gavage feeding, the client or a family member can pass the tube and carry out the feeding.

If gagging or vomiting occurs, stop feeding immediately. If possible, have a suction machine and tubing available to prevent aspiration should this occur. Otherwise, turn the client on his side and clear the mouth of vomitus.

---

### Performance Checklist
### Gavage Feeding

1. If possible, have the client in the upright position to prevent regurgitation.
2. Before each feeding, check for correct position of tube.
3. Generally, aspirate stomach contents to determine amount of residual feeding. If there is a large amount (more than 100 ml), do not feed but return aspirate to stomach and notify doctor.
4. Use either an Asepto syringe without the bulb as a feeding funnel, or a disposable bag hung on an IV pole.
5. Instill about one ounce of warm water to clear the tube.
6. To prevent distention, clamp or pinch tube to prevent air from entering.
7. Add formula slowly (either a commercial or balanced, blended house diet) by regulating drip from bag or by filling the funnel. To slow the flow, lower funnel or pinch tubing for a short time. To prevent air from entering stomach, refill funnel before it empties. For single feeding, 150 to 200 ml q 3 to 4 hours is adequate (or as ordered).
8. Add one ounce of water after formula has been given to clear tube.
9. Clamp tube and remove or secure to client's clothing.
10. Make the client comfortable. Oral hygiene is important.
11. Record amount of feeding (plus water) and client's response.

---

**Gastrostomy**  In this procedure, feedings are performed in a manner similar to the one above, although the feeding tube is inserted through an abdominal opening into the stomach. The skin around the incision requires care to prevent excoriation, which sometimes occurs from leakage. Various methods of skin protection are used. Karaya powder or karaya products in other forms that cover the skin are frequently used.

## Hyperalimentation

Hyperalimentation is a method for providing the essential nutrients intravenously when gastrointestinal intake is insufficient or impossible. It is used for persons whose gastrointestinal tract needs rest or those who are in danger of aspirating. Those who need additional calories and cannot tolerate them by the gastrointestinal route are also candidates for hyperalimentation.

Hypertonic dextrose (containing approximately 1,000 cal/liter) is commonly used. Amino acids, electrolytes, vitamins, and trace elements are added. The solution is prepared either commercially or in the laboratory. Standard intravenous fluids do not provide the calories or nitrogen required for adequate nutrition. For example, a liter of 5 percent dextrose in water contains approximately 200 calories. The average adult male would require 8 liters per day to obtain the calories required. This amount of fluid cannot be given intravenously because of the effect it would have on the blood volume.

The person who is to receive hyperalimentation needs to be carefully prepared. He needs to know what he is to do when the catheter is inserted (usually through the left subclavian vein into the superior vena cava). His body position and breathing during insertion are important. He needs to know that he *can* move after the tube has been properly placed and the position verified by chest x-ray. Because of the meaning food has to people, not to be able to eat can affect the client. He may also be concerned about the suppression of his appetite caused by hyperalimentation. He should also be informed that the size of his stool will be decreased.

These clients need frequent mouth care. The insertion site must be checked for signs of infiltration and infection (swelling, pain, redness, heat). Ointments and dressings aré prescribed to correct these conditions.

## SUMMARY

Nutrition is affected by one's culture, religion, psychological background, socioeconomic status, and health. Nutritional needs vary throughout the life cycle. The young, the old, and the ill have special needs. So do those with little knowledge or understanding of nutrition. In selecting an adequate diet, it is good to remember that no single food has all the nutrients required for health. Therefore, many different kinds and combinations of food lead to a well-balanced diet. All the nutrients required by the body are available through foods. No supplements are necessary if the diet is adequate. Skill and patience are required in assisting a client who has a problem related to nutrition. By increasing the interest and understanding of health professionals in nutrition, the public as well as the individual client will be better served.

## LEARNING ACTIVITIES

1.  In the laboratory, have a classmate feed you a breakfast of cold cereal, soft-boiled egg, toast, orange juice, and coffee while both your arms are immobilized. Describe your reactions—pleasant and unpleasant.

2.  Evaluate your own diet for one day by listing all the foods eaten and compare your list with RDA.

3.  Discuss the problem of overnutrition and suggest some ways to prevent or control it.

4.  Describe the functions of each nutrient group.

5.  Suggest ways to increase the interest in food in an elderly woman who lives alone.

6.  After consultation with a nutritionist, teach a client how to adapt his usual diet to a low sodium diet.

## REFERENCES AND SUGGESTED READINGS

Borgen, Linda.  Total parenteral nutrition in adults. *American Journal of Nursing*, February, 1978, pp. 224–228.

Bush, James.  Cervical esophagostomy to provide nutrition. *American Journal of Nursing*, January, 1979, pp. 107-109.

Caly, Joan.  Helping people eat for health: assessing adults' nutrition. *American Journal of Nursing*, October, 1977, pp. 1605–1609.

Dansky, Kathryn.  Assessing children's nutrition. *American Journal of Nursing*, October, 1977, pp. 1610–1611.

Dwyer, Lois and Fralin, Florence.  Simplified meal planning for hard-to-teach patients. *American Journal of Nursing*, April, 1974, pp. 664–665.

Hoffman, Norman, 1977.  *A new world of health.*  New York: McGraw-Hill.

Krogg, Emily.  Helping people stretch their grocery dollars. *American Journal of Nursing*, April, 1975, pp. 646–648.

Lappé, Frances, 1970.  *Diet for a small planet.*  New York: Ballantine Books.

Latham, Michael, et al., 1975.  *Scope manual on nutrition.*  Kalamazoo, Michigan: Upjohn Company.

Mallison, Mary.  Updating the cholesterol controversy: verdict—diet does count. *American Journal of Nursing*, October, 1978, p. 1681.

Markesbery, Barbara and Wong, Wendy.  Helping people eat for health: points for maternity patients. *American Journal of Nursing*, October, 1977, pp. 1612–1614.

Noback, Charles and Demarest, Robert, 1975.  *The human nervous system.*  2nd ed. New York: McGraw-Hill.

O'Toole, Thomas. Tooth decay rampant in U.S., scientist says, citing sugar. *Washington Post*, January 7, 1979.

Robinson, Corinne, 1972. *Normal and therapeutic nutrition, 14th ed.* New York: Macmillan.

Snell, Barbara and McLellan, Connie. Whetting hospitalized preschoolers' appetites. *American Journal of Nursing*, March, 1976, pp. 413–415.

Williams, Eleanor. Making vegetarian diets nutritious. *American Journal of Nursing*, December, 1975, pp. 2168–2173.

Williams, Sue, 1977. *Nutrition and diet therapy.* 3rd ed. St. Louis: C. V. Mosby.

# 17

# Elimination: Bowel and Bladder

Introduction
Structure and Function of the Bowel
Nursing Interventions in Common Bowel Problems
Structure and Function of the Urinary System
Nursing Interventions in Common Urinary Problems
Summary
Learning Activities
References and Suggested Readings

## Behavioral Objectives

Upon completion of this chapter, the student will be able to:

1. Describe the normal structure and function of the bowel and urinary system.
2. Assess a client's bowel and urinary elimination.
3. Describe the characteristics of normal feces and urine.
4. Plan, implement, and evaluate nursing actions for the prevention and treatment of common bowel and urinary problems.

## Key Terms

albuminuria
anuria
cathartics
catheter
colostomy
commode: bedside
constipation
defecation
dialysis: hemodialysis,
   peritoneal
diarrhea
distention
diuresis
dysuria
enema
feces

flatus
fracture pan
frequency
gastric decompression
glycosuria
hematuria
hemorrhoids
impaction
incontinence: fecal,
   urinary, stress
laxatives
Levin tube
meatus
meconium
micturition
naso-gastric tube

nocturia
oliguria
polyuria
proteinuria
pyuria
residual urine
retention; retention with
   overflow
sphincter
stoma
stool
suppositories
urgency
urinal
voiding

## Introduction

While some elimination occurs through the skin and lungs, we shall be concerned here only with bowel and bladder elimination. When elimination processes are normal, we pay little attention to them. However, there are physical, social, and emotional implications when elimination problems exist.

Normal bowel and bladder structure and function will be reviewed briefly. Health assessment as it relates to the bowel and bladder will be described.

Nursing may be required when a client seeks assistance in promoting normal elimination, as well as when elimination problems exist. The nurse's role, for example, might be to teach the importance of proper diet, excercise, and the proper environment to prevent constipation. Or it might be the nurse's role to perform a procedure to facilitate bowel or bladder elimination. These techniques will be described.

The person who has limited or no control over the nerves and muscles that empty the bowel and bladder needs assistance, whatever his age. The infant and toddler who have not developed continence need care as well as the older person who is temporarily or permanently incontinent. Nursing interventions for elimination problems such as these will be described.

## STRUCTURE AND FUNCTION OF THE BOWEL

The functions of the colon are to absorb water and electrolytes from the digestive chyme and to store fecal matter until it can be expelled. The proximal half of the large intestine functions chiefly in absorption and the distal half in storage. In adults, the large intestine is approximately 5 feet long and 1 to 3 inches in diameter. The large intestine consists of the ascending, transverse, descending, and sigmoid colon, the rectum, and the anus. The rectum is approximately 4 to 6 inches long and the anal canal constitutes the distal 1 to 2 inches. About 800 to 1,000 ml of liquid is absorbed daily by the intestinal tract. If too much liquid is absorbed, the stool becomes hard and dry and the person is constipated. If too little fluid is absorbed, the stool becomes liquid and the person has diarrhea.

Mass movements in the colon propel the fecal contents toward the anus. These movements usually occur just a few times a day—usually for about 15 minutes during the first hour after breakfast. Mass movements can occur in any portion of the colon, although they usually occur in the transverse or descending colon. When they have forced a mass of feces into the rectum, the urge to defecate occurs. Defecation is defined as the process of evacuating waste products from the large intestine. Muscles in the intestine, abdomen, and pelvic floor contract, the sphincters relax, and feces are expelled.

Ordinarily, defecation is triggered by the defecation reflex. Feces enter the rectum and the distention of the rectal wall initiates afferent signals that spread through the myenteric plexus to initiate peristaltic waves in the descending colon, sigmoid, and rectum. This forces feces toward the anus. As

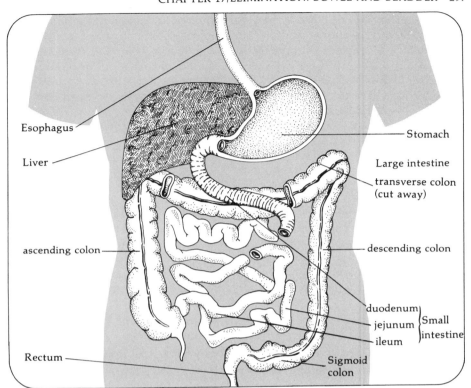

**Figure 17-1.** *The intestinal tract.*

the peristaltic wave approaches the anus, the internal anal sphincter is inhibited by receptive relaxation and, if the external sphincter is relaxed, defecation takes place. This reflex, however, is extremely weak. There is another reflex involved in defecation. When the afferent fibers in the rectum are stimulated, signals are transmitted to the spinal cord and then reflexly back to the descending colon, sigmoid, rectum, and anus by way of the parasympathetic nerve fibers.

Still other conditions are needed before defecation actually occurs. The external sphincter must be relaxed. The sphincter is under conscious control and if the time is not right for defecation, contraction is maintained and the defecation reflex dies out and does not return until more feces enter the rectum. This may be several hours later. Failure to respond to this reflex may result in constipation.

## Characteristics of Normal Feces

Normally, the feces are composed of three quarters water and one quarter solid (by weight). The solids are composed of approximately 30 percent dead bacteria and 70 percent undigested roughage, fat, protein from food, and inorganic matter. The brown color of the stool is caused by a transformed bile pigment, urobilin. The odor of the stool is the result of bacterial action on the food ingested. The color and odor of the stool may be changed by certain drugs or foods; for example, iron preparations and licorice color the stool black.

For the first two to three days of life, the newborn's stool (meconium) is dark, greenish-black and semisolid. Then the breast-fed baby has an orangish-yellow stool with a strong odor, while the bottle-fed baby's stool is brownish-yellow if his formula contains malt sugars.

The normal stool is a semisolid mass in the shape of the rectum. Change in the shape of the stool is significant. Thin, pencil-like stools that persist may indicate a change in the lumen of the colon which might be caused by a tumor.

## Assessment Guide: Bowel Elimination

The following questions are appropriate when a cleint has problems of bowel elimination. They could also be included in a general health assessment.
1. How often do you have a bowel movement? Is this normal for you?
2. Do you have any routines that encourage elimination? Are these related to opportunity, privacy, diet or liquid intake?
3. What method of bowel elimination do you use? Toilet, bedside commode, bedpan, other?
4. Describe your normal bowel movement: color, amount, shape, consistency, odor, presence of foreign matter (blood, etc.).
5. Have you noticed any recent change in your bowel movements?
6. Do you have any elimination problems? Gas/distention, constipation, diarrhea, pain, cramps, hemorrhoids, incontinence?
7. If you have any of these problems, what do you do for relief?
8. Do you take any medications (either prescribed or over the counter) to lessen the problem?
9. Has there been any recent change in the amount of stress in your life?

## Collecting and Testing Stool Specimens

Examination of stool specimens is a valuable aid to medical diagnosis. Nurses instruct clients in the method of stool collection and in some instances test the stool for abnormalities. Specific directions for collecting stool specimens and testing them are supplied by the laboratory. However, a few of the common stool abnormalities will be discussed here.

The stool is collected, when possible, directly into the waxed cardboard specimen container. When a bedpan is used the stool is transferred to the specimen container with a tongue blade or similar instrument. Stool specimens are examined, among other things, for occult blood, fat, parasites and ova, and urobilin.

Occult Blood   Blood is not a normal constituent of feces. Its appearance in the stool is indicative of bleeding somewhere in the gastrointestinal tract. Obvious bleeding can be detected by sight; occult blood by various chemical agents. Directions for testing will depend upon the chemical used, and these directions are provided on the bottle or package.

Fat    Lipids of various types are present in the normal stool. Infants with celiac disease, however, have huge, pale, bulky, foul-smelling, greasy stools that are definitive in diagnosis.

Parasites and Ova    Some examples of parasites are roundworms, tapeworms, and pinworms. The specimen to be examined for parasites must be free from oil, barium, and bismuth (ingredients often used in x-ray studies) so the client should not be given enemas or mineral oil before the specimen is collected. Parasites will not die quickly if not kept at body temperature (McGuckin, 1976). Therefore, the specimen can be either placed in a refrigerator, kept at room temperature, or preserved in transport medium until it can be taken to the laboratory.

Pinworm specimens are collected early in the morning before the client has bathed or had a bowel movement, by placing clear cellulose tape on the perianal area for less than one minute. Then the tape is removed and attached to a slide.

Urobilin    Urobilin is normally present in the stool and gives the feces its brown color. A decrease in or the absence of urobilin (stool is clay-colored) is indicative of biliary obstruction.

## Assisting a Client with Bedpan, Urinal, Bedside Commode, or Toilet

When a person is confined to a bed, a bedpan or urinal is used for elimination. The female uses the bedpan for both bowel and bladder elimination; the male uses, ordinarily, a urinal for voiding and a bedpan for defecating. Because metal bedpans are cold to the touch, they are rinsed with warm water and dried before being placed under the person. Nylon and plastic utensils do not need to be warmed.

Privacy is provided by pulling the curtains or closing the door. Unless contraindicated, the head of the bed is raised as high as the person desires after the bedpan is placed. If the person needs no assistance, he is given the toilet tissue and the call bell is put within his reach. The nurse then leaves the room until she is called to return.

The client may require help in getting on the bedpan. The nurse instructs him to flex his knees, dig in his heels, and raise his buttocks while she slips the pan in place. If he cannot lift up, the nurse instructs him to roll onto the side opposite her while she places the pan against his back. Then he is rolled back onto the pan. Some adjustment of the pan for comfort and correct positioning is usually necessary.

The nurse who is seeing a bedpan for the first time needs to examine it in view of its function; the wider part goes under the buttocks and the narrower part under the perineum. More than one student has placed her first bedpan incorrectly.

Fracture pans (a flatter pan which was used initially for persons with hip fractures) are available for use when a person has difficulty getting on a regular bedpan.

Using the bedpan is easier when the body position closely resembles the one usually used for eliminating. If possible, the client should sit on the side of the bed with his feet on a chair while he uses the bedpan. Lying flat in bed to use the bedpan or urinal is almost always ineffective because of the structure of the bladder and intestines and the lack of gravity to assist elimination.

Health professionals need to respond promptly to the call of the client who needs a bedpan or urinal. If the person cannot cleanse his perineal area, the nurse does it as matter of factly as possible. A wash cloth or basin of water is offered to the person who has cleansed himself so that he can wash his hands. Air freshener is provided for the room.

After the client is made comfortable, the contents of the bedpan are examined for amount, shape, color, odor, and any unusual characteristics of the stool. This information is then recorded.

A bedside commode is provided for the person who can get out of bed but cannot walk to the bathroom for elimination. A bedside commode is a chair with a cut-out seat. A bedpan is inserted on a ledge under the opening. Usually a pad covers the opening when the commode is not in use. The legs on the commode are equipped with locks and, to prevent accidents, it is essential that the locks be engaged before the client is assisted onto the chair.

When the client can use the toilet facilities but may need assistance, the nurse should stay nearby so that she can help when necessary. For safety, bathrooms should not be locked. They are also equipped with call bells so that help can be readily obtained. The nurse should instruct the person in the use of the call bell and direct him not to flush the toilet if she needs to examine the products of eliminations.

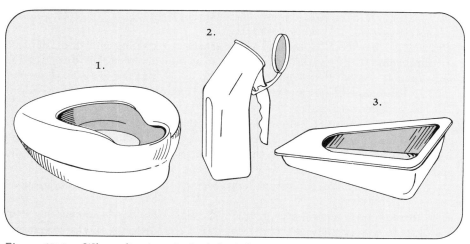

**Figure 17-2.** *When a client is confined to bed, a bedpan or urinal is used for elimination. (1) Bedpan. (2) Urinal. (3) Fracture pan.*

**Offering the Use of Toilet Facilities**    Unless the person cannot indicate when he needs to eliminate, the nurse can expect him to ask for help when he needs it. If the person is very ill, sedated, or incontinent, a plan for regular offering of the bedpan is introduced. This will be discussed in the section on bowel training programs.

## NURSING INTERVENTIONS IN COMMON BOWEL PROBLEMS

### Client Beliefs about Elimination

If the client believes it is essential to have a daily bowel movement, he might be helped by knowing this is not everyone's normal pattern. There is considerable variation in the frequency with which a normal person moves his bowels. For example, some people have one bowel movement a day; others have two or three movements. On the other hand, some healthy persons defecate only two or three times a week. The stool's consistency and quantity are more important indicators of normal evacuation than the number of times defecation occurs. The food and fluids eaten and the emotional state of the person are important factors in increasing or decreasing stool output. Other factors include activity, disease, medications, privacy, or opportunity.

Because the need for privacy during elimination is so much a part of many peoples' culture, an environmental change that decreases privacy may be responsible for changes in the defecation pattern. Privacy is decreased when a room is shared, a bedpan is used, or when one is dependent upon another for assistance. Waiting to use a bathroom may also affect the frequency of stools. It is important to try to maintain the person's normal environment if normal elimination habits are to be retained.

### Constipation

Constipation is the presence of hard, dry stool. Frequently no stool is passed for a prolonged period of time. Constipation results from reduced peristalsis and prolonged retention of feces in the large intestine. The longer the stool is retained, the more water is absorbed from the fecal matter and the harder and drier it becomes. Distress, discomfort, and pain result from the straining required to expel the constipated stool.

The factors previously mentioned account for constipation in many healthy persons. In addition, constipation can occur in those persons with decreased mobility because of aging, surgery, or enforced bed rest. Excessive use of laxatives, other drugs, mechanical obstruction, and muscular weakness can also cause constipation.

**Prevention and Treatment**    A teaching plan to prevent or treat constipation is based on the data previously obtained in the assessment of elimination. Does the diet and fluid intake encourage normal bowel elimination? A well-balanced diet with sufficient roughage (fresh fruits, fruit juices, vegetables, unprocessed bran, and other cereals) and low in highly refined carbohydrates promotes normal bowel elimination. A minimum liquid intake of 2,000 ml per day is recommended.

Does the person respond immediately to the urge to defecate? Is the required privacy available? Are toilet facilities available when needed? Can physical activity be increased as a means to promote normal elimination? Early ambulation after surgery, and exercising while bedridden, may help prevent constipation. Can anxiety be lessened? It has been suggested that excessive stimulation of the sympathetic nervous system results in constipation because peristalsis is inhibited and muscle tone decreased. Is the person taking any medications that decrease motility in the small and large intestines? Does the person use laxatives excessively? When the bowel is suddenly emptied after the use of a laxative or cathartic, a period of several days when there is no stored feces in the intestine may follow. The person may then take another laxative. Eventually, the overstimulation of the bowel results in an inability of the bowel to respond to the defecation reflex. Therefore, people can become dependent upon laxatives for bowel evacuation.

A disease or congenital defect causing an obstruction in any part of the gastrointestinal tract will delay or prevent the passage of feces. Constipation also occurs when there is a neurogenic condition (paralysis, for example) and the bulk of feces does not initiate the defecation reflex. In these instances, mechanical intervention (such as suppositories or enemas) may be necessary to relieve the constipation.

Pain caused by rectal surgery or hemorrhoids (enlarged veins in the rectal area) can also cause constipation by inhibiting the response to the normal defecation reflex.

If constipation cannot be prevented or corrected by diet, fluids, exercise, privacy, lessening of anxiety, and decrease in constipation-causing medications, more drastic means may be required until regularity can be established. Emotional support is needed as the person attempts to change long-standing habits.

*Use of Laxatives and Cathartics*    Generally a laxative is described as a medicine with a mild and gentle effect that loosens the bowel contents and encourages evacuation. A medicine with a strong effect is referred to as a cathartic. Normal bowel habits may be reestablished with the use of laxatives or cathartics if they are carefully monitored. These medications are gradually withdrawn when the bowels have begun to function normally.

The nurse should be knowledgeable about the various laxatives and cathartics available. These include medications that increase the bulk of the stool (e.g., osmotically active Milk of Magnesia, Metamucil, and Serutan, which contain colloids); stool softeners (e.g., Colace, which lubricates the fecal mass and prevents water loss); and chemical irritants which stimulate motility (e.g., Dulcolax and Cascara Sagrada). Further information is available in pharmacology texts.

*Suppositories*    A rectal suppository is a bullet-shaped soft substance containing a chemical that is inserted into the rectum to initiate a bowel movement. The suppository is about 1½ inches long and designed to melt at body temperature. Suppositories are designed for insertion into other body orifices, but only rectal suppositories will be discussed here. Suppositories are refrigerated until ready for use and they are handled very little before insertion because they quickly lose their shape and become difficult to insert. Rectal suppositories either soften fecal material, chemically stimulate peristalis, or increase bulk. When the stool is very hard, fecal softeners are used; when there is poor muscle tone and innervation, chemical stimulators are helpful. Bulk increasers act by liberating a gas, which causes distention and increases the urge to defecate. Defecation usually occurs between 15 and 60 minutes after suppository insertion.

The client or family member sometimes must be taught to insert supposi- tories. The person must lie on his left side, the suppository is lubricated with vaseline (or some other lubricant) to decrease friction and discomfort. The client then breathes through his mouth to relax the anal sphincter. And then, using the entire length of the index finger, the person guides the suppository (pointed end first) past the external and internal sphincters until the suppository is lost in the rectal canal. The client is encouraged to retain the suppository as long as possible for effective evacuation.

*Enemas*   An enema is the introduction of fluid into the rectum and/or colon for the purpose of emptying and cleansing the colon, relieving distention, or softening the fecal mass. The client needs to be physically and psychologically prepared for this procedure. Some people have never had an enema and they must be encouraged to ask questions about the procedure and their role in it, and to express their feelings about this invasive procedure. If possible, the client should be allowed to decide when he will receive the enema. If he must receive "enemas until clear," he needs to know that this is a lengthy, energy- consuming procedure and that he will be permitted to rest afterwards.

There are two types of enemas: cleansing and retention. A cleansing enema may consist of tap water, soap solution, normal saline, or a commercially prepared solution, which is usually 90 to 100 ml of a sodium phosphate solution. A retention enema usually consists of oil, given to soften the fecal mass. Commercially packaged oil enemas are available, but approximately 90 to 100 ml of warmed mineral oil can be used. The oil must be retained for about one hour if it is to be effective. The oil enema may be followed by a cleansing enema.

A cleansing enema, then, may be a commercially prepared solution of so- dium phosphate, which is hypertonic and draws fluid into the bowel to soften and lubricate the feces. It causes irritation and, therefore, peristalsis and emptying of the bowel. Its advantages include the small volume which can be rapidly administered (in approximately one minute) and more easily retained than a larger volume. The commercial preparations cause less discomfort, distention, and electrolyte depletion than tap-water enemas. The nurse selects the appropriate box from the supply closet, warms the plastic bottle and solution to body temperature, removes the cap on the prelubricated tip, inserts the tip its entire 2-inch length, and slowly squeezes the plastic collapsable bottle with one hand until all the solution has been inserted in the rectum. The tube is removed and the unit disposed of in its original container. The urge to defecate is usually felt within 2 to 5 minutes, at which time the client is assisted to the toilet facility as needed.

## Special Considerations: Enema

A cleansing enema consisting of 500 to 1,000 ml (or more if enemas "until clear" have been ordered) of tap water, soap solution, or normal saline may be ordered. The amount of fluid inserted stimulates peristalsis and causes massive evacuation. Tap water is used most often because it is less likely than a soap solution to irritate the colon and cause strong peristalsis. Normal saline solution which does not upset the fluid and electrolyte balance is prescribed when a large number of enemas is required or when the person is very young, old, or debilitated.

---

### Performance Checklist
### Giving an Enema

1.  Inform the client of the procedure.
2.  Collect the equipment for type of enema to be given.
3.  Prepare the solution (right kind, right temperature, right amount).
4.  With the solution in the container in which it is to be administered, open the clamp and clear the air from the tubing.
5.  Clamp the tube and lubricate the tip of the rectal tube.
6.  Hang the bag on an IV pole (or other support) so that it is 18 to 24 inches above client's hips.
7.  Have client assume appropriate position.
8.  Insert the lubricated rectal tube 3 to 4 inches.
9.  Unclamp tubing and give prescribed amount of fluid.
10. If the client becomes uncomfortable and is having difficulty retaining the fluid, use any of the following techniques:
    a.  temporarily clamp tubing
    b.  press the buttocks together
    c.  have the client breathe slowly through his mouth
    d.  lower bag of fluid to level of anus
11. When all solution has been inserted, clamp tubing and remove tube.
12. Encourage client to maintain assumed position and retain fluid as long as possible (approximately 10 minutes).
13. Assist client with toilet, bedpan, tissue, etc. as needed.
14. Evaluate quantity of feces and flatus expelled; describe color and consistency of stool.
15. Assist client in making himself comfortable (cleansing and preparing to rest).
16. Clean equipment or discard it as indicated.
17. Record: solution used, amount, results.

While enema equipment varies somewhat from agency to agency, and, from agency to home, a bag (or other container) is required for holding the solution, tubing, rectal tube, lubricant, metal clamps, waterproof protection for the bed, and bedpan or available toilet facilities comprise the list of needed materials. The solution is warmed to just slightly more than body temperature (100 to 105 degrees).

While the left Sims' position (lying on the left side with the uppermost leg sharply flexed so that it does not rest on the lower leg) is usually suggested as most appropriate for enema administration, the person may lie on his back, his right side, or he may take the knee-chest position. Occasionally the client will say that he prefers to sit on the toilet while the enema is administered. This is not acceptable because the fluid is then inserted against gravity. It is difficult to retain, and, therefore, not effective.

The procedure for administering the enema is based upon the following principles:

1. Pressure and heat stimulate nerve endings.
2. Additional fluid in a body cavity stimulates nerve endings and causes increased peristalsis.
3. Chemicals that irritate the mucous membrance of the bowel increase peristalsis.
4. Friction is reduced by lubrication.
5. Fluids flow from an area of greater pressure to an area of lower pressure.
6. The rate of flow and amount of pressure are influenced by the tubing lumen and size of the opening in the rectal tube as well as the height of the fluid.
7. Having the client assume a sitting position after the enema has been administered encourages contraction of the abdominal and perineal muscles that aid in emptying the lower colon.

*Fecal Impaction*    An impaction occurs when a hard, dry stool, which the person cannot expel, collects in the rectal canal. For example, the person who has had barium for x-ray examination, has received constipating drugs, or is immobilized can develop impaction. Such a client says he is constipated, has the urge to defecate but can't, and has pain in the rectal area. Some clients may have a neurogenic bowel—the nervous system does not recognize the presence of stool in the rectal canal and there is no stimulation to initiate the defecation reflex. The stool then becomes impacted. Liquid fecal contents may be expelled around the impacted fecal mass, which sometimes causes the inexperienced health-care worker to suspect, incorrectly, that the client has diarrhea. Digital removal of the stool is required. A gloved, lubricated finger is inserted into the rectum and fecal material is removed a little at a time until the entire mass has been evacuated. The size, shape, and consistency of the feces is noted and recorded. An oil retention enema followed by a cleansing enema may either precede or follow the impaction removal. However, enemas do not help if the person has no control over the rectal muscles and cannot retain the fluid. In this instance, digital removal alone is the appropriate intervention.

## Diarrhea

Diarrhea is the passage of loose, watery stools and an increase in the number of bowel movements, often accompanied by cramps. Diarrhea occurs when excessive, strong, and frequent peristalsis moves the chyme rapidly through the intestines, thus reducing the amount of time available for fluid absorption. Diarrhea may be caused by diet, stress, malabsorption, allergies, pathogenic inflammatory diseases, and drugs. Diarrhea should not be ignored even in its very early stages. Fluid and electrolyte imbalance can be severe, especially in the very young and the very old (Ch. 18). Severe diarrhea in these clients is best treated by giving nothing by mouth and feeding intravenous fluids. In all clients with diarrhea increased rest, fluids, and meticulous skin care are essential. A lubricant skin cream should be applied to the perianal area to prevent excoriation. The call bell and the bedpan should be within close reach of the client. Some medications used to control diarrhea include: Lomotil, a synthetic drug related to Demerol but with a low potential for dependence; Pectin or Kaolin, which act locally in the gastrointestinal tract as absorbents and demulcents (soothing, bland medicine); Paregoric, an opiate which is given orally several times a day to help decrease excessive intestinal motility.

## Flatus/Distention

Flatus is the presence of excessive gas in the alimentary tract. When flatus is expelled rectally there is no problem with distention. However, when the gas accumulates in the bowel, distention with resultant discomfort and cramping can occur.

Decreased peristalsis caused by certain drugs, anesthetic agents, and decreased physical activity predispose a person to distention. Fifty to seventy-five percent of gastrointestinal gas results from swallowed air. Bacterial action on incompletely digested foods accounts for the additional flatus.

To decrease the client's problem with flatus or distention, the nurse should encourage mobility, because walking stimulates peristalsis. If the client is lying in bed, his position should be changed frequently, side-lying or prone positions help. Tight-fitting garments should be avoided. Habits such as mouth breathing, taking fluids with a straw, chewing gum, and drinking carbonated beverages, which cause excessive air intake, should be discouraged. The intake of any foods that are gas-producing should be limited.

One procedure for relief of distention that the nurse may be asked to perform is the insertion of a rectal tube. A lubricated tube is inserted about 4 inches into the rectum and taped in place. The free end of the tube is placed in a container—a specimen container or an emesis basin, for example. After 20 to 30 minutes the tube is removed and the remaining distention is evaluated.

## Assessment of the Abdomen

Auscultation, percussion, and palpation are valuable parts of the assessment of bowel functioning. With a stethoscope placed lightly against the abdominal wall, bowel sounds can be detected. These are difficult to describe. They are best learned by listening to many normal abdomens. The bowel sounds can be heard anywhere on the abdomen, but are clearest near the umbilicus—above and on either side is best. It is usually necessary to listen for several minutes in each spot. Absent or infrequent sounds indicate an immobile bowel (as in paralytic ileus or peritonitis). Increased sounds with loud, rushing, high-pitched tinkling may indicate mechanical obstruction.

The gas pattern in distention can be detected by percussion. A distended bowel will by tympanitic (a relatively high-pitched, musical tone).

On deep palpation, the sigmoid colon may be felt in the left lower quadrant of the abdomen. A bolus of feces is sometimes detected in the freely movable and often tender sigmoid.

Peristalsis can be best seen by looking across the client's abdomen (inspection). Observe for several minutes. In very thin persons, peristalsis is normally quite evident. Increased peristaltic waves may indicate intestinal obstruction.

## Fecal Incontinence

Fecal incontinence occurs when a person cannot control his rectal sphincters. The cause may be developmental, as with infants and children who are not yet toilet trained, or the result of temporary or prolonged disorientation, spinal cord trauma or neurological injury, disease, or poor muscle tone.

The attitude of the nurse toward a client who needs help because of incontinence is extremely important. The nursing interventions are basically the same regardless of the cause of the incontinence: scrupulous skin cleansing and protection of the skin with a lubricant cream. The baby who has neither the physical nor emotional maturity for toilet training is accepted by those who care for him. However, incontinence in any one past the toddler age is often more difficult to accept. The older person who soils himself may be very upset by the incident. While diapering is not usually acceptable to the adult client or his family, some sort of padding may be necessary to help keep the bed dry. A bowel training program such as that described below may help in the care of a person who is incontinent.

## Bowel Training Plan

Rehabilitation and pediatrics textbooks describe in detail toilet training plans for toddlers and adults. Some basic suggestions for training follow:

1. Decide upon the appropriate mode for elimination: toilet, commode, or potty chair.
2. Determine the time when defecation usually occurs. Have the person sit on the commode at that time for about 20 minutes.
3. Sometimes a suppository is inserted shortly before the time when defecation usually occurs; for example, shortly before the morning meal.

4. Provide a diet high in roughage and a fluid intake of 2,500 to 3,000 ml for an adult and 1,000 ml for a child.

5. Establish a balance between exercise and rest.

Medications or enemas are sometimes used temporarily to establish bowel patterns. Enemas are more effective than medications. Stretching the anal sphincter by digital stimulation may also be instituted.

Successful bowel training has obvious advantages. However, the hazards include the emotional trauma to the client when the plan does not succeed. Certainly, consistency, persistence, and patience are needed if any bowel training program is expected to succeed.

## Colostomy

A colostomy is a surgical opening from the large intestine through the abdominal wall and skin, for the purpose of fecal elimination when defecation through the normal route is not possible. A colostomy is either temporary or permanent.

Nursing Interventions    Teaching, supporting, and, initially, caring for, are the nurse's methods of assisting the person with a colostomy. The client may need help in adjusting to his changes in elimination.

In many instances, control of the frequency and consistency of fecal drainage is not possible. If the colostomy is located in the descending colon or the sigmoid, however, control is maybe achieved. Colostomy irrigations may be used to empty the bowel and control elimination and soiling between irrigations. However, if control is not possible, irrigations are not used. Some surgeons also discourage the use of irrigations because of the possible trauma to the colon when the irrigating tube is inserted repeatedly.

Usually, immediately after the surgical formation of the colostomy, a plastic pouch that adheres to the skin is applied to collect the intestinal drainage. The pouch has an open end that is secured with a clamp until it is to be emptied. The bag (pouch) needs to be replaced about every 2 to 3 days, or when it no longer adheres to the skin. A tight seal depends, in part, upon the location of the stoma (the external opening of the colostomy), body contours, and dry skin. When the seal is inadequate and there is leakage of feces, skin irritation can occur; the client's self-esteem certainly suffers.

When the bag is replaced, the skin is first washed with soap and water and dried. This is *not* a sterile procedure. Many persons consider it offensive for the nurse to wear gloves when she cleans and replaces the colostomy bag. One enterostomal therapist insists that only if the nurse wears gloves when she performs her own toileting should she wear gloves when caring for a client's colostomy.

Products to protect the skin include Stomahesive and karaya, which act as barriers to protect the skin from the fecal drainage. Tincture of Benzoin is no longer used to toughen and protect the skin, because of its tendency to cause irritation. Odors can be avoided by frequent emptying of the bag and by use of various deodorizers such as Nilodor and Odoway. Oral Bismuth Subgallate, a tasteless powder, and charcoal products that absorb odor can be taken orally.

Assisting a client to adapt psychologically to the change in elimination is an important goal. Ostomy clubs, which are self-help groups for colostomy clients and their families, have proven helpful as the person with a new colostomy moves back into the community.

## Assisting with Gastric Decompression

There are times when the nurse is required to assist in caring for a person whose stomach or small intestine needs to be kept empty and free from distention. A tube is passed into the stomach or small intestine, and mechanical suction provides decompression. Decompression is used following surgery on the stomach and small intestine, for example, and when there is an intestinal obstruction. Basically, the insertion of the tube through the nose into the stomach or the intestine follows the same procedure. The tubes, however, are different. Those going into the intestine are weighted and are longer than the naso-gastric tube (Levin or Salem Sump) which is used for stomach decompression. The Levin tube is also used for gavage feeding. This

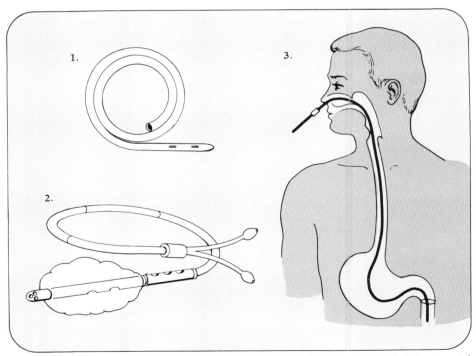

**Figure 17-3.**   *Decompression tubes such as the Levin tube (1) and Miller-Abbott tube (2) are inserted into the stomach or small intestine when it is necessary to keep the stomach or small intestine empty and free from distention.*

has been decribed in the chapter on nutrition. The method of assisting with insertion and irrigation of a naso-gastric tube will be described.

The Levin tube (used to empty the stomach of its contents) is made of rubber or plastic and is about 3 feet long. In the first 6 to 9 inches of the tube, there are a number of holes along the sides. The distal end of the tube is attached to a mechanical suction machine.

## Special Considerations

The principles related to insertion of the tube are directed toward safe insertion into the stomach with the least discomfort to the client.

---

### Performance Checklist
### Assisting with Insertion of Naso-Gastric Tube

1. Obtain a chilled rubber or unchilled plastic Levin tube (or similar tube, as ordered), emesis basin, tissues, water-soluble lubricant, a 20 to 50 ml aspirating syringe, suction machine, glass of water, and drinking straw.
2. Doctor or nurse explains purpose and method of tube insertion.
3. Position the client in Fowler's position for ease and safety of tube passage.
4. Depending upon agency policy, either doctor or nurse inserts tube.
5. Measure the tube (nose to proximal earlobe and then down to the umbilicus) and mark this distance with tape.
6. Use water-soluble lubricant (to prevent aspiration pneumonia) to lubricate tip of tube.
7. Pass tube gently up one nostril.
8. Have client swallow water (if permitted) as tube is passed to assist in its passage.
9. Push tube slowly but gently until it is in stomach (distance measured).
10. If client becomes cyanotic, dyspneic, or cannot hum upon request, the tube is in the trachea and must be removed immediately.
11. Check for proper positioning of the tube by using any one of the following methods:
    a. Attach syringe to end of tube and aspirate to see if stomach fluids are present.
    b. place end of tube in glass of water; if there is little or no bubbling, the tube is in the stomach or esophagus.
    c. place a stethoscope over the stomach and listen for a rushing sound as 20 ml of air is injected into the tube.
12. When tube is in correct position, tape it to the nose.
13. Attach free end of tube to low intermittent suction furnished by either machine or wall device.
14. Record the time of tube insertion, person inserting tube, and client's reaction.

---

Comfort measures are very important for the person who has a naso-gastric tube in place. The nostrils must be lubricated with a water-soluble lubricant every few hours and the person helped with oral hygiene. Care must be exercised to see that the client does not swallow water or mouth wash during oral hygiene.

Drainage in the collection container must be checked at frequent intervals. Suction is intermittent, but if no stomach contents appear, the following procedure should be introduced:

1. Change the client's position.
2. Have him breathe deeply several times and cough.
3. "Strip" the tube by pulling gently lengthwise.
4. Check to be sure that all connections are tight, tubing is not kinked, and electric switch is turned on.
5. If there is still no drainage the tube may be occluded and, if irrigations are ordered, an irrigation is performed.

---

### Performance Checklist
### Irrigating Levin Tube

1. Check doctor's order to determine whether or not irrigation is ordered; if so, determine frequency of irrigation, amount, and type of solution ordered (usually normal saline solution to prevent electrolyte imbalance).
2. Disconnect tubing from suction machine.
3. Attach syringe containing 10 to 15 ml of solution to tubing.
4. Pull back on plunger and withdraw solution (both irrigating solution and stomach contents). Discard. (Sometimes solution is allowed to flow out by gravity.)
5. Repeat steps 3 and 4 until amount of irrigating solution ordered has been inserted.
6. Record on intake and output record amount of irrigating solution used as well as any stomach contents. Also record color, odor, and any unusual characteristics of stomach returns.

---

The drainage bottle is emptied at times designated by agency policy (usually every eight hours). The amount of drainage is recorded on the intake and output record. The problems of fluid and electrolyte imbalance when a stomach tube is in place are discussed in Chapter 18.


## STRUCTURE AND FUNCTION OF THE URINARY SYSTEM

The kidneys act as a complex filtration unit that selectively filters out and eliminates water and other substances not needed by the body. These end products of metabolism include urea, creatinine, uric acid, phosphates, sulfates, nitrates, and phenol.

The nephrons, after they have filtered the blood plasma and reabsorbed the necessary substances, deposit urine in the pelvis of the kidney. The urine

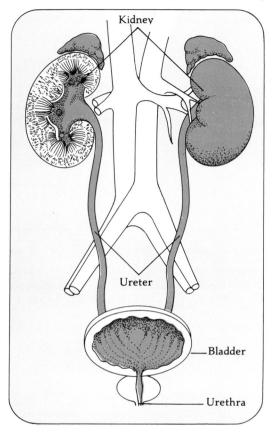

**Figure 17-4.** *The urinary system.*

passes through the ureter from each kidney to the bladder where it is stored until the bladder is emptied. Micturition and voiding are terms that are used interchangeably to described bladder emptying. When 300 to 500 ml of urine are stored in the adult bladder, the urge to void occurs. However, the normal adult bladder can stretch to accommodate much more urine. The urine passes from the bladder through the urethra and is excreted through the urinary meatus.

*Micturition* is the process by which the bladder empties itself when it is filled. The bladder progressively fills until the tension in its walls rises above a threshhold value; a micturition reflex is then elicited, greatly exacerbating the pressure in the bladder and causing a conscious desire to void. The internal sphincter relaxes, then appropriate signals from the central nervous system cause relaxation of the external sphincter, allowing voiding. Since this is under voluntary control, voiding can be postponed. For conscious bladder control, the micturition reflex is partially inhibited all the time except when the person desires to void. Then the cortical centers initiate the micturition reflex, *inhibit* the external urinary sphincter, and urination occurs (Guyton, 1976).

## Characteristics of Normal Urine

The total volume of urine excreted per day varies with the fluid intake and with fluids lost by other routes (perspiration, vomiting, diarrhea). Normally, a healthy adult will excrete between 1,000 and 1,700 ml of golden yellow to amber colored urine in 24 hours. Darker urine is more concentrated, and lighter urine is more dilute. Urine has a characteristic odor that can, however, be affected by certain foods. Food and drugs can also change the color of the urine. Clients who have this information can be spared considerable concern.

While urine is usually slightly acid, certain foods can change this. Ordinarily urine is free of bacteria because the urinary tract is sterile. Bacteria are normally found at the tip of the urethra and can be washed into the urine specimen unless the meatus is cleansed before specimen collection.

### Normal Urine

| | |
|---|---|
| color: golden yellow to amber | Protein: (in 24 hr. specimen—none) |
| clear (if freshly voided) | in random sample: male, none |
| pH: 4.5–7.5 | to a slight trace; female: none to a |
| | trace |
| Specific Gravity: 1.010–1.025 | |
| Glucose: None | Bilirubin: none |
| Ketones: none | Urobilinogen: -0.3–2.0 |
| | Ehrlich units: 2/hr |

## NURSING INTERVENTION IN COMMON URINARY PROBLEMS

### Collection and Testing of Urine Specimens

In general, persons who are able are given instructions in collecting their own urine sample. In many instances, voiding into a clean container is the method used. If there is a possibility a urine culture will be performed, a clean-catch midstream specimen is obtained. In this procedure, after the external genitalia are washed, a portion of the urine is expelled, the urinary stream momentarily interrupted, and the remainder of the urine collected in a sterile container.

**Special Considerations**

When the client is male, the only difference in the clean-catch procedure is the cleansing. Before the urethral area is cleansed, the foreskin on the uncircumsized penis is retracted. It is sometimes necessary to obtain a urine specimen from a woman who is menstruating. Temporarily inserting a cotton tampon into the vagina will usually be sufficient to obtain a specimen free from vaginal secretions. As a last resort, a catheterized specimen might be obtained.

---

## Performance Checklist
## Clean-Catch Midstream Urine Collection

Female Client
1. Obtain the following equipment: cotton balls or sponges, antiseptic liquid or sterile water, sterile urine container.
2. Instruct client to wash hands.
3. Using language the client understands, explain that the labia are kept separated with one hand until after the specimen is obtained. With the other hand, first one side of the vulvar area is washed from front to back. Using a fresh cotton sponge for each area, the other side of the vulvar area is cleansed. Finally, with the third sponge, the area directly over the urinary meatus is cleansed.
4. Sponges are discarded in wastebasket.
5. A small amount of urine is voided into toilet.
6. Holding the specimen container by the outside, the client voids remainder of urine into container.
7. Container is covered.
8. Urethral area is dried.
9. Hands are washed

---

While there are many diagnostic urine tests, only a few that are frequently performed by the client or nurse and not sent to the laboratory will be described.

Specific gravity indicates the concentration of the urine. Older instruments for measuring specific gravity include the urinometer. The urinometer is a glass instrument consisting of a mercury bulb attached to a stem that is measured on a graduated scale that indicates a concentration from 1.000 to 1.060. The principle by which this instrument functions is displacement: the more concentrated the solution, the more the instrument floating in the solution is displaced upward. The disadvantage of the urinometer is that at least 20 ml of urine is required.

The refractometer is a more sophisticated instrument available for measuring specific gravity. One drop of urine is placed on a slide on the front of the instrument. The scale measuring from 1.000 to 1.035 is read by holding the instrument up to the eye.

Chemical reagent strips or tablets are available for performing other common urine tests including tests for the presence of glucose, ketones, protein, blood, bilirubin, and urobilinogen. Abnormalities are detected by color changes. The directions printed on the container are carefully followed and the findings compared with the color chart. The chemical agents remaining in the container must be protected from moisture. Replacing the top of the container will help provide this protection.

When a 24-hour specimen is required, the collection begins after the bladder is emptied and that urine is discarded. Then all the subsequent urine is saved until the 24-hour period ends. Preservatives, refrigeration, or ice may be required for preservation of the specimen. The laboratory provides specific instructions.

## Assessment of Urinary Elimination

Valuable information for the client's total health assessment can be obtained by asking him questions about his urinary elimination. The following list can serve as a guide:

1. How frequently do you pass your water (urinate, empty your bladder, void)? While there is considerable variation in voiding patterns, persons usually void first thing in the morning, possibly 4 to 5 times during the rest of the day, and before retiring.
2. What color is your urine?
3. Describe its odor.
4. Have you noticed anything unusual about your urine?
5. What method of eliminating do you use?
   a. toilet, commode, bedpan
   b. other
6. If the client is a toddler, is he toilet trained?
7. Do you have any problems passing your urine?
   (retention, incontinence, pain, burning, or other discomfort)
8. Do you have any related problems that might affect your urination (recent surgery, enlarged prostate, vaginal infection)?
9. If you have any urinary problems, how do you cope with them?

## Urinary Retention

Urinary retention describes the condition of the urinary bladder that is unable to empty or empties only partially. Retention may be a problem when the person has a neurogenic bladder, has suffered the trauma of surgery, has a swollen urinary meatus following childbirth, is on prolonged bedrest, or has an obstruction such as that caused by an enlarged prostate. With retention, the bladder continues to fill even though it does not empty. The distended bladder causes pain or discomfort. In addition, urinary tract infections are frequent when the bladder does not empty completely.

A distended bladder can be palpated in the suprapubic region. Percussion will indicate dullness when the bladder is full.

When there is urine in the bladder but the person is unable to void, every effort is taken to encourage voiding. Ask the client what usually helps him. With his response as a guide, one or more of the following methods may be tried:

1. The bed-ridden female may be helped to sit on the bedpan on the side of

the bed with her feet dangling. The male may be helped to stand, when there is no contraindication.

2.   Privacy should be ensured if the client desires it.

3.   A warm bedpan may be offered.

4.   Warm fluids of the person's choice (within medical constraints) may be offered.

5.   The sound of running water may help some clients.

6.   The client's hands may be placed in warm water.

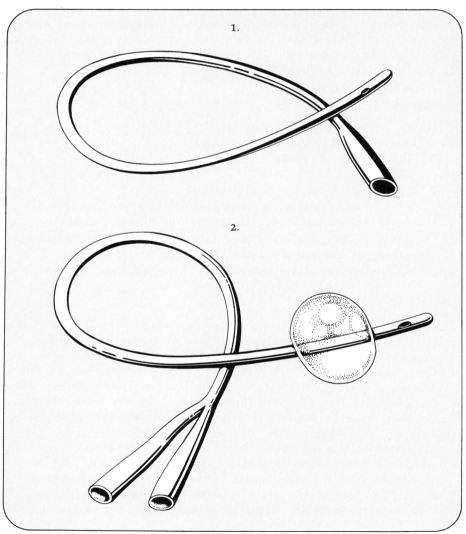

Figure 17-5.   *Catheters: (1) Straight urinary catheter. (2) Indwelling Foley catheter with balloon inflated.*

7. Warm water may be poured over the perineum.

8. Pain medication may be offered.

**Retention with Overflow**   When the person has retention with overflow, he is able to void but the bladder does not empty completely. Normally, after

---

### Performance Checklist
### Straight Urinary Catheterization

1. Explain the procedure.
2. Obtain the catheterization kit, a light, and a bath blanket.
3. Wash hands.
4. Provide privacy.
5. Drape person with bath blanket.
6. Position light for good visualization.
7. Open the sterile package.
8. Put on sterile gloves.
9. With drapes folded around your gloved hands to keep them sterile, place sterile drapes under person's hips and over the vulva or penis.
10. Pour cleansing solution on cotton wipes in container.
11. Lubricate catheter (2 to 3" for female; 5 to 7" for male).
12. Open specimen container if appropriate.
13. Expose urinary meatus.
14. Cleanse as follows, using cotton wipes held in forceps.
    a. female: keeping labia separated with nondominant hand, cleanse each side of vulva with a down stroke, one sponge for each stroke; cleanse over meatus last
    b. male: use circular motions starting at the meatus and moving outward; continue 2 to 3" down the shaft of the penis.
15. Discard each cotton wipe in a container placed away from the sterile field.
16. Insert catheter, touching nothing except the meatus.
    a. female: insert up and back 2 to 3" until urine flows
    b. male: holding the shaft of the penis almost straight up (for ease in insertion), insert 5 to 7" until urine flows
17. Hold catheter in place with one hand while urine drains into container provided with kit (place distal end of catheter in container before inserting proximal end into meatus).
18. When urine flow begins to diminish, withdraw tube about ½ inch at a time until urine barely drips.
19. Make client comfortable.
20. Dispose of equipment.
21. Record:
    a. type and size of catheter used
    b. time of procedure
    c. volume and description of urine
    d. client's response to procedure
    e. if specimen obtained, record laboratory test prescribed

voiding the bladder contains only 1 to 3 ml of residual urine. In retention with overflow, pressure within the bladder causes a few ml of urine to be voided, usually at frequent intervals, while the bladder remains distended and the person continues to feel discomfort.

**Relief of Retention** If all the other methods to encourage voiding have failed, a catheter (a hollow tube) may be inserted into the bladder to empty it. The catheter may be left in the bladder (indwelling) or, after the urine has been drained, removed (straight catheter).

Catheterization is performed, in addition to relieving retention, in preoperative preparation, postoperatively to relieve the discomfort of a distended bladder, to obtain a sterile urine specimen, to obtain an accurate output measure (in diabetic coma, for example), or to keep the incontinent person dry.

**Special Considerations**

The procedure is performed so that sterility is maintained. The client is kept relatively comfortable, and privacy is protected. Perhaps the most significant point is the correct identification of the female urinary meatus so that the catheter can be inserted without contamination.

## Modifications for Indwelling Catheter Insertion

A Foley catheter (a tube with an inflatable balloon surrounding its tip) is inserted in the same manner as that described for straight catheterization with the following changes:

After step 17—

1. When urine flow has diminished to dripping, attach the syringe prefilled with sterile water (usually 8 ml to fill a 5 ml balloon and the tubing leading to it), to the other part of the tube. Insert the solution.
2. Test the catheter's position in the bladder by pulling slightly on it and noting the client's response when fluid is inflating balloon (if balloon is in the urethra, client will feel pain and catheter should be advanced further).
3. Attach the part of the tube from which urine drains to the collecting device if this was not done before the catheter was inserted.
4. Tape catheter in place.
5. Continue with steps 19 through 21 in straight catheter procedure.

## Emptying Urine Bag

It is important to follow the directions printed on the bag; they are usually self-explanatory. In general, a clamp attached to tubing at the corner of the plastic bag is released, the bag tipped to empty the contents, and the contents measured. Then the tube is reclamped and the tip of the tube reinserted into its pocket. Some collection bags are calibrated and the urine measurement can be taken before the bag is emptied. Otherwise, a graduated container is used to collect the urine when the bag is emptied. The time for urine measurement is assigned by the agency (usually once every 8 hours unless more frequent measurement is required).

The drainage bag is attached to the side of the bed and kept below the level of the bladder to promote drainage and prevent backflow of urine, which could cause bladder infection.

## Specimen Collection When Catheter Is in Place

A 3-cc syringe and a 21 to 25-gauge needle are used to aspirate a specimen of urine. First, the port on the rubber catheter or a spot near the distal end is cleansed with an antiseptic solution. Then, the needle slanted toward the drainage tube is inserted and the urine aspirated. This method will prevent accidental puncturing of the lumen leading to the balloon. If no urine is available, the tubing is carefully lifted to return a small amount for aspiration. If there is still no urine, the distal portion of the catheter is clamped for a short time (10 to 15 minutes) until urine is available. Then the urine is transferred to a sterile specimen container, labeled, and sent immediately to the laboratory. If immediate transport is not possible, the specimen is refrigerated to decrease bacterial growth.

**Cleansing the Urinary Meatus**  In order to prevent infection when an indwelling catheter is in place, the area around the urinary meatus is cleansed two or three times daily, or as determined by the doctor or the agency. A washcloth, soap, and water can be used if a special kit is not available. Cleansing begins at the meatus and proceeds distally. In some agencies, an antiseptic or antibiotic ointment is applied after the cleansing.

## Bladder Irrigation

Bladder irrigations may be ordered to decrease infection when the catheter is indwelling or to decrease blood clotting (e.g., after a prostatectomy). Antiseptic or antimicrobial solutions are used. A three-way urinary catheter, which has one lumen leading to the inflatable balloon, one to the drainage tube, and another from the irrigation solution to the bladder, permits continuous drip irrigation by a closed drainage system. The rate of irrigation and type of solution is ordered by the physician.

When a bladder irrigation is ordered and the catheter in place is not a three-way catheter, the following procedure may be used. Maintaining aseptic technique is essential if bladder infection is to be avoided.

1. The junction between the catheter and connecting tubing is cleansed with an antiseptic solution.
2. Then the catheter is disconnected from the tubing.
3. A sterile 50 to 60 ml syringe filled with the sterile irrigating solution is attached to the end of the catheter. (Care is taken not to touch the sterile end of the catheter or the tubing with the hands throughout the procedure).

4. The patency of the catheter is checked by aspirating. The irrigating solution is then injected.
5. The irrigating solution drains from the catheter by gravity into a sterile container.
6. Irrigation continues until the return flow is clear (or as otherwise ordered).
7. Catheter and tubing ends are again cleansed with antiseptic solution before they are reconnected.
8. The amount of irrigation solution is not included in the measurement of the urinary output.

It goes without saying that the nurse's hands must be scrupulously clean for all of these procedures if her client is to be protected from bladder infection.

## Catheter Clamping and Removal

After long-term catheter use, a period of clamping and releasing is often prescribed before the catheter is removed. The alternate stretching and relaxing of the bladder walls help maintain or restore bladder tone. Initially, clamping may be tolerated for about 30 minutes. Gradually, the length of time is increased until clamping for a 2-hour period is tolerated.

The client's tolerance of this procedure must be carefully assessed. For example, the unconscious client with an indwelling catheter cannot say when he is uncomfortable, but increased restlessness might indicate poor tolerance.

Increased fluid intake is encouraged while the indwelling catheter is in place. The client should also be encouraged to continue this after the catheter is removed. Some mild burning or frequency may occur for a short time after catheter removal. The client should be instructed to tell the nurse the first time he voids after the catheter is removed, the amount, and whether or not

---

### Performance Checklist
### Removing the Catheter

1. Obtain scissors and a basin.
2. Cut off the distal portion of the inflatable lumen of the catheter.
3. When the water has emptied into the basin (5 to 8 ml), gently rotate the catheter while removing it.
4. Discard.
5. Cleanse the meatus with soap and water or an antiseptic solution.
6. Record time of removal and amount of urine in bag. In some agencies, the internal tip of the catheter is cut off, placed in a sterile specimen container, and sent to the lab for culture. If this is done, record it.

---

## Urinary Incontinence

The problem of urinary incontinence may be overcome by clean self-catheterizaton, Credéing (pushing or massaging over the bladder), bladder training programs, and the use of external male catheters. More specialized textbooks can be consulted for information on most of these techniques. Only the use of external male catheters will be discussed in this text.

Skin irritation, tissue breakdown, and infection are major problems when the skin is wet with urine. The use of a male external catheter (e.g., Texas Catheter) helps prevent these problems. The condom-like shield is placed over the penis and held in place with a velcro strip. Tubing and a collection device are attached. At least once a day the device is removed, the penis washed and dried, and the shield replaced. The tubing is kept from kinking, which would obstruct the urinary flow and cause the urine to pool in the shield.

## Effects of Immobility on the Bladder

Immobility can create bladder problems of incontinence, incomplete bladder emptying with stasis and the tendency towards infection, and formation of calculi. Some of the nursing measures which help alleviate (or prevent) these problems include encouraging the client to get dressed in street clothes and to move about. This not only discourages incontinence but also discourages urinary stasis or retention with overflow. Moving the person from side to side in bed and from flat to elevated position also helps prevent urinary stasis in the bladder. Weight-bearing exercises and increased water intake help prevent urinary calculi (stones) which tend to form because of inactivity, as calcium is removed from the bones.

## Anuria

Strictly speaking, anuria means the complete absence of urinary output, but the term is also used to indicate marked reduction in daily urinary output. Anuria, therefore, may indicate a severe oliguria or a urinary tract obstruction. If the oliguria or anuria result from end-stage renal failure, dialysis may need to be employed to remove toxic waste products. Peritoneal dialysis, which is a temporary process, may be used in poisoning or in end-stage renal failure when hemodialysis is not available. Chronic dialysis requires regular dialyzing for life or until a kidney transplant is performed.

Dialysis artificially performs the excretory and regulatory functions of the kidney by diffusion and osmosis. In hemodialysis, the blood is circulated through a compartment formed of a semipermeable membrane. In peritoneal dialysis, the dialysate is inserted into the abdomen, remains there a set period of time, and then is drained off. Complete information related to dialysis is available in more specialized textbooks.

## SUMMARY

This chapter has presented basic information related to the elimination functions of the bowel and bladder. Assessment techniques were described as well as nursing interventions for some common problems of elimination. Prevention of constipation was emphasized. The nursing procedures required when elimination is a problem were presented in detail. These included assisting with toileting, collecting specimens, administration of suppositories, enemas, removal of impactions, insertion of rectal tubes, assisting with gastric decompression, catheterizations, irrigations, and the application of external catheter in the male client.

## LEARNING ACTIVITIES

1. Plan a program for the relief of constipation in a healthy young adult.
2. Discuss appropriate nursing interventions for a person who is incontinent of feces.
3. Assess a client's bowel activity by using inspection, auscultation, percussion, and palpation.
4. Teach a family member how to give a cleansing enema.
5. A client's major health problem is flatulence of long standing. Plan a program to assist him in overcoming this problem.

## REFERENCES AND SUGGESTED READINGS

Bass, Linda. More fiber—less constipation. *American Journal of Nursing,* February, 1977, pp. 254–255.

Blackwell, Ardith and Blackwell, William. Relieving gas pains. *American Journal of Nursing,* January, 1975, pp. 66–67.

Corman, Marvin L.; Veidenheimer, Malcolm C.; and Coller, John A. Cathartics. *American Journal of Nursing,* February, 1975, pp. 273-277.

DeGroot, Jane. Urethral catheterization. *Nursing 76,* December, 1976, pp. 51–55.

Guyton, Arthur, 1976. *Textbook of medical physiology.* 5th ed. Philadelphia: W. B. Saunders.

Hogstel, Mildred. How to give a safe and successful cleansing enema. *American Journal of Nursing,* May, 1977, pp. 816–817.

McConnell, E. All about gastrointestinal intubation. *Nursing 75,* May, 1975, pp. 30–37.

McGuckin, Maryanne. Microbiologic studies, part 4: what you should know about collecting stool culture specimens. *Nursing 76,* March, 1976, pp. 22-23.

Rodman, Morton J. and Smith, Dorothy W., 1974. *Clinical pharmacology in nursing.* Philadelphia: J. B. Lippincott.

Tudor, Lea T. Bladder and bowel retraining. *American Journal of Nursing,* November, 1970, pp. 2391–2393.

Watt, Rosemary C. Colostomy irrigation: yes or no? *American Journal of Nursing,* March, 1977, pp. 442–444.

# 18

# Fluid and Electrolytes

## Behavioral Objectives

Upon completion of this chapter, the student will be able to:

1. Explain the basic elements of fluid and electrolyte balance.
2. Identify the person with a potential or existing fluid and electrolyte problem.
3. Plan, implement, and evaluate nursing measures to prevent or correct fluid and electrolyte problems.

## Key Terms

| | | |
|---|---|---|
| acidosis | extracellular fluid | perspiration, insensible |
| acid-base balance | filtration | pH |
| active transport | fistula | phagocytosis |
| adenosine triphosphate | fluid volume deficit | phlebitis |
| alkalosis | fluid volume excess | pinocytosis |
| anions | homeostasis | plasma |
| antidiuretic hormone | interstitial fluid | potassium deficit |
| anuria | intracellular fluid | potassium excess |
| cations | ions | sodium deficit |
| diffusion | milliequivalent | sodium excess |
| drop factor | oliguria | solutes |
| edema, pitting | osmosis | venipuncture |
| electrolytes | paralytic ileus | |

## Introduction

We assume that the student comes to the nursing courses with a knowledge of fluid and electrolytes obtained in courses in the basic sciences. A brief summary of the basic elements of fluid and electrolyte balance is included, however, as a review. Six commonly encountered fluid and electrolyte problems are: fluid volume excess, fluid volume deficit, sodium excess, sodium deficit, potassium excess, and potassium deficit. An assessment guide is presented to help the student identify the person with an existing or potential fluid and electrolyte problem. Nursing measures to prevent imbalance are suggested. Methods for assisting the client to focus on oral and intravenous fluid intake are presented.

It is the rare illness that poses no threat to fluid and electrolyte balance. Many of the nursing measures related to specific fluid and electrolyte problems are addressed in other sections of the book (e.g., under body temperature, respiration/circulation, and elimination).

## BASIC ELEMENTS OF FLUID AND ELECTROLYTE BALANCE

All living organisms require water and electrolytes for homeostasis. Water is the most essential nutrient for life. No living thing—plant or animal—can exist for very long without it. Humans can survive only a few days without water. While the daily requirement for water varies with age, size, environment, and activity, 6 to 8 8-ounce glasses will meet the health needs of the average adult.

Body fluids, then, consist of water and important dissolved substances including electrolytes and nonelectrolytes such as dextrose, urea, and creatinine. Water has unique chemical and physical characteristics. Its boiling point is 100°C; its freezing point, 0°C. It is the closest substance known to a universal solvent.

Body water has two major components: extracellular fluid (that outside the cell) and intracellular fluid (that contained within the billions of body cells). Although age, sex, and body fat influence the amount of body water, in the average adult male 60 percent of body weight is water. Twenty percent is extracellular fluid (ECF) and 40 percent is intracellular fluid (ICF). In the average adult female, 50 percent of body weight is water of which 15 percent is ECF and 35 percent ICF. Therefore, about 1/3 of total body water is extracellular fluid and the remaining 2/3 is intracellular. The rest of body weight (40 percent) is made up of protein and related substances, minerals, and fat. Because fat contains a small amount of water, the less fat present in the body, the greater the percentage of body weight composed of water.

The cells making up the bodies of all but the simplest multicellular animals exist in an "internal sea" of extracellular fluid. The composition of this fluid closely resembles that of sea water, in which, presumably, all life began.

Extracellular fluid is divided into two types: plasma and interstitial fluid. Plasma (fluid within the vascular system) is 5 percent of body weight, and interstitial fluid (outside the blood vessels between the body cells) makes up 15 percent of body weight. Total blood volume is about 8 percent of body weight (Ganong, 1977).

Usually, lymph and cerebrospinal fluid are regarded as interstitial fluid. Other essential body fluids are secretions (such as those fluids manufactured in the stomach, pancreas, liver, and intestine) and excretions (urine, feces, and perspiration).

The distribution of body water, electrolytes, and dissolved substances (solutes) from compartment to compartment depends primarily upon the concentration of the solutes present.

## Electrolytes

Electrolytes are substances whose molecules split into ions when placed in water. Some ions develop a positive charge and some a negative charge. Cations are positively charged ions. When an electric current is passed through the solution, these ions migrate to the negative pole—the cathode — from which they take their name. Sodium ($Na^+$) is an example of a cation. Ions with a negative charge are anions. Under the influence of an electric current they migrate to the positive pole (the anode). Chloride ($Cl^-$) is an example of an anion. When salt is placed in water and an electric current is passed through the solution, the sodium chloride molecule separates into two charged particles (ions): sodium moves to the negative pole (cathode) and chloride to the positive pole (anode). All electrolytes in solution dissociate in a similar manner.

Some ions that develop positive charges include sodium ($Na^+$), potassium ($K^+$), calcium ($Ca^{++}$), and magnesium ($Mg^{++}$). Some that develop negative charges are chloride ($Cl^-$), bicarbonate ($HCO_3^-$), sulfate ($SO_4^-$), phosphate ($HPO_4^-$), proteinate Pr.$^-$), and organic acids (Org. Ac.$^-$).

## Milliequivalents

Electrolytes are measured in terms of their potential for chemical activity. Cations and anions measured in this way always balance each other. Therefore, a given number of milliequivalents (mEq) of a cation always react with exactly the same number of milliequivalents of an anion. It does not matter what the anion or cation is.

## Composition and Function of Body Fluids

Each specific body fluid is composed of certain electrolytes and water. The intracellular fluid contains large amounts of potassium (its major cation) and phosphate (its major anion). Small amounts of the other electrolytes are present. In the extracellular fluid, sodium is the principal cation and chloride the principal anion. The chief difference between plasma and interstitial fluid is the much greater amount of the electrolyte proteinate in plasma, which acts as a sponge to prevent excess plasma from seeping into the intestitial fluid.

The chief function of body fluids is to maintain optimal living conditions for the cells of the body. The cellular fluid normally contains all the nutrients the cells need. It also serves as a supply source to replenish the nutrients that are used. In addition, the cellular fluid must be cleared of the breakdown products of protein as well as carbon dioxide. The extracellular fluid does this. Nutrients and other materials seep from the plasma into the interstitial fluid at the arterial end of the capillary beds, and are carried to the cells by way of the interstitial fluid. Wastes pass from the cellular fluid into the interstitial fluid and back to the plasma by way of the venous capillaries. The plasma sorts the waste products for excretion or storage and carries them to their destination. Extracellular fluid also transmits additional substances, including enzymes and hormones.

## Transport Between Compartments

Materials are transported between cellular and extracellular compartments by several processes, including osmosis (the most important), diffusion, filtration, active transport, pinocytosis, and phagocytosis.

**Osmosis**   When two solutions are separated by a semipermeable membrane, the solution with the greatest electrolyte concentration draws water from the solution with less electrolyte concentration. Osmosis occurs when the ECF develops an electrolyte content lower or higher than normal. If you remember that "water goes where salt is," you will have a description of osmosis.

**Diffusion**   Diffusion occurs through the movement of ions and molecules to provide an equal concentration in all parts. They pass from regions of high concentration to regions of low concentration. For example, oxygen and carbon dioxide exchange occurs through diffusion.

**Active Transport**   Active transport occurs when it is necessary for ions to move from areas of lesser concentration to areas of greater concentration. Adenosine triphosphate (ATP) is released from a cell to enable certain substances to acquire the energy needed to pass through the cell membrane. The mechanism of transfer is not fully understood at this time.

**Filtration**   This is the transfer of water and dissolved substances through a permeable membrane from a high pressure area to a low pressure area. Hydrostatic pressure produced  by the pumping action of the heart is the mechanism behind filtration. For example, fluid and electrolytes pass from the arterial end of the capillaries to the interstitial fluid by the process of filtration. The force opposing hydrostatic pressure is oncotic pressure, as found in the plasma proteins, which tends to hold the fluid and electrolytes within the blood vessels.

**Pinocytosis and Phagocytosis**   Pinocytosis is a process by which substances of large molecular weight enter body cells by invagination (telescoping) of the cell membrane. Phagocytes digest or engulf microorganisms, cells, or foreign material in the process of phagocytosis.

## Regulation

The body regulates movement of fluid and electrolytes to maintain homeostasis—a normal body fluid state. The principal homeostatic regulating mechanisms are the pituitary, parathyroid, cardiorenal, pulmonary, and adrenal mechanisms. Practically every organ and body system is used to maintain homeostasis; but the lungs, kidneys, heart, adrenals, pituitary, and parathyroid are the most important. The lungs regulate the oxygen and carbon dioxide level in the blood. They help to maintain the acid-base balance of the extracellular fluid. The kidneys are most important in determining the volume and composition of the extracellular fluid. They depend for their action on the heart, which pumps the blood to them for cleansing. Of approximately 180 l of blood filtered through the kidneys daily, approximately 1.5 l of the filtrate is excreted as urine while the rest of the filtrate is absorbed.

The adrenals secrete numerous hormones that function in retention and excretion of fluid and electrolytes. The pituitary secretes an antidiuretic hormone (ADH), which directly affects the body's conservation of water. The parathyroids regulate the calcium level of extracellular fluid. If any of these regulating mechanisms malfunctions, a serious fluid and electrolyte problem results.

## Acid-Base Balance

Normal body fluid composition depends not only upon electrolyte concentrations but also upon acid and base (alkali) concentrations. When acid-base balance is maintained, the body fluid is neutral and normal. When the balance is upset, the fluid becomes either acid or alkaline. The number of hydrogen ions in the fluid determines whether the reaction is acid, neutral, or alkaline.

A substance that releases hydrogen ions when dissolved is called an acid. A substance that combines with hydrogen when dissolved is called a base. One example of an acid is carbonic acid ($H_2CO_3$). It is called an acid because it releases $H^+$ ions. It also releases bicarbonate ($HCO_3^-$), which is capable of recombining with $H^+$.

The hydrogen ion concentration in body fluid is expressed by the symbol pH. A low pH means a high concentration of hydrogen; a high pH means a low concentration. The normal pH of arterial blood is 7.4. When it drops below this point, the person is acidotic; when it is above 7.4 he is alkalotic. The extracellular fluid range of pH conducive to life is very limited. It is maintained by buffering systems and by the kidney and lung functions.

In general, the ratio of carbonic acid to base bicarbonate determines the hydrogen ion concentration of the extracellular fluid. Carbon dioxide combines with water in the extracellular fluid to form carbonic acid. The cations sodium, potassium, calcium, and magnesium unite with the anion bicarbonate to form base bicarbonate. While other buffers enter into the acid-base balance, carbonic acid and base bicarbonate are the most important. The normal ratio of carbonic acid to base bicarbonate is 1:20. As long as there is 1 mEq of carbonic acid for every 20 mEq of base bicarbonate in the extracellular fluid, the pH is normal.

It may help to consider acid-base balance as a see-saw with carbonic acid on one end and base bicarbonate on the other. In health the see-saw is balanced. Any health problem that tilts the balance toward the carbonic acid side causes acidosis (acidemia), and anything that tilts it toward the base bicarbonate side produces alkalosis (alkalemia). Imbalances caused by alterations in base bicarbonate concentrations are called metabolic disturbances. The kidneys are largely responsible for regulating bicarbonate concentration. The lungs are largely responsible for increasing or decreasing the carbonic acid concentration of the extracellular fluid. Imbalances caused by carbonic acid alterations are called respiratory disturbances.

## Fluid Balance

The healthy person who eats a balanced diet and drinks 6 to 8 glasses of liquid a day satisfies his fluid and electrolyte needs. The sick person who has difficulty eating a balanced diet and taking adequate fluids risks fluid and electrolyte imbalance.

In health, fluid is gained through the water present in liquids, in solid foods, and that derived from metabolism. The amount of water gained averages 2,600 ml per day. Losses occur through urine (1,500 ml), feces (100 ml), and insensible perspiration (1,000 ml) which is unavoidable vaporization from the lungs and skin. The total amount of water lost averages 2,600 ml.

Fluid imbalances occur when there are discrepancies between the fluid intake and fluid output. Fluids and electrolytes are lost from the central, nervous system (in cerebrospinal fluid); the respiratory tract (excessive ventilation, pulmonary edema); the lymphatic system (fistulas of lymphatic ducts); the gastrointestinal tract (saliva, vomiting, suction drainage, exudate, fistula, diarrhea, gastric washing, or faulty absorption); the kidneys; the skin (lactation, sweating, draining fistulas, paracentesis, burn exudate, or massive urticaria); and by hemorrhage. The electrolyte loss varies with the source of the fluid loss.

## PREVENTION OF IMBALANCE

It was suggested earlier that any health deficit poses a threat to fluid balance. Similarly, any prolonged time period without adequate intake is a hazard. Consider the person who fasts (NPO) before surgery and receives only tea, juice, and broth for the next 24 hours. While there may not be a fluid deficit, if such a diet continues there is inadequate nutrient intake to prevent an electrolyte imbalance.

Any person who is losing excessive fluids from the body is threatened with imbalance. Any person who has difficulty eating the proper liquids and other nutrients needs close observation to prevent imbalance between intake and output. Thirst normally indicates the need for fluid. If the client is thirsty and fluids are available, he will maintain a balance.

Anorexia, nausea, and vomiting make it difficult for the person to get adequate nutrients. Specific nursing measures to increase intake in these instances are discussed in Chapter 16.

Encouraging fluids or restricting them when necessary helps prevent imbalances. The nurse encourages oral fluids when there has been an excessive loss of body fluids. Parenteral fluids are carefully monitored so that they are administered at the correct rate. The client and his family are important participants in the prevention of fluid and electrolyte imbalance. They should be taught about medications that may cause an imbalance and foods that will restore balance. For example, persons receiving antihypertensive medication may be instructed to take in extra potassium by drinking a glass of orange juice or tomato juice or eating a banana or whole orange every day. When the client understands the reason for the instruction and the variety of foods that can be used, he will be likely to follow the instruction.

Laxatives and cathartics may also be a frequent cause of imbalance. The nurse should instruct her clients in more appropriate ways to overcome constipation (Ch. 17).

## ASSESSMENT OF FLUID AND ELECTROLYTE BALANCE

The nurse observes and questions her client in order to identify changes that indicate a body fluid disturbance. Does he have a known health problem that can disrupt fluid balance? Is he taking any medication that threatens balance? Is his diet restricted in any way? Does he have an abnormal loss of body fluids? Does his intake balance his output?

Reading the client's record to see if the laboratory reports indicate balance is an important part of the nursing assessment. If, for example, the urine specific gravity is high, this might indicate fluid deficit. If the hemoglobin and hematocrit are high, this too might indicate fluid deficit; whereas, if the urine specific gravity, hemoglobin, and hematocrit are low, excessive fluid may be present.

Many fluid and electrolyte alterations develop gradually and early manifestations are quite general. Weakness, dizziness, or tiredness may indicate the beginning of a fluid and electrolyte problem. The nurse must be alert to changes the client reports. Is he more weak or tired than usual? Is he more irritable or depressed?

His usual pattern of eating and drinking should be established as a basis for comparisons. If he drinks a large amount of fluids, for example, he will have more difficulty when his fluids are restricted than the person who is accustomed to drinking less.

The following assessment guide poses questions that help identify the person with a potential or actual fluid and electrolyte disturbance. The following questions may be used as a guide:

1. Why is the client seeking health care?
2. Is he taking any medications? If so, which ones?
3. Has there been any change in his food or fluid intake within the past week?
4. Has there been any change in urine amount or color?
5. Has there been any change in the client's appetite? Thirst?
6. Has he noticed any weight change?
7. Is his diet restricted in any way?
8. Are food and water readily available to him?
9. Is there any nausea, vomiting, or diarrhea? If so, for how long?
10. Is there a change in energy level: more sleep, activity, or apprehensiveness than usual?
11. Is there any dizziness?
12. Inspect for signs of dehydration: dry skin and mucous membranes, furrowed tongue, sunken eyes, poor skin turgor (when skin is pinched it returns slowly to normal position). Inspect the peripheral veins for changes in fluid volume. Raise and lower the hand (normally the veins empty or fill in 3 to 5 seconds). With decreased volume it takes longer for the veins to fill. With increased volume the hand veins take longer to empty when the hand is elevated. Inspect for signs of increased volume: soft, puffy tissue around the eyes, fingers, lower part of back, ankles. Does the tissue "pit?" (When thumb is pressed into tissue, indentation remains.) Has the voice become hoarse?
13. Inspect for signs of muscle weakness, tenseness, active twitch, or cramps.
14. Assess the vital signs for any change: (check temperature for fever, pulse for volume, respirations for rate or moisture, increase or decrease in blood pressure).
15. Is there fluid loss from any abnormal source?
16. Is he receiving parenteral fluids?
17. Is he on measured intake and output? If so, how do they compare?

## ASSISTING THE CLIENT WHO HAS FLUID AND ELECTROLYTE PROBLEMS

### Encouraging Oral Fluid Intake

A person of any age who cannot get the fluids he needs is in danger of a fluid and electrolyte imbalance. The elderly bedridden person, for example, must be able to reach the water on his bedside table. If the client seldom drinks water but likes another beverage, he should be given what he likes within medical

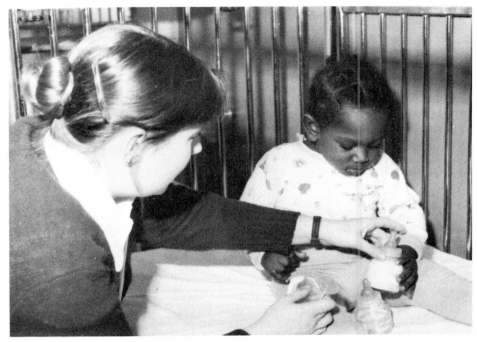

**Figure 18-1.**   *Encourage a baby who may not be thirsty to increase her fluid intake by offering her a choice.   (Photo by Frank R. Engler, Jr.)*

allowances. Fluids should be offered to the client on a regular basis. A schedule should be posted in the room so that everyone knows, for example, that on the hour the client should be given 2 ounces of a specified fluid. The schedule should be planned for 24 hours, allowing periods when sleep is encouraged and the client will not be awakened for fluids.

Ingenuity is needed to encourage the person who is not thirsty to increase fluid intake. For children the use of pretty cups, straws, and some reward (such as a gold star pasted on the chart each time liquids are taken) may help. The parent can often identify ways used at home to encourage fluid intake.

Sometimes it is necessary only to explain why extra fluid is needed. Foods that are high in water content, such as salads and fruits, ice cream, and jello, should be included on the diet.

If the client has difficulty swallowing, he needs to be protected against aspiration by placing him in an upright position before he begins to eat or drink. An intact swallowing reflex can be determined by watching to see if he swallows saliva. If he can swallow but he has not yet been given fluids, he must be started slowly, with a sip of water first. A suction apparatus should be available, if possible. Teaspoons, straws, syringes, and special drinking cups with spouts or covers are some devices that may be useful in increasing fluid intake.

## Oral Fluid Intake When Fluids Are Restricted

When we are thirsty and fluids are restricted, we are tempted to acquire fluids by any possible means. Hospitalized clients have been known to drink water from an ice cap, borrow liquids from a roommate's tray, walk to the nearest water fountain, and send relatives to vending machines to buy liquids to satisfy their thirst. Clearly, then, it is important to explain to the client and his family why fluids must be restricted. It is also essential to evaluate frequently the success of the restriction.

Spacing and Diversion Techniques   The clients who will have fluid restrictions include those scheduled for surgery, for tests on the gastro-intestinal tract, and for other tests requiring anesthesia. People with kidney failure who are on dialysis must severely restrict fluids between dialysis treatments. Many persons with cardiac problems must restrict intake. After surgery nothing by mouth (NPO) is a frequent necessity.

The nurse, whenever possible, should work with the client to make a 24-hour schedule for the dispersal of the allotted fluid. In the plan is included the fluid served at mealtime as well as that dispensed with medications and served at bedtime. Ice, too, is calculated in the fluid intake. One cup of ice chips equals ½ cup of water. This should be explained to the client.

When fluid intake is limited, the client should be encouraged to keep occupied. Some activity of interest to him may help take his mind off his desire for liquids. Unless contraindicated, gum or hard candy can be offered to keep the mouth moist and decrease thirst. It is important to avoid foods that increase thirst. Dietary restrictions often accompany fluid restrictions, so foods high in sodium are probably restricted. The client should be taught the importance of following diet restrictions as well as the fluid restrictions.

Comfort Measures   When fluids are restricted, frequent mouth care is one of the most important comfort measures. The client should be helped to brush his teeth and his tongue and rinse his mouth with either water or mouthwash. The client may need to be reminded only to rinse his mouth and not to swallow the water.

## Measuring Intake and Output

Measurement of fluid intake and output is required frequently, whether the person is at home or in the hospital. Intake and output records may be ordered by the physician but, nevertheless, should be initiated on any client when nursing judgment deems it important. For example, intake and output should be measured after major surgery, when the client is on intravenous therapy, when the diet or medication can be expected to alter fluid and electrolyte balance, when there is a heart or kidney problem, and when there is any abnormal loss of body fluid.

The importance and reason for accurate intake and output measurement must be explained to the client and his family. If the client is able and willing to

University Hospital

Bedside Intake and Output Sheet                Date: *10/8*

| | | Intake | | | | Output | | | | | | | |
|---|---|---|---|---|---|---|---|---|---|---|---|---|---|
| | Time Added | Parenteral Fluids Type | Up | In | Oral | | Urine | Gu Irrigant Up | In | Levin In Out | | Emesis | Chest | Stool |
| 7 | *8am* | | | | *240ml* | 8 9 10 | ← *200ml* | | | | | | | |
| To | *11am* | | | | *500ml* | 11 12 1 | ← *150ml* | | | | | | | |
| 3 | *2³⁰pm* | | | | *200 ml* | 2 3 | ← *140ml* | | | | | | | |
| | 8 Hours Total | | | | *940ml* | | ← *490ml* | | | | | | | |
| 3 | ᵖᵐ | *1000ml* → | | | | 4 5 | | | | | | | | |
| | *4pm* | *D₅W* | | | *100 ml* | 6 7 | *400ml* | | | | | | | |
| To | | | | | | 8 | *300ml* | | | | | | | |
| | *9pm* | | | | *140 ml* | 9 | | | | | | | | |
| 11 | | | | *1000* | | 10 11 | *300ml* | | | | | | | |
| | 8 Hours Total | | *1000* | *240 ml* | | | *1000 ml* | | | | | | | |
| 11 | | *D₅W* | *1000* | | *NPO (0)* | 12 1 2 | *150ml* | | | | | | | |
| To | | | | | | 3 4 5 | | | | | | | | |
| 7 | ᵃᵐ | | | *1000* | | 6 7 | *300ml* | | | | | | | |
| | 8 Hours Total | | *1000 ml* | | *0* | | *450ml* | | | | | | | |
| | 24 Hours Total | | *2000 ml* | *1180 ml* | | | *1940ml* | | | | | | | |

Light Blue Plastic Cup .................. 180 cc
Turquoise Cup From Carafe Set ......... 240 cc
Clear Plastic Juice Cup .................. 100 cc
Carton of Milk .......................... 240 cc
Can of Coke or Fresca ................... 360 cc
Bottle of Pepsi ......................... 195 cc
Bottle of Gingerale ..................... 210 cc
Hottle of Coffee ......................... 260 cc
Cup of Coffee ........................... 150 cc
Paper Cream Cup ........................ 15 cc
Bowl of Soup (Full) .................... 240 cc

One Serving of Jello ..................... 120 cc
Fruit Ice ................................. 80 cc
Ice Cream ................................ 60 cc
Sherbet .................................. 60 cc
Heavy Whipping Cream  ... 1/2 of Volume Served
Cup of Cracked Ice ....................... 90 cc
   Full Container of Ice is one-half of the
   Liquid Volume, EG.:
   Plastic Cup of Water ............... 180 cc
   Plastic Cup of Ice ..................... 90 cc
One Ice Cube ............................. 7 cc

**Figure 18-2.**  *Sample bedside intake and output sheet.*

do so, he should be encouraged to keep his own intake and output record. A table can be posted for him showing the amount that a cup, glass, bowl, and other container hold. He should be instructed to record the liquid after it is drunk, not when it is offered. If the liquid is measured in ounces, conversion to ml can be made easily before the record is charted.

Any food that is liquid at room temperature (e.g., ice cream and jello) should be measured and recorded as liquid intake. Both the amount and kind of fluid intake must be recorded. There is usually a column on the form for oral intake, parenteral intake, and output. The kind and amount of intravenous fluid is also charted (e.g., 250 ml packed red cells).

The type, amount, and method of fluid loss is recorded. The client uses the bedpan or urinal if his output is being recorded. If the client is incontinent of urine, the amount should be estimated and recorded. Vomitus is measured or estimated and recorded as output, as are diarrheal stools. Perspiration is also estimated and recorded as output.

The bedside record is usually tallied every 8 hours and totalled every 24 hours, and recorded on the permanent record. Totals may be recorded on the graphic sheet (where vital signs are recorded) or on a separate fluid sheet.

Hourly urine measurements may be needed when kidney function is being closely monitored. An output of less than 30 ml per hour is considered indicative of inadequate kidney function.

Intake and output inaccuracies are encountered frequently, as exemplified by doctor's orders requesting "accurate intake and output." One cause of inaccuracy is forgetting to record the intake or output at the time it occurs. In addition, some people (both clients and hospital personnel) may not know intake and output is to be recorded. A large sign prominently displayed on the door of the person's room and improved verbal communication help increase accuracy.

Weight  Body weight is a valuable measure to validate fluid intake and output. The client's daily weight is an accurate indication of fluid loss or gain when it is difficult to obtain an accurate measurement by other means. When serial weights are used, the person must be weighed under the same conditions each time. The same scale is used at the same time of day, and the client must wear similar clothing. A popular time for weighing is first thing in the morning, after the person has voided and before he has eaten. However, just before any meal would be equally appropriate as long as the client is weighed at the same time every day. If the person to be weighed can stand on the upright scale, he removes his robe and slippers and stands on a paper towel. If he has an intravenous in place and an attached arm board, this weight must be subtracted.

Bed scales are used to weigh the person who cannot stand. A special board or sling is placed under the person's body, which is then suspended by use of a hydraulic lift. The weight is read and the person returned to his former position in bed. Directions for use are provided with the bed scales.

When a baby is weighed, he is usually undressed, placed supine on a balanced scale, and protected from falling while the weight is read. An alternative is for the nurse to weigh herself; then, holding the baby, she weighs herself and the baby and finds the baby's weight by subtracting her own weight.

## Intravenous Therapy

When the doctor orders intravenous therapy for a client, the nurse must often explain what is meant by "being fed through the vein." If he has had an intravenous some time in the past, the person has some idea of what to expect. However, many clients will be receiving intravenous solutions for the first time. It may be frightening because the person believes only the very ill receive IVs. The nurse can explain, for example, that the IV is needed to give a specific medication or that after surgery many persons receive intravenous therapy for a short time. The procedure should be explained to the client before the technician, nurse, or doctor arrives with the equipment needed to perform the venipuncture.

The intravenous is started, whenever possible, in the nondominant arm so that independence is retained. A needle or catheter of appropriate size for the vein is selected. The smaller the number, the larger the size of the needle (e.g., 16 gauge is a large needle and a 25 gauge is small). For an adult, a size 19 or 21 is generally chosen. Pliable intravenous catheters are popular because immobilization is unnecessary and freedom of movement makes the IV more acceptable. After the skin is appropriately cleansed and the needle (or catheter) inserted, gauze pads and tape secure the needle in place. Arm boards are used if indicated.

Calculating the Rate of Flow    Calculating and monitoring the intravenous flow are frequently the nursing student's responsibility. When an intravenous therapist starts the IV she will regulate the flow. It is important, nevertheless, for the student to be able to calculate flow rate.

When an intravenous order is written, it usually specifies the amount of fluid to be absorbed per hour. The nurse, then, must calculate the number of drops per minute required to deliver the hourly volume prescribed. For example, the order reads "1,000 ml D5 in water at 125 ml per hour IV." The nurse needs more information before she can calculate drops per minute. How many drops are there in an ml? This *drop factor* differs according to the administration set being used. In most macro (large) drop sets the drop factor is 10 to 16 drops per ml. In micro (small) drop sets, such as the Buretrol or Volutrol, the drop factor is 60 drops per ml. The information (the drop factor) is printed on the box containing the administration set. When the drop factor is determined the following formula calculates the number of drops per minute required to give the amount ordered per hour.

1

**Example:**    drop factor (d.f.) = 12

$$\times \text{ (drops per minute)} = \frac{\text{volume to be given/hour} \times \text{d.f.}}{\text{time of infusion in minutes}}$$

$$\times = \frac{125 \times 12}{60} = 25 \text{ drops per minute}$$

**Example:**    d. f. = 60

$$\times = \frac{125 \times 60}{60} = 125 \text{ drops per minute}$$

As we can see, when the drop factor is 60, no written calculation is necessary. The ml/hr and the drops/min are the same.

After the flow rate has been calculated and adjusted, it is monitored frequently. The nurse should check the IV every time she goes into the room, or at least once each hour, because the rate of flow may change. The following factors affect flow rate: position of the needle in the vein, which may be altered if the client changes his position; the height of the IV bag or bottle; patency of the needle; plugging of the air vent on the tubing; and venous spasm caused by an irritating solution. If the rate has changed from that desired, it must be corrected.

Some complications of intravenous infusions include infiltration, phlebitis, air embolus, and circulatory overload. The needle insertion site is inspected for temperature, swelling, and tenderness to touch. If the needle has slipped out of the vein and the fluid is infiltrating the surrounding tissue, the area will generally be cool, swollen, and tender, and the flow rate will be decreased. Correct needle placement can generally (but not always) be verified by lowering the infusion container below the injection site. If there is a back flow of blood in the tubing, the needle is usually correctly situated.

The insertion site is also inspected frequently for any sign of redness, tenderness, heat, or swelling that might indicate infection or phlebitis. The danger of infection and phlebitis is lessened with the use of plastic catheters, frequent tubing change (usually q 24 hours), and changing insertion sites (approximately q 48 hours).

When IV fluids are continuous, the infusion source (bag or bottle) is checked so that it does not empty completely before the next one is added. If this were to happen, air would enter the tubing and adding the next bag would push the column of air into the vein. This problem is easier to prevent than to correct. The danger of air embolus exists when air enters the vein. Most authorities agree that 10 ml of air in the vein is a hazard.

Circulatory overload can occur if excessive IV fluids are given. Coughing, shortness of breath, increased respiratory rate, and dyspnea are signs suggesting circulatory overload. If these signs occur, the infusion must be stopped or slowed immediately and the physician notified. The possibility of this complication is the reason that no attempt to "catch up" to the ordered amount of fluid should ever be made.

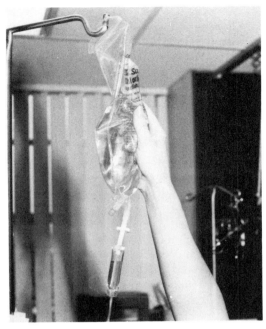

**Figure 18-3.** *Check the intravenous fluids frequently so that the source does not empty before another can be added. (Photo by Frank R. Engler, Jr.)*

**Recording**   The type of intravenous solution, rate of flow, amount absorbed, and any applicable client reactions are recorded on the appropriate sheet.

**Removing the IV needle**   When the IV is to be restarted or terminated, the needle is removed according to the following technique: the tubing is clamped to stop the fluid flow. The tape holding the needle or tubing in place is carefully and quickly loosened while the needle is stabilized to keep it from injuring the wall of the vein. Then a dry sponge or band-aid (alcohol burns) is placed over the insertion site as the needle or catheter is slowly removed. Light pressure is applied to assist clotting and, if the arm was the needle site, the arm is elevated temporarily.

## COMMON FLUID AND ELECTROLYTE IMBALANCES

### Fluid Volume Excess

An excess of extracellular fluid reflects an increase in interstitial fluid, as well as an increase in electrolytes. Excessive fluid in the interstitial spaces interferes with the transfer of nutrients and wastes between the blood and the cells. Some of the causes of imbalance include the following: excessive infusion of isotonic sodium chloride solution (this contains 154 mEq/l of sodium and 154 mEq/l of chloride; the body's extracellular fluid contains 142 mEq/l of sodium and 103 mEq/l of chloride, so it is relatively easy to cause a fluid volume excess). Congestive heart disease, chronic kidney disease, and chronic liver disease also cause fluid excess. In these disorders, the body homeostatic mechanisms are not functioning properly. Excessive administration of steroids (e.g., cortisone) can also cause fluid volume excess.

If the client has edema, it may be local (in areas such as the soft tissue around the eyes, the fingers, the ankles, the sacrum) or generalized. The tissues are soft and puffy. There is a weight gain greater than 5 percent. Moist râles will be heard in the lungs and there will be shortness of breath. The pulse will be full and bounding, the blood pressure elevated, the peripheral veins engorged. Urinary output may be decreased; hemoglobin and hematocrit are also decreased because of the large volume of fluid.

Treatment requires correction of the cause of the problem. Intake may be reduced and diuretics given to increase sodium excretion.

Nursing interventions include emotional support for the person who is having difficulty breathing and who is required to undergo frequent blood tests. The person who has edema should be turned or encouraged to move frequently to increase circulation and prevent tissue breakdown. If there is fluid in the abdomen (ascites), pressure is exerted on the diaphragm and abdominal organs. Daily weights, intake and output records, frequent checking of vital signs, and skin care are included in nursing interventions specific for this problem.

## Fluid Volume Deficit

Fluid deficit is a deficit of both water and electrolytes in approximately the same proportion as they exist in the normal extracellular fluid. Some of the causes of fluid deficit include an abrupt decrease in fluid intake, an acute loss of secretions and excretions, or a combination of decreased intake and increased output. The person will have experienced vomiting, severe diarrhea, fistulous drainage, a systemic infection with fever and increased use of water and electrolytes, or intestinal obstruction in which both water and electrolytes are unavailable for metabolic use.

This deficit is frequently difficult to identify because so many of its symptoms appear in any person who is seriously ill. Depression of the infant's anterior fontanel indicates fluid volume deficit. In other persons, the skin is dry and so are the mucous membranes; the tongue has longitudinal furrows; there is oliguria or anuria; there is acute weight loss (greater than 5 percent). The blood pressure (systolic) is 10 mm Hg lower when the person stands than when he is supine. Pulse and respirations are elevated and the temperature is normal. Venous pressure is decreased. The hemoglobin and hematocrit may be elevated.

The aim of treatment is to restore the fluid volume to normal without altering the electrolyte composition of the fluid. Balanced solutions are given either orally or parenterally. When balanced solutions are given, the body's homeostatic mechanisms selectively retain or excrete water and electrolytes as needed.

Nursing interventions include taking daily weight, intake and output records, and frequent vital signs, and giving skin care. Urinary output is carefully monitored and includes specific gravity readings. Adequacy of urinary output is determined before solutions containing potassium are given (the balanced solutions usually contain potassium). Fluid intake by mouth or vein is closely watched.

## Sodium Excess

Sodium excess is an excess of sodium in the extracellular fluid. The extracellular fluid becomes hypertonic because water is lost from it without salt loss. This condition results from decreased water intake or increased output of water, or from increased ingestion of sodium chloride or decreased output of sodium. It may occur in any condition when more water is lost than electrolytes. This occurs in rapid and deep breathing, in febrile illnesses, and in profuse watery diarrhea. The person who cannot take fluids because he is unconscious may develop sodium excess; so may the person who has ingested sea water.

The client will have dry, sticky mucous membranes, flushed skin, elevated body temperature, rough and dry tongue, and feel extreme thirst. Oliguria or anuria is present. Tearing is depressed. He appears agitated and restless. His tissue turgor is firm and rubbery. Laboratory findings include a plasma sodium above 147 mEq/l; plasma chloride above 106 mEq/l; and urine specific gravity above 1.030.

The goal of treatment is to dilute the concentration of electrolyte excess. Balanced solutions that provide free water to dilute the electrolyte concentration excess as they replenish maintenance amounts are administered. In this way, normal water to electrolyte ratio is reestablished.

Nursing measures, in addition to those previously stated for the client with a fluid and electrolyte imbalance, include measures to lower the body temperature and to alleviate thirst. Safety measures are necessary to protect the agitated and restless person from injury.

## Sodium Deficit

Sodium deficit occurs when the concentration of sodium in the extracellular fluid is below normal. Either water accumulates more rapidly than sodium, or sodium is lost more rapidly than the water in the extracellular fluid. This condition may be caused by drinking plain water after excessive sweating, gastric suctioning and irrigation of the tube with plain water, potent diuretics, plain water enemas, or infusions of electrolyte-free solutions.

At first, the person with sodium deficit is anxious and apprehensive; this is followed by a feeling of impending doom. He is weak, confused, and may become stuporous. He may have abdominal cramps and muscle twitching or even convulsions. Urinary output is depressed or absent. Fingerprinting is visible over the sternum. When pressure is applied with a finger over the sternum, the fingerprint remains because of the transfer of the water from the extracellular fluid into the cells. The plasma sodium is less than 137 mEq/l and chloride is below 98 mEq/l. Urine specific gravity is less than 1.010.

The treatment goal is to restore the sodium concentration to normal as quickly as possible without producing excessive fluid.

Nursing actions are aimed at helping to prevent this problem, for example, by careful attention to replacing fluids lost after excessive perspiration with electrolyte solutions and irrigating naso-gastric tubes with saline solution rather than plain water.

## Potassium Excess

Potassium excess, or hyperkalemia, is an excess of potassium in the extracellular fluid. It can be caused by: renal disease, as a result of which the kidneys fail to excrete potassium normally; adrenal cortical insufficiency; burns; tissue trauma (when potassium escapes from the cells into the extracellular fluid); excessive potassium intake; rapid administration of stored blood; and respiratory or metabolic acidosis.

The client may experience nausea or diarrhea and intestinal colic (indicative of gastrointestinal hyperactivity); muscle weakness and paresthesias; muscle pain and cramps; dizziness; oliguria; and cardiac arrhythmias, which can be fatal. The electrocardiogram shows high peaked T waves and depressed S-T segment. The serum potassium is above 5.6 mEq/l.

In uncomplicated potassium excess, the treatment consists of avoiding additional potassium either orally or parenterally. This treatment method assumes normal kidney function. Other more complex methods used to remove excess potassium include dialysis and ion exchange resins.

Nursing measures for the client with potassium excess consist of attempts to lessen nausea and provide relief and comfort if there is diarrhea. Measuring urine output and reporting laboratory findings promptly are important functions. Preventive measures include educating the client about potassium intake, especially when there is a kidney problem. Careful administration of stored blood at a slow rate also will help prevent potassium excess.

## Potassium Deficit

Potassium deficit, or hypokalemia, is a deficit of extracellular potassium. It occurs in a great variety of conditions. It is caused by excessive loss of potassium in secretions and excretions, increased use of potassium by the body, or by decreased intake of potassium.

Administration of powerful diuretics without potassium supplementation is considered a leading cause of potassium deficit. Surgery involving the gastrointestinal tract with loss of potassium-rich fluids is another cause of potassium deficit. Vomiting, diarrhea, draining fistulas, excessive sweating, and fever also cause potassium deficit. These are only a few of the conditions likely to cause potassium deficit.

The symptoms of potassium deficit are caused largely by muscle weakness. At first the person just does not feel well. Then skeletal muscles become weak, with decreased or absent reflexes. Cardiac muscles are affected and the pulse becomes weak, heart sounds faint, blood pressure falls, and there is increased sensitivity to digitalis. Intestinal signs include anorexia, vomiting, gastric distention, and paralytic ileus. Respiratory muscle weakness produces shallow respirations, and death can occur from respiratory arrest. Laboratory findings include serum potassium, below 3.5 mEq/l. Electrocardiograph findings include low, flat T wave, depressed S-T segment, and prominent U wave.

Treatment is not difficult. Losses are counteracted by providing a high potassium diet or by oral administration of a potassium supplement. Intravenous solutions containing potassium are also given.

Again, nursing measures to prevent potassium deficit are of great importance. Persons taking diuretics must be taught the importance of eating foods that contain additional potassium. Because potassium cannot be stored it is necessary for everyone to take in an adequate amount of potassium daily. People who work under high environmental temperatures should be taught the importance of replacing both sodium and potassium lost in perspiration.

## SUMMARY

The basic elements of fluid and electrolyte balance were presented as a review. Preventing imbalance as well as nursing interventions to overcome imbalances were presented. Suggestions were made for encouraging fluid intake as well as methods to use when intake is restricted. Measuring intake and output, weighing, calculating intravenous flow rate and monitoring IV were discussed. Finally, there was a brief discussion of some common imbalances.

## LEARNING ACTIVITIES

1. Examine a hospitalized client's intake and output record for a 24-hour period and decide whether or not he is in fluid balance.

2. Explain to a client the meaning of fluid and electrolyte balance.

3. Describe what you would do if you walked into a room and found the intravenous bag was empty.

4. Identify the condition and implement nursing actions that are appropriate for a client with the manifestations of one of the fluid and electrolyte problems presented in the chapter.

## REFERENCES AND SUGGESTED READINGS

Aspinall, Mary Jo.   A simplified guide to managing patients with hyponatremia. *Nursing 78*, December, 1978, pp. 32–35.

*Baxter Guide to Fluid Therapy*, 1969. Morton Grove, Illinois: Baxter Laboratories.

Beaumont, Estelle. The new infusion pump. *Nursing 77*, July, 1977, pp. 31–35.

Burgess, Ann W., 1978. *Nursing: levels of health intervention.* Englewood Cliffs, N. J.: Prentice-Hall.

DuGas, Beverly, 1977. *Introduction to patient care.* Philadelphia: W. B. Saunders.

Fuerst, Elinor; Wolff, LuVerne; and Weitzel, Marlene, 1974. *Fundamentals of nursing.* 5th ed. Philadelphia: J. B. Lippincott.

Ganong, W. F., 1977. *Review of medical physiology.* 8th ed. Los Altos, Cal.: Lange Medical Publishers.

Lee, Carla; Stroot, Violet; and Schaper, C. Ann. Extracellular volume imbalance. *American Journal of Nursing*, May, 1974, pp. 888–891.

Metheny, Norma and Snively, W. D., 1974 *Nurses' handbook of fluid balance.* 2nd ed. Philadelphia: J. B. Lippincott.

Metheny, Norma and Snively, William. Perioperative fluids and electrolytes. *American Journal of Nursing*, May, 1978, pp. 840–845.

Piper, Mary. Fluid and electrolyte balance. *Nursing Mirror*, 143 (October 28, 1976), 55–57.

Reed, Gretchen. Confused about potassium? Here's a clear, concise guide. *Nursing 74*, March, 1974, pp. 20–27.

Reed, Gretchen and Sheppard, Vincent, 1977. *Regulation of fluid and electrolyte balance: a programmed instruction in clinical physiology.* 2nd ed. Philadelphia: W. B. Saunders Company.

Snider, Malle. Helpful hints on IV's. *American Journal of Nursing*, November, 1974, pp. 1978–1981.

Ungvarski, Peter. Parenteral therapy. *American Journal of Nursing*, December, 1976, pp. 1974–1977.

# 19

# Medication Preparation and Administration

Introduction
The Use of Medications
Medication History
The Medication Order
Medication Administration
Summary
Learning Activities
References and Suggested Readings

## Behavioral Objectives

Upon completion of this chapter, the student will be able to:

1. Take a medication history.
2. Instruct a client in the use of medications.
3. Calculate drug dosage.
4. Administer medications by the routes described to persons of all ages.

## Key Terms

allergy
ampule
Antabuse
anticoagulants
anticonvulsants
antidiabetic
antihistamine
antihypertensive
buccal
capsule
compliance
conjunctival sac
deltoid
drugs
generic
gluteus maximus
gluteus medius

grain
Hochstetter's site
intradermal
intramuscular
intravenous
liniment
lotion
medications
meniscus
milligram
narcotics
ointment
oral
over-the-counter
parenteral
pill

Povidone-Iodine
prescription
rectus femoris
sedatives
subcutaneous
sublingual
tablet
topical
tracking
tranquilizer
unit dose system
vastus lateralis
ventrogluteal
vial
viscosity
z-track

## Introduction

One important aspect of the nurse's role related to medications is to teach the client about his medication regimen. This includes drug actions and interactions, drug-food interactions, and drug-alcohol interactions. The hazards of over-the-counter medications are included in the teaching program.

Another essential nursing responsibility is the medication history; guidelines to taking such information are presented in this chapter.

The nurse prepares medications and administers them in many ways. The unit dose system (preparation of individual drug dose by the company or the pharmacist) is discussed, as well as the more traditional method of preparation from a stock supply.

Administration of medications orally, subcutaneously, intramuscularly, intradermally, intravenously, and topically are described. A method for calculating drug dosage is presented. It is hoped that some of the ritual surrounding the medication procedure, and the anxiety produced in the student as she learns, will be lessened by the approach taken in this chapter.

The nurse evaluates the effect of the drugs administered. However, in this chapter, information about specific drugs and their effects—both desired and adverse—is not included. The student should consult a pharmacology textbook for this information.

## THE USE OF MEDICATIONS

As the trend towards self-care continues, the need increases for clients to be knowledgeable about the medications necessary for their well-being. Bryar (1977) believes that self-care is being encouraged, intentionally or unintentionally, by increased home care and earlier hospital discharge. Certainly, as the focus turns to prevention rather than treatment of illness, the hazards of using any medication need to be made known.

### Over-the-Counter Medicines

Use of over-the-counter medications (those available without a prescription) for treatment of self-diagnosed symptoms is widespread (Bryar, 1977; Parker, 1976). Parker reports that nearly 40 percent of the population uses over-the-counter medicines. Knowledge of the known hazards of a medication, as well as the possibility of unknown dangers, should be available to the public in easily understood language. The ever-increasing scientific findings seem to suggest that no medication is without some danger. Aspirin, antacids, laxatives, and bromides are cited as the over-the-counter drugs most frequently involved in drug-induced illnesses requiring hospitalization (Caranasos, Stewart, Cluff, 1974).

While some over-the-counter drugs are harmless to most people in most instances when used as directed, some people cannot use them safely. There may be unknown reactions which can cause future problems. This can be seen in recent studies of the harmful effects of drugs and alcohol on developing fetuses.

Clients can be taught to relieve discomfort by means other than the use of medications: relaxation to lower tension; fluids and rest for a cold are examples. Probably the most important teaching goal is to change the attitude that a pill will cure almost anything.

## Using Someone Else's Medicines

The use of medications prescribed for someone else is widespread (Caranasos, Stewart, Cluff, 1974). Especially within the family, medications that have been left over from one member's illness are often given to another with similar symptoms. Dangers involved in this practice include all those of self-diagnosis and self-treatment. The second person's health problem may be different from the first person's, and the medicine may do harm as well as delay treatment. One person may not be allergic to the drug; another may. In addition, as the drug ages, its chemical properties change. It may have become either weaker (and ineffective) or stronger (and possibly toxic).

## Drugs/Medications

The terms *drugs* and *medications* are used interchangeably. However, not all lay people consider them synonymous. A person may say he takes a medication for a cold and a *drug* for sleep. Therefore, when we ask a person if he takes any medicines, we may get one answer and when we ask him if he takes any drugs, an entirely different one. The better question may be "Do you take any medicines? Prescribed? Over-the-counter?"

## MEDICATION HISTORY

Parker (1976) states that a medication history provides valuable information about past medical problems, the basis for planning present and future therapy, and a readily available drug profile for use by consultants. Information is sought about prescription as well as nonprescription medications, those taken currently as well as in the past, reactions to drugs and drug allergies, and compliance. Parker (1976) found that from 25 percent to more than 50 percent of all out-patients had failed to take medications as prescribed. Missed doses and failure to take the entire prescription occurred even more often.

The client should be asked the following questions about his medication history. These questions and their responses can be recorded on a convenient form for use by all health-care workers:

1. **Prescription Drugs**   What are the names of the medicines you are taking now that your doctor prescribed? If you don't know their names, do you have them with you? If not, can you describe them and tell why you were given them? What strength are they and how often each day do you take them?

2. **Nonprescription Medications**   Do you take any over-the-counter medicines or home remedies? For example, do you take anything for pain, stomach upsets, constipation, insomnia, colds, allergies? Do you take any vitamins? If you do, how many do you take and how often do you take them?

3. **Medicines Taken in the Past**   Some medicines have long-lasting effects. What prescribed medicines have you taken in the past? What non-prescribed ones?

4. **Reactions**   Whether the medicines were prescribed or not, how did your body react to each one?

5. **Allergies**   Define: do any drugs cause you problems? Do you have any known allergies to medicines? If so, describe them. Do you know how they were treated? Do you wear or carry identification stating your allergy?

6. **Compliance**   How often do you take your medicines? What do you do if you miss a dose? Did you take the pills as long as they lasted?

## Setting Up a Teaching Program

In setting up a specific teaching plan for a client concerning his prescribed medications, the nurse determines whether or not the client has accepted the need for the medication. The degree of motivation present plays an important role in how he learns (DeBarry, Jefferies, and Light, 1975).

The teaching sessions should be structured to fit in well with other scheduled events. The client should select the appropriate time for teaching whenever possible. Family members should be encouraged to be present during the teaching, because this tends to motivate the person to learn and reinforces the teaching. However, the fewer teachers involved, the better. Ideally, the staff nurse on the unit does the teaching. Since most of this information must be presented while the client is under the stress of hospitalization, it should be reinforced at a later time, either in the home or during an outpatient visit.

What should the nurse teach? DeBarry, Jefferies, and Light (1975) found that the name of the medicine was often difficult for their patients to learn. Some people never learned to pronounce or remember the names of their medications. These researchers believe that it would be sufficient if clients could pick out the specific pill from a group of pills. They suggest that the pharmacist might label the bottle with the purpose of the medication as well as its name; e.g. Digoxin: heart pill.

These researchers also discovered that the people in their sample had difficulty learning the actions of their medications, though the teachers admitted having difficulty explaining the difference between *purpose* and *action* in terms that could be easily understood (p. 2193). The authors believe that if the person knows why he is taking his medication, it is not essential for him to know its action.

The nurse should teach the dose of the medication, the frequency, and the way the medication is taken. She should also tell the client always to take the prescribed number of pills, as directed on the pill container, at the times directed, and as directed. Does he let the pill dissolve under his tongue (as with Nitroglycerin) or does he swallow it and drink a full glass of water?

Another important consideration in compliance—whether the client takes the medications when and as directed—is whether or not he has ready access to the medications. Does he have the money to pay for them? Can he get to the drug store to pick them up? Another question to be considered is whether he understands the directions. If a medication is ordered after each meal and at bedtime, it is usually assumed that four pills will be taken each day. Not everyone eats three meals a day and, therefore, less than the prescribed dose will be taken. When pills are ordered once or twice a day, they can be taken in the morning and at bedtime unless contraindicated. It is easier for the working person to take his pills at home than at work where he is apt to forget them.

A drug calendar is especially valuable when drugs are taken several times a week rather than daily. Another method is to put the day's supply of pills in full view so that the client will know that he needs to take them. These are a few suggestions. The individual client may have a system that works much better for him.

The nurse teaches the client where and how to store his medications. The pharmacist will indicate on the label if a medicine requires refrigeration, as well as the date after which the supply should not be used. Remind the client not to repackage his medications. While it seems handy for traveling to put all the pills in one container, for safety each medication should be kept in its original container.

It is important to keep all medications out of reach of children. Safety tops, which help protect children from access to medications, are difficult for some elderly persons to remove. If there are no children in the household, the pharmacist might be requested to use easy-off tops on the medication containers.

If there is anything the client must do before he takes his medication, he should be instructed in the procedure. For example, some persons must count their pulse to be sure it is 60 or above before they take a prescribed heart medication.

The client should be taught the pill's expected effects as well as the side effects of his medication. An antihistamine to relieve itching may also cause drowsiness. This has safety implications for the person who drives a car or works around dangerous machinery. He should also know clearly what side effects he should report immediately to the doctor.

The nurse should teach the client the interactive effects of the prescribed medication and any others (prescription or nonprescription) he may be taking. For example, a person taking Coumadin (Warfarin) is in danger of bleeding if he also takes aspirin.

The nurse needs to be continually aware of the potential for drug-food interactions and alert her client. Certain foods should be eaten when some medications are taken and avoided with others. For example, many diuretics require foods high in potassium (such as oranges and bananas) in the diet. Many antibiotics are poorly absorbed when there is food in the stomach and should be taken two hours before or after meals. Mixing drugs and liquids to mask the taste can alter the pH and thereby alter the absorption of the medicine.

Alcohol may either increase or decrease the action of medications. Serious problems have resulted because people were not aware of this interactive effect. Some dangerous combinations are listed below:

Alcohol + sedatives and tranquilizers
Alcohol + oral antidiabetic agents
Alcohol + anticoagulants
Alcohol + antihistamines
Alcohol + aspirin
Alcohol + narcotics
Alcohol + anticonvulsants
Alcohol + non-narcotic pain killers
Alcohol + Antabuse
Alcohol + antihypertensives

The effect of any combination that might involve a particular client should be clearly explained. Is the effect of the medication exaggerated or diminished, for example, by another substance? Caffeine and nicotine affect the way some medications work.

Because not all interactions are known, the client should be instructed to call the doctor immediately if any new symptom occurs.

In summary, the nurse should take the following steps to teach her clients about medication:

1. Explain the dangers of over-the-counter medications and their interactive effects with prescribed medications.
2. Define and describe the medication prescribed, the dose, frequency, method of administration, and anything special the client should do before, during, or after taking the medication.
3. Explain the medication's purpose.
4. Describe any side effects that should be reported immediately.
5. Instruct in proper storage of the medication.
6. Describe the interactive effects, if any, of foods, alcohol, caffeine, or nicotine when taken with the prescribed medication.
7. Instruct the client to take only the medication prescribed for him, in the dosage and manner prescribed.

8. Instruct him to keep an accurate count of his daily dose so that under- or over-medicating will not occur.
9. Instruct him to take the medication as long as it lasts (entire course of medication).

The hospitalized client is helped by taking his own medications under supervision before discharge. Written instructions, such as a separate drug card for each medication, including the important points about each, are given him. If injected medications are required, sterile techniques as well as the injection process are taught according to the technique described for nurses later in the chapter.

## THE MEDICATION ORDER

The doctor prescribes medication by writing the order on the doctor's order sheet or on a prescription blank. Under certain circumstances defined by the specific agency, telephone orders may be accepted by a registered nurse. She then writes the order, identifies it as a telephone order, signs the doctor's name and her own. The doctor signs the order at the first opportunity (or within the time period specified by the agency). In emergency situations, registered nurses follow verbal orders for medications. The inherent hazards in taking verbal orders in stressful situations are obvious.

In many agencies, the doctor's order sheet is duplicated and a copy sent to the pharmacist who prepares the medication. If there are any questions about the order, the pharmacist or the nurse contacts the doctor. In other agencies, the nurse or ward clerk transcribes the doctor's written order, places the drug order with the pharmacy, and makes the medication card. Computers are also being used to expedite medication ordering. When the nurse prepares medications, the drug card is compared with the original order, which is on the doctor's order sheet.

The drug order includes the date, the client's name and location, name of drug, dosage, method of administration, time for administration, a stop date if there is one, any special directions for administration, and the doctor's signature. If the order is written on a prescription pad, it will also include the number of permitted refills and any other pertinent labeling directions.

Sample medication order written on doctor's order sheet:

16 August 19—                 Joe Doe                 Room 267B

Peritrate 80 mg. p.o. b.i.d. p.c.

signed: Paul Junner, M.D.

*interpretation:* p.o., by mouth; b.i.d., twice a day (e.g., 9 a.m. and 5 p.m.); p.c., after meals.

Increasingly, the generic drug name rather than the trade name (e.g., Peritrate) is written. Usually the prescription can be filled at a lower cost if the drug is available generically. Despite the pros and cons surrounding the provision of drugs under their generic names, consumers are becoming more and more vocal in their demand for them.

## Abbreviations

Only standard abbreviations are used in writing prescriptions. A table of common abbreviations is printed inside the back cover.

## Sources of Drug Information

The nurse can find the prescribed drug's purpose, usual dose, desired action, effect, and side effects from a nursing textbook in pharmacology, the *Hospital Formulary*, or a similar publication. The *Physician's Desk Reference* (PDR) is made available by funds from the drug companies and is a compilation of information found in the drug inserts which accompany all medications. Because of its drug company affiliation some practitioners consider it to be an unreliable source. When information cannot be obtained from a readily available printed source, the pharmacist is usually able to provide it.

## Safety

The nurse is legally responsible for her own actions. She is expected to question a doctor's order if she suspects that it is contrary to the usual drug, dose, or method of administration. She is also responsible for observing and reporting the medication's effect. Is the drug producing the desired effect? Are any side effects displayed? Levine (1970) has found that, despite this agreed-upon responsibility, the effect of drug therapy is seldom reported by nurses.

The largely accepted rule, called the *Five Rights*, is considered an important safety measure: the right drug, the right dose, the right route, at the right time, to the right patient. The unit-dose system has helped increase the safety in administering the right drug, dose, and route. The right patient is correctly identified by asking the person his name and then, in most agencies, by checking his identification band. The right time for medication administration is designated by the agency: it is usually between 15 and 30 minutes of the time stated on the order. While some medications clearly must be given at a precise time, it is impossible for each medication to be given at the exact time ordered unless the nurse-client ratio is 1:1. For example, a medication ordered once a day is usually given at 9 or 10 A.M. However, there is usually no reason why it cannot be given later. One author suggests that allowing more leeway in the time would allow drugs to be administered at a more appropriate time based on the drug's action.

Many authorities insist that, when the nurse is preparing medications, she read the label three times. This is part of the medication ritual that has *not* increased the safety of the procedure. The best procedure to select the right drug from a stock supply is to *compare* the label on the medication container with the medication card or the Kardex. In this way, drugs that are spelled similarly will not be confused.

Medications are stored securely and appropriately. The medication cupboards or carts are locked. Medications requiring refrigeration are stored in a medication refrigerator. Narcotics are always strictly controlled. Specific regulations for the storage and recording of controlled drugs are spelled out by the agency and regulated by the law. Counting drugs regularly to verify the written drug record and installing special locked storage areas are among the safeguards established.

For safety, once a drug has been poured from the stock supply, it is discarded if it is not administered. This is not necessary with the unit dose because the drug package is not opened until the nurse is at the client's bedside.

It is important, while preparing and giving medications, to avoid distractions caused by interruptions and conversing. The nurse who gives the medications is legally responsible, and for this reason the person who prepares the medications administers them. Considerable risk is assumed in giving what someone else has prepared. Again, with the unit dose this is less of a problem.

Despite all the precautions taken to avoid medication errors, errors will still occur. When this happens, the nurse's concern is for her client's safety. The doctor is notified immediately and the error is described on the chart. Any necessary remedial measures for the client's welfare must be carried out. Agencies frequently require that an incident report be filed when there is a medication error. The situation is fully explained on the report and the action taken to remedy the problem is recorded. The doctor's signature, as well as that of the nurse, is required.

## Preparation of Medications

As the pharmacist becomes more involved in the total preparation of medications for administration, the nurse is freed increasingly from this task. Unit dose (premeasured, individually packaged and labelled medications) is one method of medication preparation currently in use. Pouring a certain number of pills from a stock bottle to a pill cup is fast becoming obsolete in agency settings, and with this change, medication errors are decreasing. It is possible that some of the rituals surrounding the medication procedure will become less necessary.

Unit-Dose System   In this system, the pharmacist or drug company is responsible for the preparation of drugs in premeasured, prepackaged, and labelled individual doses. A carbon copy of the doctor's order is sent to the pharmacy where it is interpreted, filled, and delivered to the nursing unit. Refills and charges are also taken care of in the pharmacy. Drugs are delivered on a scheduled basis (usually twice a day) as well as on a *stat* (immediate) basis.

The nurse or ward clerk transcribes the order to the medication Kardex.

Usually it is here that the medication is recorded after it is given. This becomes a part of the client's permanent record.

Advantages of the unit-dose system include accuracy, speed, and convenience for the nurse who administers the medication. Medication errors should decrease because both nurse and pharmacist scrutinize the records. The process takes less of the nurse's time and therefore more time is available for direct client care. According to the study conducted by Steward, Kelly, and Dinel (1976), under the unit-dose system, team leaders spent 8 percent of their time on medication functions. Under the traditional system they spent 21 percent of their time on medications. Additional advantages include the decreased cost of medications on "stand-by," because the stock of medications kept on the floor or ward are markedly decreased. There is also less waste and pilferage, which decreases cost. Other materials such as charge slips, medication cards, and medication cups are nearly eliminated.

## MEDICATION ADMINISTRATION

Included among the factors determining the route of drug administration are the nature of the drug, the site of its desired action, and the rapidity of the desired effect. Drugs are administered by mouth, parenterally (in general practice means by injection), and topically.

### Oral

The oral method is a convenient, safe, and economical way to give medications when it is appropriate to do so. Medications cannot be given orally, for example, when a person cannot swallow, is unconscious, is vomiting, or is fasting. In addition, some medications cannot be given orally. Oral medications may have a local effect on the gastrointestinal mucosa. If absorbed into the blood stream, they have a systemic effect. Because of their slower action, drugs given orally are more easily controlled than those given parenterally.

Oral medications may be in the form of tablets, capsules, pills, or liquids. Tablets (a compressed dry form of the drug), if scored, may be carefully divided to obtain the ordered dose. Tablets may be crushed, if necessary. Capsules cannot be emptied, nor can pills be crushed or divided without altering their known dosage or action. For example, enteric coated pills are covered with a substance that delays the drug's release until it reaches the intestines. If these are crushed, the onset of action occurs earlier. A pill is a globe-shaped solid form of a drug. A capsule is a medication enclosed in a gelatinous container. A capsule may be used to disguise the taste of a medication or to alter its absorption rate, as in a spansule. A few drugs are dissolved and absorbed while in the mouth. A buccal medication is placed in the cheek; a sublingual medication under the tongue.

Some liquid medications are suspensions. They must be shaken well before administration to distribute the particles evenly in order to ensure an accurate dose. The bottle will be so labeled.

If a person vomits after taking his medicine, the doctor should be consulted about the possibility of administering the drug by another route. If a person has trouble swallowing a tablet, it may be crushed. The doctor or pharmacist is consulted about supplying the medication in liquid form.

Any special instructions for drug administration should be clearly indicated on the medication Kardex or medication card. For example, liquid potassium products may be given with orange juice to disguise the taste; mineral oil is chilled before administration and followed with orange juice to increase palatability. Some liquid medications stain the teeth and are taken with a straw. Cough syrups are not followed with water. Cough syrups have a local effect, as do throat lozenges. Lozenges are dissolved in the mouth and not chewed, swallowed whole, or followed by water. Some persons are required to count their pulse to see if it is above 60 beats per minute before they take Digitalis. All of these special directions should be clearly outlined.

## Special Considerations: Giving oral medications

As with all procedures in which client contact is required, the nurse washes her hands before she begins, in order to prevent the spread of pathogens from nurse to client. She carefully checks the doctor's order to identify any discrepancies in medication orders (e.g., discontinuation of drug). She identifies the client accurately by asking his name rather than saying, for example, "Are you John Simpson?" Then she reads the identification band to verify the client's response. Other considerations:

1. The client should sit upright, if possible, to take the medication in order to lessen the danger of choking (aspiration).
2. Inform the client of the purpose and action of the medication he is receiving.
3. Give water or other liquids after a medication to help the client swallow, to dilute the medicine, and to enhance the palatability.
4. The unit dose tablets and liquids are individually packaged in disposable containers. The client drinks the liquid directly from the original container. This is a safety measure; it also prevents waste.

The nurse stays with the person until he has swallowed his medication as an assurance that he has indeed swallowed it. As the client is allowed more responsibility for his own care, this ritual may become unnecessary. A few medications currently are kept at the bedside for use as needed. These include nitroglycerin and antacids.

Ordinarily, the physician is contacted if the medication cannot be given for any reason. It is more important that some drugs not be omitted than others. In some agencies, the administration time is circled if the drug has been omitted (for example, a drug is omitted if a person is fasting for a diagnostic test or surgery). If the drug is refused, this is reported and recorded promptly. The nurse must try to find out why the drug was refused. A client may refuse a medication because he does not think it is meant for him. If it is a new order, it can be easily explained. However, if it is not a new order, his refusal is an indication that the drug card should be rechecked against the doctor's original order. The reason for the omission of a drug is recorded on the Kardex or the nurses' notes. If a drug has been forgotten, this fact should be reported immediately upon discovery so that the decision to give the drug or not can be made.

The medication is handled as little as possible to prevent the spread of pathogens from nurse to medication to client. The medication must be identifiable at all times. Therefore, each medication is placed in a separate cup. For example, if the drug is Digoxin, and the client's apical pulse is 50, the nurse will not give the drug. She must be able to correctly identify it by having it in its own medication cup with a medication card.

A liquid medication is poured with the label up so that dripping medication will not stain the label and make it difficult to read. The medication cup is held at eye level during the pouring for accuracy in measurement. The liquid reading is made at the bottom of the meniscus. Then the bottle top is wiped

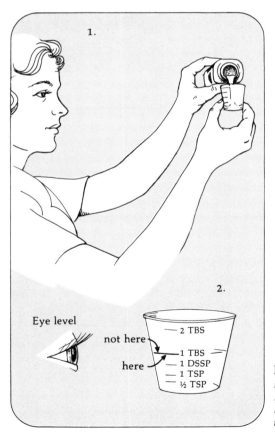

**Figure 19-1.** *Measuring liquid medication: (1) Pour from the bottle with the label held up. (2) Hold the medication cup at eye level and measure the dose from the bottom of the meniscus.*

clean before it is replaced on the shelf to keep it from sticking the next time it is used.

---

## Performance Checklist

### Giving Oral Medications when Using the Unit-Dose System:

1. Wash your hands.
2. Compare the medication order on the Kardex with that on the doctor's order sheet and the label on the medication package.
3. Take the medication cart (or medication on tray) to the client area.
4. Ask the client his name and then check his identification band as you explain the need for this procedure.
5. If necessary, assist the client to sit up.
6. Inform him of the medication's purpose, taking into account his individual desire to know.
7. Open the unit-dose package and place the pill (or liquid in its original container) in the person's hand.
8. Give water or other liquids as permitted or desired.
9. Stay with the client until he has taken his medication.
10. Record medication immediately in the appropriate place and manner as: given, refused, or omitted.

---

## Performance Checklist

### Giving Medications from the Stock Supply

1. Compare the drug card with the doctor's order.
2. Wash your hands.
3. Prepare the drug:
   a. select the correct medication from the shelf by comparing the medication card information with the medication container label
   b. pour the pill from bottle cap to medicine cup
   c. compare the medication card and bottle label again as the bottle is returned to the shelf.
   d. Keep the medication cup and card together on a tray at all times.
   e. If more than one medication is being given, place each in a separate cup.
   f. For liquid medications:
      1) calculate the desired dose
      2) with the bottle label turned up and medication cup held at eye level, pour the amount desired
      3) wipe top of bottle with paper towel before replacing cap; return container to shelf
      4) if medication is ordered by drops, place ordered amount in medication cup
4. Take the medication with the card to client's bedside and administer according to procedure for giving unit-dose medications. Substitute the following for step 7; Hand the medication cup to the person.

## Dosage Computation

While entire courses have been taught in dosage calculations, the actual computation involves problem-solving techniques familiar to most students. As the unit dose system becomes more widely used, nurses will be required to do less calculation. However, the nurse should always be able to calculate a dosage or check the calculations of others should the need arise. Some general comments related to calculation are:

1.  Only tablets that are scored can be cut in half if accuracy is to be ensured.
2.  If the calculated dose seems excessive (e.g., 4 to 5 pills), recalculate. Except in a few instances, recommended doses are manufactured so that one pill, of the required strength, can be administered. Therefore, half a tablet or two tablets might be reasonable, but four or five tablets would not. The same holds true for parenteral medications. Usually one ampule, a portion of an ampule, or two ampules may be required but seldom as many as four or five. It is a wise practice to have someone check your calculation for accuracy; it is essential if you have any questions and sometimes it is required by the agency.

**Method of Calculation**  One method of calculating the prescribed dose is to form a ratio of the prescribed dose over the available dose.

*Example:*  prescribed dose:  5 mg

available dose:  1 mg = 2 ml

$$\frac{5 \text{ mg}}{1 \text{ mg} = 2 \text{ ml}} \qquad 5.00 \div 1 = 5 \qquad \begin{array}{l} 5 \times 2 \text{ ml} = 10 \text{ ml} \\ \text{(amount required} \\ \text{to deliver 5 mg)} \end{array}$$

Another method for solving dosage problems uses dimensional analysis (Carr, McElroy, and Carr, 1976). Given amounts are multiplied by conversion factors equivalent to 1 until *only the desired units are left uncancelled in the answer.*

*Example:*  Question:  How many milligrams are there in 3 grains?

There are 2 facts: the first one is given: there are 3 grains. The second fact that 60 mg = 1 gr is obtained from a conversion table.

Write the two facts as $\dfrac{60 \text{ mg} = 1}{1 \text{ gr}}$

or

$$\dfrac{1 \text{ gr}}{60 \text{ mg}} = 1$$

Select the ratio that will cancel the gr unit in the numerator. Grain in numerator can only be cancelled by grain in denominator.

For example,        3 gr × $\dfrac{60 \text{ mg}}{1 \text{ gr}}$

$$3 × 60 \text{ mg} = 180 \text{ mg}$$

$$3 \text{ gr} = 180 \text{ mg}$$

More information related to dimensional analysis is available in the article cited.

## Parenteral Medications

Parenteral medications are those given by injection. Injections are prescribed when the client cannot take medication by mouth, when the digestive juices would counteract the drug's effect, when a more rapid action is desired, when medication is to be concentrated in a specific part of the body, and when a local anesthetic action is desired.

Nurses are involved in administering subcutaneous, intramuscular, and intravenous medications. They also may be called upon to give intradermal injections, which are usually diagnostic. Agency policy defines what medications may be given parenterally by nurses.

Subcutaneous, intradermal, intramuscular, and intravenous injections will be described as well as the preparation of injections.

**Special Considerations: Preparing Injections**

Unit dose injections are delivered from the pharmacy already prepared. Therefore, no calculations or preparations are necessary. When other systems are used, the medications for injection are contained in vials, ampules, or cartridges. Sterile technique is used for giving injections because, while the unbroken skin is a barrier against infection, anything that breaks the skin (e.g., a needle) breaks that barrier. The need for clean hands and sterile equipment is clear.

A sterile syringe and needle are obtained. Usually one-time use, disposable sterile needles and syringes are available. Even in the home, people usually find the convenience and comfort (needles are always sharp) of disposable equipment worth the cost. Students often find that at first their hands shake a little as they prepare an injection. If the needle or any part of the inside of the syringe or plunger is touched, it is contaminated and must be discarded and replaced with sterile equipment. The student should begin again with the knowledge that almost every nurse has experienced similar problems.

Syringes are packaged with or without needles, in paper packages or plastic containers. The size (caliber and length) of the needle depends upon the site of the injection, the size of the client, and the viscosity of the medication. For example, a 25 G, ⅝ inch needle may be used for a subcutaneous injection; a 21 G, 1½ inch needle for an intramuscular. The gauge of the needle refers to the width of the internal diameter. The larger the number of the needle gauge the smaller its size; for example, number 25 and 26 needles have a small internal

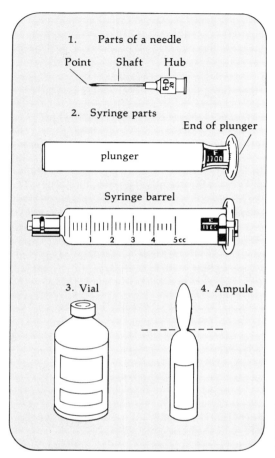

1.   Parts of a needle

Point    Shaft    Hub

2.   Syringe parts

End of plunger

plunger

Syringe barrel

1   2   3   4   5cc

3. Vial                    4. Ampule

**Figure 19-2.**   *Equipment for injections: (1) Parts of a needle. (2) Parts of a syringe. (3) A vial is a closed system. (4) An ampule is an open system.*

diameter and number 19 and 20 needles have a large internal diameter. The shorter length needles (e.g. ⅝ inch or ½ inch) are used for subcutaneous or intradermal injections. Longer needles are used for intramuscular or intravenous injections. The size of the syringe chosen will depend upon the volume of the medication. Syringes are usually available in 1, 3, 5, 10 ml, and larger sizes.

The syringe and needle are examined for close fit (needle securely attached to syringe), or else medication will be lost and the equipment contaminated. Because this is a sterile procedure, all attempts are made to assure a sterile system. The rubber stopper on the vial is cleansed with an antiseptic solution before the needle is inserted, and only the end of the plunger is manipulated. Air is inserted into the medication vial to increase the pressure within the vial and make withdrawal of the medication easier. The air is injected into the air space in the vial rather than into the medication to prevent formation of air bubbles and, therefore, difficult measurement. Any air in the syringe alters the amount of medication. If the dose level is read when there is air in the syringe, the person will get less medication than that prescribed.

When medication is contained in an ampule, it is important to consider the following: Any medication that stays in the top of the ampule is lost for usage; therefore, it must be flicked to the bottom of the ampule before the top is snapped off. Ampules are cleansed at the site where the top will be snapped off to assist in keeping this a sterile procedure. Glass ampules can cut the fingers unless precautions are taken. Ampules are easy to upset; holding them as the medication is withdrawn prevents spills. There is no need to add air to the open system (the ampule) as there is in the closed system (the vial). Care is taken to insert the needle directly into the ampule so that sterility is maintained. If the total amount of medication in the ampule is not used, it is discarded, because there is no suitable way to maintain its sterility. Agency policy may require special recording of the amount discarded, especially if the substance is a narcotic.

---

### Performance Checklist
### Removing Medication from a Vial

1. Compare medication card with doctor's order for medication, dosage, and route.
2. Wash hands.
3. Obtain syringe and needle of proper size as well as skin cleansing agent.
4. Test to see that needle is tightly attached to hub of syringe by pushing it straight on.
5. Cleanse the rubber stopper on the vial with antiseptic solution.
6. Remove and retain plastic needle cap.
7. Manipulating only the end of the plunger, draw into the syringe the amount of air equal to the amount of medication to be withdrawn from the vial.
8. Pick up the vial, inject the air into the air space in the vial.
9. Withdraw the prescribed amount of medication into syringe. If there are any air bubbles in syringe, hold syringe vertically and push them out until a drop of medication appears at needle lumen.
10. Withdraw the needle from the vial.
11. Replace protective cap on needle.
12. Place syringe with medication, medication card, and antiseptic wipe on tray.

---

## Administering a Subcutaneous Injection

Medications are given by the subcutaneous route (into the tissue layer under the skin) when slow absorption is desired. Intramuscular and intravenous routes provide quicker absorption. Irritating medications are not given subcutaneously because of poor tissue tolerance.

### Special Considerations
While any subcutaneous tissue can be used for injection, the usual sites are:

## Performance Checklist
### Removing Medication from an Ampule

1. Compare medication card with doctor's order sheet.
2. Wash hands.
3. Use your fingers to flick down any medication contained in the top of the ampule.
4. Using an antiseptic wipe, cleanse the neck of the ampule at the scored line.
5. With one hand holding the ampule top, antiseptic wipe wrapped around its neck, and the other hand holding the bottom of the ampule, snap the top away from you.
6. Either hold the open ampule in your nondominant hand or set the ampule on the medication tray.
7. With no air in the syringe, insert the needle directly into the ampule.
8. Withdraw the amount of medication required.
9. After needle is withdrawn from ampule, replace protective needle cover.
10. Place medication-filled syringe and antiseptic wipe on tray with medication card.
11. Discard any unused medication remaining in the ampule.

## Performance Checklist
### Using a Tubex Syringe

1. Compare medication card with doctor's order sheet.
2. Wash hands.
3. Obtain medication cartridge, metal tubex syringe, and antiseptic wipe.
4. Grasp the barrel of the syringe in one hand; pull back on the plunger with the other hand until entire plunger section swings downward at a 90 degree angle.
5. Insert cartridge into barrel, needle end first.
6. Rotate cartridge several turns clockwise until front end is threaded in place.
7. Swing plunger into place and rotate it clockwise 3 or 4 turns until back end of cartridge is threaded in place.
8. If entire medication is not required, remove rubber needle sheath, discard medication not needed, and replace sheath.
9. Place filled syringe and antiseptic wipe on tray with medication card.
10. Administer medication by the route ordered according to procedure on pages 363 and 366.
11. Remove cartridge from syringe by reversing insertion process: turn counterclockwise, plunger end first to release back end of cartridge, then turn front of cartridge counterclockwise. Break off needle and dispose of cartridge as indicated by agency policy.
12. Return metal syringe to storage area.

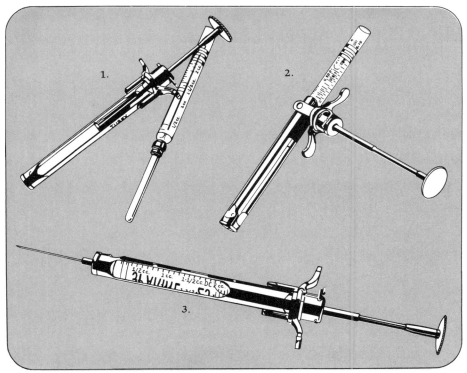

**Figure 19-3.**  *Using a Tubex syringe.*

the dorsilateral aspect of the upper arm, the abdomen (except around the beltline and about an inch around the umbilicus), and the anterior and lateral thighs approximately 3 inches above the knee. Sites free from scars, freckles, or bruises are chosen.

When frequent injections are given, the injection site is rotated in an orderly fashion to facilitate absorption and lessen discomfort. When a proper site is chosen, it is seldom that a blood vessel is entered. Aspirating (pulling back on the plunger) is a safeguard to ascertain that the needle has not entered a blood vessel.

Good judgment will determine whether spreading the skin or picking it up will be more likely to have the needle reach subcutaneous tissue. The size and health condition of the client help determine amount of subcutaneous tissue. This tissue is abundant in well-hydrated, well-nourished persons but not in those who are poorly nourished and dehydrated. Nursing judgment determines how far and at what angle the needle should be inserted.

To cleanse the skin, a circular motion from the inside out and friction at the injection site lessen the danger of injecting organisms into the tissues. A skin cleansing agent such as Providone-iodine solution or alcohol is used. The wipe is held where it will be easily accessible when the needle is withdrawn. Most

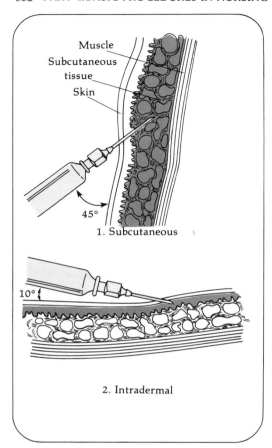

**Figure 19-4.** *(1) The needle is inserted at a 45-degree angle for a subcutaneous injection. (2) The needle is inserted just under the skin for an intradermal injection.*

authorities suggest that a bit of the shaft of the needle be visible in case the needle breaks; then the needle can be removed by grasping the shaft. Needles seldom break off after they have been inserted. Before the needle is removed from the tissue, the site is covered with the antiseptic wipe so that the medication will not seep out. Then the needle itself is quickly covered as a protective measure. Massaging the tissue aids in distribution and absorption of the medication. Massage, however, is contraindicated when some medications are given (e.g., Heparin). It is important to record the injection site so that an orderly system of rotation can be followed. The needle and syringe are destroyed by cutting just below the hub so that they cannot be used again.

## Intradermal Injections

Intradermal injections are most often used for diagnostic purposes to determine the presence of disease, allergies, or drug sensitivities. Absorption

## Performance Checklist
### Giving a Subcutaneous Injection

1. Take the prepared medication to the client.
2. Identify him by asking his name and then reading his identification band.
3. Explain the purpose of the medication.
4. Select an appropriate injection site.
5. Using a circular motion, cleanse the injection site.
6. Place the antiseptic wipe between the 4th and 5th fingers of your nondominant hand.
7. Either pick up and hold the skin and subcutaneous tissue to be injected or spread the tissue.
8. Remove the needle cover.
9. Inject the needle, usually at a 45 degree angle.
10. Release your hold on the tissue.
11. Withdraw the needle a little so that some of the needle shaft can be seen.
12. While supporting the syringe with one hand, aspirate (pull back on the plunger) with the other.
13. If no blood appears, slowly inject solution.
14. Place antiseptic wipe over needle site, quickly withdraw needle, and cover it with protective cap.
15. Gently massage area unless contraindicated.
16. Make client comfortable.
17. Record injection in appropriate place: include drug, amount, route, and site. Sign record.
18. Dispose of needle and syringe appropriately.

takes longer from this method of injection than from any other. The usual injection site is the medial aspect of the anterior surface of the forearm approximately 2 inches below the elbow. Other sites can be used as long as they can be readily observed for reactions.

**Special Considerations**

The skin is drawn taut before the needle is inserted so that it more easily enters the tissue just under the skin. The welt (wheal or elevation) produced indicates that the medication is in the proper location, just under the skin. Some reactions to be watched for after injection include redness, itching, pain, increased size of the wheal. These reactions, which occur if the person is allergic to the injected substance, may occur suddenly or after several days.

Equipment includes a tuberculin syringe for accurate measurement of the small amount of solution used (0.01–1 ml). The needle is 25–27 gauge, ¼ to ⅝ inch long. Preparation of the needle, syringe, and solution is the same as that described for other injections.

---

### Performance Checklist
#### Intradermal Injections

1.  Take the prepared injection to the client.
2.  Identify him and explain the procedure.
3.  Select and cleanse the injection site.
4.  Expel any air that remains in the syringe.
5.  Draw the skin taut over the proposed injection site.
6.  Insert the needle, bevel up, almost parallel to the skin (10-15 degree angle) so that the needle shaft is under the skin to a depth of 1/16 to 1/8 inch.
7.  Slowly inject solution. If medication seeps out, insert needle deeper; if welt does not appear, withdraw shaft slightly.
8.  Place antiseptic wipe over needle site, quickly withdraw needle. Do no apply pressure.
9.  Make client comfortable as you observe for reactions.
10. Record injection.
11. Dispose of equipment.

---

## Intramuscular Injections

The intramuscular injection provides fairly rapid but sustained drug action. Potentially irritating and painful drugs are better tolerated by the muscle than by the subcutaneous tissue. Absorption from both the intramuscular and subcutaneous sites depends upon the blood supply to and from the site. For example, areas of edema or paralysis are not used for injections.

### Special Considerations

The maximum amount of solution given into large muscle is 2 to 3 ml. When the required volume exceeds this amount, half the solution is given in one site and half in another. This prevents the discomfort of pressure caused by a large amount of fluid in the tissues.

The age, build, and physical condition of the client will help determine the muscle chosen for injection. In the adult, the muscle sites most frequently chosen are the posterior gluteal, the ventrogluteal (Hochstetter's site), the vastus lateralis, and the deltoid. These muscle sites provide safe areas for administration, as they are removed from major blood vessels, bones, and nerves. Because injections into tense muscles cause pain, the nurse encourages relaxation techniques. For example, for a posterior gluteal injection, the client lies in prone position with toes turned in.

The deltoid muscle provides a relatively small area for injection. As indicated in Figure 19–5, this area is bounded on the top by the lower edge of the acromion process, on the bottom by the axilla, and by the lateral third of the arm. No more than 1 ml of solution is injected at this site and no oily preparations are injected here.

The *gluteus maximus* and *medius* are two frequently chosen sites for intramuscular injections. Guidelines for injection into the *gluteus maximus* are as

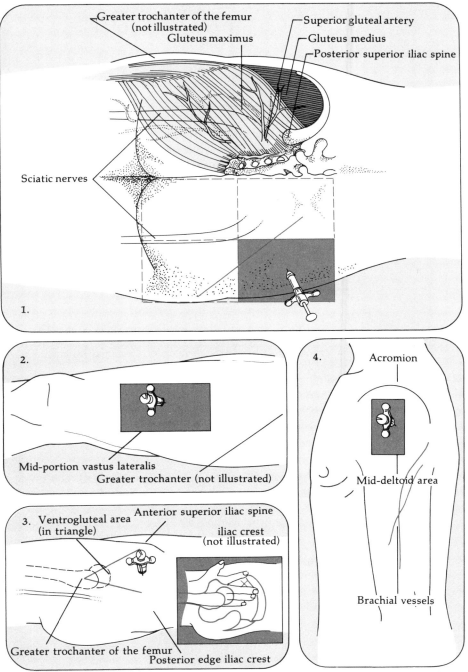

**Figure 19-5.** *Intramuscular injection sites: (1) Posterior gluteal, needle inserted into the gluteus medius. (2) Vastus lateralis. (3) Ventrogluteal (Hochstetter's site). (4) Deltoid.*

follows: draw an upper line across the iliac crest; draw a lower line at the lower edge of the buttock; draw lateral lines at the division of the buttocks and the outer edge of the body. Divide this area into four equal parts. Give the injection in the upper outer quadrant, 2 to 3 inches below the top of the iliac crest.

Injection into the *gluteus medius* is above and outside a diagonal line connecting the greater trochanter with the posterior superior iliac spine (see sketch).

For injections into the posterior gluteal muscles, the client should be lying prone with toes turned in for relaxation. While modesty is to be preserved, the area must be well-exposed so that landmarks can be properly identified.

The *ventrogluteal* muscle (Hochstetter's site) has a very small fatty layer and a thick muscle layer. It is a good site for injection for persons of any age. The person may be in either the prone, supine, or side-lying position. The nurse identifies the site by placing her palm on the greater trochanter, index finger on the anterior superior iliac spine, middle finger spread as far as possible along the iliac crest. The center of the triangle formed by the index and middle fingers is the injection site.

---

### Performance Checklist
### Giving an Intramuscular Injection

1. As for any other medication, verify the drug order by comparing the medication card or Kardex order with the doctor's order sheet.
2. Wash your hands.
3. Prepare medication from ampule, vial, cartridge, or obtain unit-dose injection. Select needle size dependent upon person's body size and medication viscosity.
4. Add 0.2 ml of air to the medication in the syringe to prevent tracking.
5. Take medication to client; identify him and explain the purpose of the medication.
6. Help client assume the correct position for the site chosen for injection.
7. Cleanse site with antiseptic wipe; place wipe between the 4th and 5th fingers for later use.
8. Spread (or "pick up") tissue at injection site.
9. Rest the heel of the hand holding the syringe on the person's skin.
10. Holding the syringe vertically with the needle at a 90 degree angle, plunge the needle quickly into the tissue until only a small portion of the shaft is visible.
11. While steadying the syringe with one hand, pull back on plunger with other hand (aspirate). If blood returns, remove needle, prepare new injection, and select another injection site.
12. Slowly inject the medication and the air bubble.
13. Place wipe at site of needle insertion, quickly remove needle, and apply pressure. Massage area only if absorption is to be hastened.
14. Record: medication given, time, dose, route, location. Sign entry.

The *vastus lateralis* muscle, on the side of the leg, is a thick muscle with no large blood vessels or nerves near it. The person may lie on his back or sit.

Additional considerations when an intramuscular injection is to be given include the following: The length and gauge of the needle are selected so that the needle will reach the muscle layer and the needle gauge is large enough to permit the medication to flow freely through the needle opening. Whether the skin is spread or picked up depends upon the size of the muscle and the needle length. If possible, the client should be allowed to help decide where the injection will be given. If the heel of the nurse's hand rests on the client's skin, it provides some reassurance and also provides good positioning for the needle thrust.

To prevent "tracking," air is added after the medication is drawn into the syringe. This air forces the solution through the needle and then seals it in the tissue where it was injected. If medication remains in the needle, "tracking" of the medication through the tissue occurs as the needle is withdrawn. Pain and damage to underlying tissues may then occur.

## Z-Track Injections

The Z-track method of injection is used when the medication causes staining or irritation of the superficial tissues if it "tracks" out of the muscle where it is injected. Imferon (an iron preparation) is one drug given by the Z-track method.

### Special Considerations

This method differs from other intramuscular injections in the following ways: The tissue is displaced before the needle is inserted; a 0.5 ml air bubble is introduced; the area is not massaged; the posterior gluteal muscles are used

---

Performance Checklist

Z-Track Injection

1. After withdrawing required amount of medication, add 0.5 ml air.
2. Change to a fresh 2-inch needle.
3. Select the posterior gluteal site.
4. Cleanse skin.
5. Pull the skin toward the lateral aspect of the buttock.
6. Insert needle at 90 degree angle.
7. Aspirate.
8. Slowly inject medication and air bubble.
9. Wait 10 seconds.
10. Withdraw needle.
11. Release the skin.
12. Do not massage area of injection.
13. Record medication, dose, and site.
14. Discard equipment appropriately.

for injection sites; and a needle 2 inches long is used. All of the above steps are used to prevent "tracking" and to keep the medication in the deep muscle tissue where it was injected.

## Intravenous Medication

In this chapter, techniques for adding medication to existing intravenous lines are described. In chapter 18 on fluids and electrolytes, the procedure for monitoring an intravenous was presented.

Agency policy, based on the state law, defines the nurse's role in administering intravenous medication. What drugs she can give and under what circumstances she can give them are outlined in the agency policies. It is, of course, essential that the nurse know what is permitted in the state where she is practicing.

Drugs are given intravenously if they are irritating or ineffective if given by another route, when rapid action is required, and when consistent drug levels are required.

### Special Considerations

Geolot and McKinney (1975) outlined several important points to be considered before a drug can be given safely by the intravenous route. These include dilution, rate of administration, and drug compatibility.

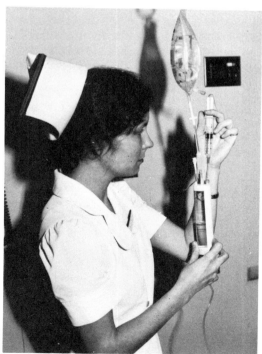

Figure 19-6. *Adding medication to a volume-control chamber. (Photo by Frank R. Engler, Jr.)*

The dilution decision is based on the properties of the drug, the desired action, and the condition of the person receiving the drug. The doctor's order (or the medication insert) will indicate if the drug is to be diluted, and how. When quick action is desired, drugs may be diluted in a small fluid volume and given directly into the vein (sometimes referred to as intravenous push). Other drugs require greater dilution and a longer administration time and are placed in a volume-controlled device such as a Buretrol or a Soluset. Still other drugs are placed directly in the infusion bag.

The amount and kind of solution to be used for diluting the intravenous medication are determined by the doctor or the directions accompanying the packaged medication. Drugs are never combined in an intravenous solution unless they have been proven compatible. Lists of drugs that can be mixed in intravenous fluids are available from the pharmacy and should be posted in a

---

### Performance Checklist
### Giving Intravenous Medications

Adding Medication to a Volume-Control Chamber:
1. Check the infusion site for any signs of infiltration or inflammation.
2. Open the clamp between the medication unit and the fluid reservoir (bag or bottle) to allow 10-15 ml of fluid into the chamber.
3. Close the clamp.
4. Cleanse the rubber top on the medication injection site (called the port) with the antiseptic wipe and inject the medication from the syringe into the volume-control chamber.
5. Open clamp again to rinse any trapped medication into the chamber and fill to desired level to provide proper dilution.
6. Close clamp and gently shake or squeeze chamber to help distribute drug throughout the chamber.
7. Regulate flow as ordered. Label chamber to indicate drug and dose being administered.
8. When medication chamber is empty, flush remaining medication from tubing by running solution from the intravenous reservoir through the tubing.
9. Clamp off medication unit and proceed with usual intravenous therapy as ordered.

Adding Medications to Intravenous Bag or Bottle:
1. Cleanse medication port on IV bag.
2. Insert sterile needle through rubber (or opening in bottle) and push plunger of syringe to place medication in bag (or bottle). Mix by gently squeezing or turning receptable.
3. Remove needle. Dispose of needle and syringe appropriately.
4. Place label on container to indicate medication, dose, date and time added, and name of person adding medication.

conspicuous place.

When there is an existing intravenous, it is important to be certain the needle is in the vein before intravenous medication is given. It would be dangerous and irritating to the surrounding tissue if the medication infiltrated the tissue. The medications are mixed in a sterile manner and inserted so that they are evenly distributed throughout the receptacle. Labeling is a safety measure that identifies a medication that is being infused over a prolonged time.

### Giving Medications to Infants and Children

Marlow (1969) states that, because the dose of medication ordered for an infant or child is relatively small, an error in the amount of drug given makes a greater proportional error. Often the dose is based on the child's weight. Considerable care, then, is required when medications are given to infants and children. Drug reactions are carefully watched for because the child's reaction is less predictable than the adult's.

The following points are important when giving oral or parenteral medications to children:

#### Oral

1. The form of the medicine is often modified to make it easier to administer; for example, tablets are crushed, or liquids in the form of elixirs or suspensions are provided.
2. Oral medications are given by using either a small spoon, a rubber-tipped glass or plastic dropper, a medicine cup, syringe (without the needle), or a nipple.
3. Place the medicine in the buccal region in the back of the mouth so that it is not pushed out of the mouth, but swallowed.
4. For ease in swallowing and to prevent choking, have the baby in a sitting position or elevate his head and shoulders. If you are holding him on your lap, tuck one of his arms under yours to keep it out of the way.

#### Parenteral

1. Injection sites for infants and young children depend upon agency policy but usually are the mid-anterior muscle of the thigh (rectus femoris), mid-lateral (vastus lateralis), and the deltoid. When a child is over 2 years of age and has well developed gluteal muscles from walking, the gluteals may also be used for injections.
2. For an intramuscular injection, it is customary to use a one inch needle inserted at a 45° angle, but the needle length and angle of needle insertion depend upon the size of the child.
3. Your approach and explanation will depend upon the level of psychological and physical development of the child.

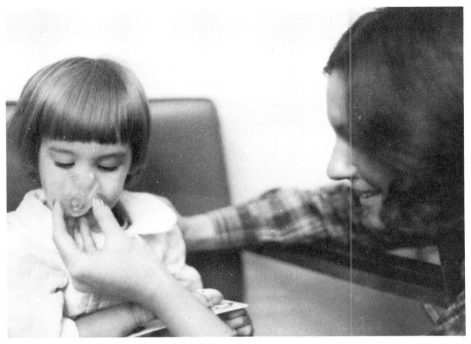

**Figure 19-7.**   *A medicine cup is one method used to give oral medication to a child.   (Photo by Frank R. Engler, Jr.)*

4.  Always identify the child by reading his identification band.
5.  Seek help when necessary to hold the child while he gets the injection.
6.  After the injection, cuddle the child; let the pre-schooler give an injection to a doll; show that you care.

## Topical Medications

Topical medications include those applied to the skin or another body surface. They are usually intended for direct action at the site where they are applied. However, the action depends upon the type of tissue and the nature of the drug.

Lotions, liniments, or ointments are applied to the skin. Lotions are drugs in liquid form applied to the skin to protect it, soothe it, or relieve itching (e.g., Calamine lotion). A liniment is a liquid drug preparation that is rubbed into the skin, dilates superficial blood vessels, and relaxes muscles (e.g., Ben Gay). Lotions are patted on to the skin by using sterile gauze or cotton balls. A sterile glove may be used on the hand that is applying the lotion. Liniments are also applied in the same manner except that they are then rubbed into the skin. An ointment is a medication prepared in a fatty base. It is usually squeezed from a tube onto a tongue blade (sterile) and applied to the site. A sterile dressing may be indicated.

Vaginal creams can be applied by using the narrow tubular applicator and attached plunger with which they are usually packaged. Suppositories may also be used in the vagina. The client is taught how to use the medication and to wear a pad to avoid soiling her clothing. Rectal or urethral suppositories may be ordered. Sterile technique is used to insert a urethral suppository. Rectal suppositories were discussed in the chapter on elimination.

## Nose Drops

### Special Considerations

The positions described for instillation of nose drops allow the solution to flow to the back of the nose. There is more chance of contaminating the solution if the dropper is inserted in the bottle after it has been placed in one nostril than if all the required medication is removed the first time. Keeping the head back prevents the escape of solution from the nose.

---

### Performance Checklist
### Instillation of Nose Drops

1. Give the client a tissue; have him sit with his head tilted back. An alternate position is to have the client lie on his back with a pillow under his shoulders.
2. Draw sufficient medication for both nostrils into the dropper.
3. Place dropper just inside nostril (about 1/3 inch) and instill prescribed number of drops.
4. Have person keep head tilted back for several minutes. Have him expectorate any medication that has run down his throat.

---

## Ear Drops

### Special Considerations

The ear canal is straightened in order for the medication to reach all parts of the ear canal. Cotton inserted loosely into the canal helps prevent the drops from escaping.

---

### Performance Checklist
### Instillation of Ear Drops

1. Expose and straighten the ear canal: pull the lobe down and back to straighten a child's ear canal; pull the auricle up and back for the adult.
2. Insert the tip of the medicine dropper into the ear canal. Inject the medication.
3. Withdraw the dropper and place a cotton ball in the external meatus.

## Eye Drops

### Special Considerations

The lids are cleaned from the area of the eye near the nose (the inner canthus) outward toward the ear. This helps prevent spread of infection. Drops and ointments are dropped into the lower conjunctival sac because direct application of solution onto the eyeball might injure the cornea. The lids are closed to help distribute the drops or ointment throughout the eye.

---

### Performance Checklist
### Instillation of Eye Drops

1. Give the client a tissue.
2. Draw up the approximate number of drops required.
3. Wipe the lids and lashes clean.
4. Expose the lower conjunctival sac as follows:
   a. ask the client to look up
   b. place your thumb near the margin of the lower lid just below the lashes and press down over the cheek
   c. as the lid is pulled down and away from the eyeball, the conjunctival sac is exposed
5. With the dropper close to the eye but not touching it, drop the desired number of drops into the sac.
6. Ask the client to close the eye and gently roll it to help distribute solution.

---

## SUMMARY

The nurse accepts as part of her role the need to teach her client about the use of his medications. Drug interactions, drug-food interactions, and drug-alcohol interactions are taught. A medication history is important in planning nursing actions. The guide included in the chapter assists in securing the medication history. Calculation of dosage is seldom necessary when medications are available under the unit-dose system. With other systems, however, some calculations are necessary. One method of drug calculation is described. The nurse prepares and administers medications to persons of all ages by many routes. Following supervised practice, she should be able to give medications efficiently.

## LEARNING ACTIVITIES

1. Select a client in your clinical agency and take a medication history based on the content presented in this chapter.
2. You have a 75-year-old client who has just had prescribed 3 new medications: one is for hypertension, one for congestive heart failure, and the other a tranquilizer. Each is ordered once a day. Instruct her in their use.

3. According to the literature cited in the chapter, what aspects of drug administration are most difficult to teach?

4. State 4 ways to prevent medication errors.

5. You need to give 20 mEq of KCl. The multiple dose vial contains 10 ml; 1 ml = 10 mEq. What volume of medication will you use?

6. State the criteria you would use to determine the site for an intramuscular injection.

## REFERENCES AND SUGGESTED READINGS

Bryar, Rosamund.   Self-medication in a student population. *Nursing Times,* January 13, 1977, pp. 52–55.

Burkhalter, Pamela.   Medication errors: let's eliminate them! *Supervisor Nurse,* November, 1972, pp. 58–62.

Caranasos, George; Stewart, Ronald; and Cluff, Leighton.   Drug-induced illness leading to hospitalization. *Journal of the American Medical Association,* 228 (May 6, 1974), 713–717.

Carr, Joseph; McElroy, Norman; and Carr, Bonita.   How to solve dosage problems in one easy lesson. *American Journal of Nursing,* December, 1976, pp. 1934–1937.

Coleman, Vernon.   Desert isle drugs. *American Journal of Nursing,* March, 1978, p. 429.

DeBarry, Pauline; Jefferies, Lenner; and Light, Margaret.   Teaching cardiac patients to manage medications. *American Journal of Nursing,* December, 1975, pp. 2191–2193.

Fuerst, Elinor; Wolff, LuVerne; and Weitzel, Marlene, 1974.   *Fundamentals of nursing.* 5th ed.   Philadelphia: J. B. Lippincott.

Geolot, Denise and McKinney, Nancy.   Administering parenteral drugs. *American Journal of Nursing,* May, 1975, pp. 788–793.

Lambert, Martin.   Drug and diet interactions. *American Journal of Nursing,* March, 1975, pp. 402–406.

Levine, Myra.   Breaking through the medications mystique. *American Journal of Nursing,* April, 1970, 799–803.

Marlow, Dorothy, 1969.   *Textbook of pediatric nursing.* 3rd ed.   Philadelphia: W. B. Saunders.

Newton, Marian and Newton, David.   Guidelines for handling drug errors. *Nursing 77,* September, 1977, pp. 62–68.

Parker, William.   Medication histories. *American Journal of Nursing,* December, 1976, pp. 1969–1971.

Romankiewicz, John, et. al.   To improve patient adherence to drug regimens: an interdisciplinary approach. *American Journal of Nursing,* July, 1978, pp. 1216–1219.

Smith, S. E.    How drugs act, 5: intolerance, idiosyncrasy, and hypersensitivity. *Nursing Times,* July 24, 1975, pp. 1170–1171.

Stewart, Diane; Kelly, June; and Dinel, Brian.    Unit-dose medication: a nursing perspective. *American Journal of Nursing,* August, 1976, pp. 1308–1310.

Wood, Lucile, 1975.    *Nursing skills for allied health services.* Vol. 3.    Philadelphia: W. B. Saunders.

# 20

# Activity, Rest, and Sleep

## Behavioral Objectives

Upon completion of this chapter, the student will be able to:

1. Explain the importance of obtaining a balance between activity and rest.
2. Perform a musculoskeletal assessment on a healthy client emphasizing range of motion.
3. Assist a client who has changes in mobility.
4. Implement physical and psychological measures to promote rest and sleep, and evaluate their effectiveness.
5. Discuss the relationship of circadian rhythm to shift rotation.
6. Implement and evaluate nursing actions based on knowledge of the stages of sleep.

## Key Terms

| | | |
|---|---|---|
| abduction | calculi | decubitus ulcers |
| active range of motion | calisthenic | delta waves |
| adduction | center of gravity | dorsiflexion |
| alignment | circadian rhythm | EEG |
| alpha rhythm | Circ-Olectric bed | endurance |
| axillae | concavity | enuresis |
| barbiturates | contracture | eosinophils |
| biofeedback | convexity | eversion |

| | | |
|---|---|---|
| extension | isotonic | plantar flexion |
| fatigue | kyphosis | posture |
| flexion | line of gravity | pronation |
| foot drop | Lofstrand crutches | range of motion |
| Fowler's position | lordosis | REM |
| gatch | mantra | scoliosis |
| good body mechanics | meditation | sleep |
| gravity | NREM | spindles |
| Hoyer lift | osteoblasts | Stryker frame |
| hyperextension | osteoclasts | supination |
| insomnia | passive range of motion | trochanter roll |
| inversion | physical fitness | Yoga |
| isometric | | |

## Introduction

When the musculoskeletal system is functioning properly, body movement is free and comfortable. Helping an individual maintain or improve function seems more realistic when the nurse herself is actively involved in good health practices. She can encourage her clients to develop good body mechanics when she is observed using her own body efficiently. The focus of part of the chapter will be, therefore, on the nurse's requirements, as well as the needs of her client. Physical fitness is based on good body mechanics and ease of movement. Fitness for nursing as well as for meeting the individual client's objectives for fitness will be presented. When the nurse examines a client's musculoskeletal system, she will find this is often an appropriate time for teaching body mechanics and range of motion exercises. This is the approach that will be described in this chapter.

The importance of maintaining a balance between activity and rest will be discussed throughout the chapter. For the client who has changes in mobility, methods of assistance are an important part of the nurse's actions. Turning, moving, positioning, and use of assisting devices are discussed.

While immobility causes changes in the entire body, only the effects on the musculoskeletal system are discussed in this chapter. The effects of immobility on other body systems are presented elsewhere in this text.

Measures to promote physical and psychological rest are an important part of maintaining the needed balance between activity and rest. Nursing measures are stressed. Yoga, meditation, biofeedback, and relaxation techniques are introduced.

Sleep requirements, patterns, and routines that the client uses to induce sleep are elicited through use of an assessment guide. Circadian rhythms, stages of sleep, and some deviations from normal sleep are described. Nursing actions to promote sleep are included.

## PHYSICAL FITNESS

Physical fitness is the state in which a person is able to complete all the required tasks of daily living without fatigue or exhaustion, with energy left over for leisure activities. Bailey et al. (1974) report that 3 out of 4 young persons they studied were unable to pass tests designed to evaluate physical fitness for their age. Young adult females aged 20 to 29 had the lowest rating of all groups tested.

Other studies suggest that students who are physically fit are more alert and tend to get better grades than those who are not (Hoffman, 1977). Individuals of all ages and at all levels of health benefit from programs to achieve physical fitness. While the interest in physical fitness appears to be growing, it is not yet widespread. Nurses can play an important role in informing others about the value of physical fitness throughout the lifespan, and about the means to achieve and maintain it.

Nursing students or their clients can assess their own general physical fitness by using the following method from Diekelmann (1977): Select a stair and step up and down on it for one minute. Step up with the left foot, then the right. Step down with the left, then the right. If you weigh between 100 and 160 pounds, repeat this exercise at the rate of 30 per minute. If you weigh between 160 and 220, reduce the rate to between 20 and 30 steps per minute.

Immediately afterwards, sit down and count your pulse. Count it for 10 seconds and multiply by 6, which will give the pulse rate at the moment of the exercise. The pulse slows down rapidly after exertion, so that a full-minute count is not accurate for this purpose.
1. If the pulse is greater than 120, you are in poor physical condition.
2. If the pulse is less than 120, repeat the one minute exercise immediately. Then, if the pulse rate is more than 120, you are in fair physical fitness.
3. If after the second exercise your pulse rate is less than 120, repeat the one minute exercise immediately for a third time. If the pulse rate is greater than 120, your physical fitness rating is good. If it is less than 120 your rating is excellent.

There are three elements of fitness: strength, flexibility, and endurance. Calisthenic exercises are most useful in developing and maintaining strength and flexibility. Bending and stretching all parts of the body through their normal range of motion without undue strain are good exercises. Strength and flexibility are developed by the lifting, pulling, walking, climbing, and carrying required throughout the performance of the activities of daily living. The use of good body mechanics is essential in the performance of bending, stretching, lifting, and carrying. This will be discussed in the next section of this chapter.

Endurance is largely a matter of developing an adequate oxygen transport system. It can be achieved by sustained whole-body exercise such as running, cycling, and swimming. It involves continuous rhythmic cardiorespiratory overload. The body responds to these demands by adapting. In time, the heart muscle develops increased tissue vascularity. The heart also becomes stronger and more efficient. It beats less often and pumps out an increased amount of blood with each beat.

It has been suggested that fitness postpones physiological aging. Regular exercise leads to fitness—it enhances strength, flexibility, and endurance. It helps regulate the appetite, release tension, protect the heart, and encourage sleep. Exercise speeds up the removal of lactic acid and other waste products by increasing the supply of blood and oxygen to the tissues.

There is an appropriate level of physical activity for everyone. Gradual resumption of exercise and continuous, regular exercise combining calisthenics with endurance training are necessary for lifetime fitness. Exercising at least 3 times a week is recommended. It cannot be emphasized too much—fitness is not a temporary need but continues throughout life.

Maltz, Zeller, and Chandler (1973) compared the physically fit young adult with one who was not. The physically fit subject had: a) a slower heart rate during exercise; b) a more rapid recovery rate after exercise; c) lower blood

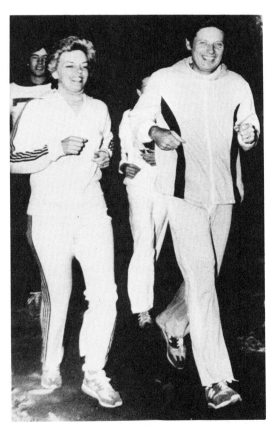

**Figure 20-1.** *More and more people are including jogging as part of a physical fitness program. (United Press International photo)*

pressure before, during, and following exercise; d) lower oxygen intake in exercise; and e) less lactic acid in the blood during exercise.

Jogging and running have become popular forms of endurance exercising. However, any adult over the age of 35 should have a complete physical examination, including a stress electrocardiogram, before beginning an exercise program. Others who should have a complete physical examination before beginning such a program are those who smoke more than one pack of cigarettes a day, have a close relative who had a heart attack before the age of 50, have hypertension and/or elevated serum cholesterol, and anyone who is more than 25 percent overweight (Deikelmann, 1977).

Certain safeguards should accompany endurance exercising. There should be a gradual increase in the amount of exercise. Throughout the entire exercise program, at least 5 minutes of warm-up time is needed to allow the heart to adjust to the increase in exercise. When the heart rate is up to 135-160, exercise should continue for 20 minutes. After this, a cooling-down period when exercise is slowly reduced is necessary. Walking, for example, should follow jogging.

An exercise program should be tailored to the individual's physical condition and adapted to his lifestyle and preference. Specific exercise programs are described in Hoffman (1977), Cooper (1970), and other widely available sources.

The advantages of being physically fit are well expressed by two nurses, Friedman and Knight (1978), who conclude their article on running by saying, "Our body image, self-respect, and self-confidence have improved significantly. By becoming active participants in good health practices, including an exercise program, we are demonstrating fitness and stimulating the interest of others. This sense of well-being is available to everyone."

## BODY MECHANICS

Basic to physical fitness is good body mechanics, which may be defined as using the musculoskeletal system effectively. For the health-care worker, as well as for her clients, standing, sitting, stooping, reaching, lifting, carrying, and moving objects can be done in such a way that the body is protected. As the nurse uses her body effectively in caring for her clients, she serves as a role model. Many clients can be helped to learn better ways to stand, sit, stoop, lift, and carry. (Some principles of body mechanics are presented in the discussion on assisting a client who has changes in mobility.) Other concepts and terms will be presented here.

### Principles of Body Mechanics

**Posture**  Posture is the position of the body and the relationship of its parts to each other. In *standing posture*, the feet are parallel, 4 to 8 inches apart with weight equally distributed. The knees are slightly flexed. The pelvis is stabilized. This is done by tightening the muscles of the buttocks and the abdomen. The chest is up, the waist extended; the shoulders are relaxed but slightly back. The head is erect, chin in.

In this standing position, the center of gravity (the point where the mass is centered) is the center of the pelvis, about halfway between the umbilicus and the pubis. The body is balanced (kept in a steady position). The body parts are in good alignment (parts are in proper relationship to each other).

*Sitting posture* is the same as standing posture except that the hips and knees are flexed approximately 90 degrees. *Side lying posture* is the same as standing except that there is 90-degree flexion at the hip and knee and both arms are flexed at the elbow and the shoulder. Support is usually supplied in the form of pillows or pads.

*Gravity* is the force of attraction between two objects. Whenever movement occurs, energy is expended to overcome gravity. Movements of the body are brought about by muscle contractions. The *line of gravity* is a vertical line passing through the center of gravity. Stability is maintained when the line of gravity falls within the base of support. The base of support is the area on which an object rests. For example, the feet are the base of support when one is standing.

*Rolling or sliding* an object is more efficient than lifting it against the pull of gravity. When sliding a large object, friction is lessened by reducing the area of contact. For example, one might tip the object onto its edge. Friction between the object and the surface on which it is being moved affect the amount of work required for movement. *Pulling and pushing* use the force of body weight to move an object. One leans toward the object being pushed and away from that being pulled.

*Stooping* is more efficient than bending. This not only broadens the base of support, but also makes use of the large and strong leg muscles, which tire less quickly than the small muscles of the back. To lift an object, one flexes the knees, stabilizes the pelvis, and gets close to the object. Then the object is carried close to the body. *Pivoting* is better than twisting when turning the body. Twisting causes muscle strain.

The nurse should flatten a client's bed before attempting to move the person in it. Objects (and, of course, people) moved on a level surface are not opposing gravity. Mechanical devices should be used to help one lift objects whenever possible. The nurse should flex her hips and knees and keep her back straight when moving a client.

## ASSESSMENT OF THE MUSCULOSKELETAL SYSTEM

An understanding of the following terms is necessary before one can assess, report, and evaluate an individual's musculoskeletal system:

*abduction*   the movement of a limb *away from* the midline.
*adduction*   the movement of a limb *toward* the midline.
*extension*   straightening or increasing the angle between two adjoining parts.
*flexion*   bending; reducing the angle between two adjoining parts.

*hyperextension*   increasing the angle between two parts so that it is greater than the normal range.

*supination*   positioning the forearm so that the palm of the hand faces up.

*pronation*   positioning the forearm so that the palm of the hand faces down.

*range of motion*   the normal extent of joint movement.

*active range of motion*   movement performed by the individual without assistance.

*passive range of motion*   movement performed by another person.

*eversion*   a turning outward.

*inversion*   a turning inward.

The examination includes the evaluation of the individual in various body positions. Proper draping is essential. A gown that is open in the back is worn as well as some type of underpants. The nurse must remember that she is examining a person, not a musculoskeletal system. In the standing position, body contours, posture, muscles, and extremities can be examined.

The spine is examined to assess tenderness, curvature, and mobility. Regarding the cervical spine, the normal position of the neck is a gentle C curve (a concavity), referred to as the normal cervical lordosis (Prior and Silberstein, 1973). The normal dorsal spine has a kyphotic curve (a convexity). This balances the cervical lordosis and lumbosacral lordosis. The lumbosacral spine normally has a forward curve (a concavity) at the lumbar region.

Any tenderness of the spine should be noted. Backache is a frequent problem in adults, with the lower back most frequently involved. Mobility of the back is assessed. A normal individual may not be able to extend his knees, bend forward, and touch the floor (one test of lumbar mobility).

Scoliosis and kyphosis are spinal curvatures seen fairly often. Scoliosis is a lateral curvature of the spine, which may be congenital or acquired. Deformities of the rib cage often accompany scoliosis. A kyphosis is a marked increase in the convexity of the thoracic spinal curve (hunchback deformity). It may also be congenital or acquired.

The extremities are inspected and palpated to determine symmetry, size, shape, muscular development, color, temperature, and movement. Is there any discomfort or pain on movement? Any swelling, redness, increased temperature? Is there complete range of motion in all joints? All joints have a circumscribed range of motion determined by their structure. The nurse should ask her client to perform the following active range of motion exercises:

1.   **Head and Neck**   While in a sitting position, ask the client to lower the head until the chin touches the chest; extend the head backward as far as it will go; tilt the head to the left side as far as it will go and then to the right; rotate the head from the left to the right.

2.   **Shoulder**   Lying flat on his back (supine), arm at his side, palm facing in, have the client move arm straight out at shoulder height (keep arm straight); continue moving arm until it is over head, palm out. This is shoulder *extension. Rotation* of the shoulder is performed with the elbow flexed, fingers on

tip of shoulder. Elbow is moved across chest, then over the head, and back to the original position.

3.  **Elbow**    With the person sitting, have him bend the elbow until the fingers touch the tip of the shoulder (*flexion*). For *extension* straighten the elbow by extending the arm.

4.  **Wrist Flexion**    With his palm facing the floor, have the client bend the wrist as far downward as possible. For *extension*: with his palm facing the floor, have him bend the wrist as far up and back as possible. For wrist *rotation*: while holding the wrist rotate the hand to the left, and then to the right around the wrist axis.

5.  **Fingers**    Have the client alternately bend and straighten each finger (*flexion* and *extension*), including all the joints. Have him *rotate* the thumb around its axis.

6.  **Trunk**    From a standing position (for *flexion* and *extension*), and with hands on hips, the client bends trunk as far forward as possible, then straightens and bends trunk back as far as possible (*extension*). To test *rotation*, have the client, moving only the upper part of the body, turn the trunk from left to right as far as possible.

7.  **Hip**    From a side-lying position, with legs straight and feet together, the client swings the upper leg as far forward as possible and returns (*anterior flexion*). Then he swings the upper leg as far back as possible and returns (*posterior extension*). Lying on back, legs straight and feet together, the client moves one leg sideways away from the other and then returns (*lateral hip flexion and extension*).

8.  **Knee**    Lying flat on back, the client bends the knee, moving the heel toward the buttocks (*flexion of hip and knee*); then straightens the leg to lie flat on the bed (*knee extension*).

9.  **Ankle**    The client bends the foot upward at the ankle (*dorsiflexion*), extends the ankle by bending the foot downward toward the floor (*plantar flexion*); and, moving only the foot, *rotates* foot from left to right around the ankle axis.

10. **Toes**    Client bends the toes toward the sole of the foot (*flexion*); bends the toes up toward the anterior foot surface (*extension*); spreads the toes by increasing the distance beteen them as much as possible.

If the client cannot perform these range of motion actions by himself, move the part for him. This is *passive range of motion*. Supporting the part with both hands, one above and the other below the joint, smoothly and steadily move the joint until there is resistance but no pain. When the client must perform range of motion exercises, he should exercise those joints that need special attention 2 to 5 times at least twice a day (Lewis, 1976) to prevent loss of muscle tone and to assist circulation to those parts of the body.

The nurse concludes the musculoskeletal assessment by observing the individual walk, after having noted his sitting, lying, and standing postures. Any activity in which the client needs assistance and the client's activity tolerance should be recorded.

## ASSISTING A CLIENT WHO HAS CHANGES IN MOBILITY

A client frequently needs assistance in turning, moving, and positioning himself. The individual who can move himself is encouraged to do so, and he is usually more comfortable when allowed to move at his own speed and exercise at the same time. The nurse might instruct the client in easier ways to move. When the client is turning in bed, the nurse can assist him by lifting the covers, and instructing him to bend his knees and then use the side rails to support himself as he turns. For the client who cannot change his own position, the nurse assumes the responsibility for regular turning and positioning in good body alignment. Family members are shown how to turn and position a person, using techniques that are effective and efficient. It is important to use principles of good body mechanics. The nurse (or family member) stands with a wide base of support, maintains her body in proper alignment, and uses strong muscle groups for movement. The question frequently arises about how often a person's position should be changed. Research indicates that pressure areas develop even in persons whose position is changed hourly. Clearly, the helpless person is at risk even if his position is changed hourly.

### Positions

Pillows are used to help a person in bed maintain a proper position. In addition, sandbags, rolled sheets or towels, and footboards may be used.

The supine position (also called dorsal recumbent) is the back-lying position. It is similar to the standing position with the legs together and the knees slightly flexed. A small pillow under the head keeps the head and neck erect. The arms are at the sides with the hands pronated (palms facing the mattress). If the hands have limited mobility, the correct position of slight finger flexion is attained (the hand is held as if it were holding a baseball) by use of splints or rolled cloths. The legs, if weakened, are positioned and prevented from rolling outward (external rotation). Sandbags and trochanter rolls (a bath blanket or sheet placed under the hips with the part remaining rolled against the leg) prevent outward rotation. The feet are supported, if necessary, to maintain them at right angles to the leg, the toes pointing to the ceiling. A deformity called foot drop occurs when the feet assume plantar flexion as a result of weight on weakened foot or leg muscles. Foot support may be given by a footboard properly placed, as described above. It is essential that the feet be in contact with the support (see Figure 20-2).

In a prone position, the client is assisted to lie on his abdomen with his head turned to one side. A folded towel or a small pillow may be placed under the head if desired. The female client may like a small pillow at her waist. The spine is kept straight, the arms are flat at the side or flexed at the elbow. The feet should occupy the space between the bottom of the mattress and the foot of the bed or else a small pillow is placed under the lower legs to keep the feet in proper alignment.

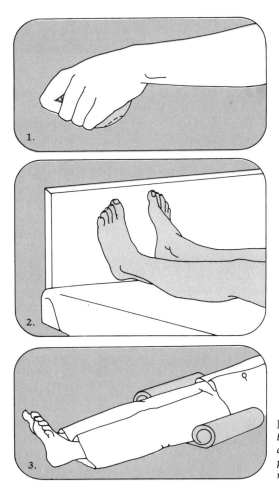

**Figure 20-2.**  *When assistance is needed to maintain correct body position, (1) a rolled cloth is placed in the hand; (2) a footboard properly placed supports the feet; (3) a blanket maintains the hips in correct position.*

For side-lying, when the client cannot turn himself, the nurse may turn him toward or away from her. To turn the client from the supine position toward her, the nurse places one hand on the far shoulder and the other on the far hip and gently rolls him toward her. She maintains a wide base of support, one foot well behind the other. As she rolls the client she rocks backward. Then she raises the side rail and goes to the other side of the bed. She places a hand under the client's shoulder and one under his hips. As she rocks back she slides his shoulder and hip to the center of the bed. The client's lower leg is slightly flexed at the knee; the top leg is flexed more sharply. The underarm is brought forward and flexed on the head pillow; the top arm is flexed in front of the body. A pillow is tucked under the back to provide support as well as to maintain the position. A pad (sheet or towel) is placed between the legs.

To turn the client away from her, the nurse must first be certain that the bedrail on the far side of the bed is up and secure. The client is asked to flex his knees and place his arms on his chest. The nurse places a hand under his shoulders and one under his hips and gently rolls him over. Then she positions him as described above.

Sitting up in bed is frequently called the semi-Fowler's position, with the head of the bed elevated 45 degrees. A small head pillow is retained. This position flexes the body at the hips. The arms may be supported on pillows to prevent pull on the shoulders. This bed position is comfortable for reading, eating, etc. Some persons need to stay in this position for ease in breathing. Because it is easy to slide down in bed from this position, there is a tendency to raise the bed's knee gatch. If this is done, the knees must be lowered (the lower part of the bed flattened) after 5 to 10 minutes. Raising the knee gatch may cause damage to the popliteal nerve and major blood vessels behind the knee if pressure is maintained.

In Fowler's position (sometimes called high Fowler's position), the bed is rolled up at the head to a 90-degree angle. The person is then in full sitting position. Breathing is often easier in this position. The same support for the arms is necessary as in the supine or semi-Fowler's position. Knees cannot be maintained in a flexed position. Using the over-bed table to lean on serves the same purpose. Several pillows are placed on the table for comfort. They help maintain the person in as erect a position as possible.

## Moving a Person Confined to Bed

**Special Considerations**

The nurse should be realistic about her ability to move a person unassisted. When the client cannot help, it is, of course, easier for two persons rather than one to do the moving. As suggested in the previous section on turning, it requires less energy to roll or turn than it does to lift. Pushing or sliding also requires less energy than lifting. Reducing friction by placing powder on the person's skin or the bed sheet also makes moving easier. Using a turn or lift sheet is another way to decrease friction.

Various mechanical devices are available for moving and turning persons. It is assumed that the nurse will learn how to operate these devices before she attempts to use them in caring for a client. The Hoyer lift, the Circ-Olectric bed, and the Stryker frame are examples of equipment designed to lessen the work of moving and turning. For the student nurse, assuming the role of client and being lifted in the Hoyer lift or turned on the Stryker frame or Circ-Olectric bed, are valuable learning experiences for the health-care worker.

Two persons can also move a client up in bed without the use of a draw sheet, although more energy is expended. With one nurse on either side of the bed, standing with a wide base of support and knees flexed, they join hands under the client's hips and shoulders. On signal they rock toward the head of the bed and simultaneously slide the client up in bed.

If the individual is light in weight, one nurse, using the above method, can

### Performance Checklist
### Moving a Person up in Bed

*Two Persons Using a Lifting Sheet*
1. Lock the bed wheels.
2. One person stands on either side of the bed.
3. Raise the bed to a comfortable working height.
4. Flatten the head and foot of the bed.
5. Remove the pillow from under the head and place it against the headboard.
6. Loosen both sides of the drawsheet and roll the edges against the client's body.
7. Ask client to bend knees and place feet flat on bed (if possible).
8. Stand with a wide base of support, facing the head of the bed.
9. Grasp the drawsheet as close to the client as possible, one hand at the top, the other at the bottom of the sheet.
10. On the agreed-upon signal, the drawsheet and the client are moved toward the head of the bed.
11. Adjust the sheet; replace the pillow and provide a comfortable position for the client.

probably do the moving with the assistance of the client who places his feet flat on the mattress and on signal helps slide toward the head of the bed.

## Moving from Bed to Stretcher

If the client can move from the bed to the stretcher unassisted, he should be encouraged to do so. First, however, the bed is raised to the height of the stretcher and both bed and stretcher are locked. Then the bed and stretcher are held firmly together. The client moves his hips to the edge of the bed, then his shoulders, and then his legs. Then, in the same manner, he moves from the edge of the bed to the middle of the stretcher. The stretcher mattress is stabilized so that it remains in place on the stretcher throughout the move. Then the seat belt is attached, unless the stretcher has side rails for safety. Usually a pillow is placed under the client's head and he lies supine unless he needs to have the head elevated for comfort. Adequate covering is provided. The stretcher is pushed feet first with a person at either end to move and guide it.

Frequently a helpless client must be moved from a stretcher to a bed or vice versa. The most efficient way to move him is to pull him carefully on the loosened bottom sheet from one surface to the other. The head and extremities are supported. The number of people required for the move depends on the size of the client and the amount of equipment being moved. When there is an intravenous infusion, a urinary drainage bag, or an extremity in a cast, more than two persons are required for the move.

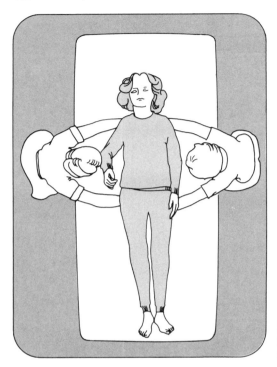

**Figure 20-3.** *Two people can slide a client toward the head of a bed by joining hands placed under the client's hips and shoulders.*

## Preparing and Assisting the Client to Get Out of Bed

A client who has been confined to bed for a long time, or one who has had surgery involving a lower extremity (e.g., an amputation), may require special exercises before he is strong enough to be out of bed. Doing push-ups and using bar-bells are two ways to strengthen the upper extremities. Quadriceps setting (contracting the muscles of the anterior thigh) will help strengthen the legs. In many settings the exercise program will be instituted by the physical therapy department. The nurse's role, then, is to help maintain the program.

*Dangling* also prepares the client for getting out of bed. The client should be helped to sit on the edge of the bed with his legs hanging over the side of the bed. The first time the client dangles (or gets out of bed), he should be assisted by a nurse who assesses his activity tolerance. His vital signs are checked and compared to his usual pulse, respirations, and blood pressure. If he feels weak or faint, he is helped to lie down.

Before a client is helped sit or stand it is a good idea to review the proper sitting and standing positions. The standing position previously described finds the person in correct position when his head is erect, his back straight, and his abdomen held in. His feet are slightly separated laterally and his weight equally distributed on them. His arms are at his sides. Proper seating is supplied by a firm chair. The trunk is supported upright with the buttocks and most of the thighs supported on the seat of the chair. The knees are together (legs not crossed) and the feet are flat on the floor or on a foot stool.

The nurse should practice sitting and rising from a chair so that she can demonstrate the proper method: standing with the backs of the knees touching the edge of the seat, one foot slightly under the chair, the pelvis is stabilized. The trunk is inclined forward, knees and hips flexed. Then she can lower herself to the chair seat.

When rising, she moves to the edge of the chair seat and places one foot slightly under the chair. The pelvis is stabilized. Then, using arm rests if necessary (or available), she places her weight on the feet and arms as she rises.

**Assisting the Client to a Chair**   The wheels of the bed are locked and a locked wheelchair or a stable straight-backed chair is placed parallel to the bed. The head of the bed is elevated to approximately 90° and the near bed rail is elevated so the client can assist himself to a sitting position on the edge of the bed. The bed is lowered to the floor and the person is helped to put on his robe and hard soled slippers or shoes if he is going to walk. Facing the client, the nurse assumes a wide base of support, one foot forward and knees flexed. She puts her hands under his arms, he places his hands on her shoulders or waist (but not around her neck) and he stands. If the client has trouble stabilizing his legs, the nurse places her legs directly in front of the client's legs and braces him as he stands. Then she allows him to stand for a few seconds and gain his balance before she pivots him onto the chair. If the chair has armrests, the client holds onto them as he assists himself to sit down. If a wheelchair is used, care is taken that the foot pedals are up and out of the way and the locks applied before the transfer is begun. Safety requires that the wheelchair be equipped with a seat belt that is fastened when the chair is in use. Newton's first law of motion indicates that the person in the chair will stay in motion after the chair has stopped unless acted upon by an external force (such as a seat belt).

**Assisting a Client Who Cannot Help Himself to a Chair**   When a person who cannot help himself is to be gotten out of bed, the following technique is useful. It is possible, and frequently desirable, to seek a second person to help. However, family members who will have no one to help them at home need to be taught the one-person technique.

The locked wheelchair or straight-back chair is placed near the middle of the bed, facing it. The upper part of the client's body is then moved to the edge of the bed. From the back, the nurse places her hands under the client's axillae, supporting his head and shoulders, if required, with her body. Leaning against the back of the chair, the nurse rocks back while pulling the person onto the chair. The chair is then grasped near its seat and pulled away from the bed until the client's feet are on the edge of the bed. His legs must be supported while his feet are lowered to the floor.

To get the client from the chair to the bed, the nurse places the chair parallel to the bed with the client facing the foot of the bed. Then standing behind the chair, she grasps the client under the arms and rolls him onto the bed. With her foot, she moves the chair out of the way. The client is helped to assume the desired bed position.

## Assisting a Client To Walk

Generally the nurse walks beside the client with her arm under his. Some persons feel more secure when the nurse holds them by their belt. Holding onto the back of the belt affords the nurse the chance to observe her client's posture as well as to support him when necessary.

A rubber-tipped cane carried on the stronger side of the body helps one to feel more secure when walking. A "quad" cane (four legged) provides more support for the person who needs it.

Walkers are lightweight metal frames with rubber tips that give valuable support to the person who has use of both arms but needs considerable support when walking.

In many settings, the nurse is responsible for teaching clients to walk with crutches. In nearly every instance, she evaluates her client's mobility on crutches. For these reasons, it is advisable for the nurse to know how crutches are fitted and the technique for efficient use of them.

Lewis (1976) cites the two following methods for measuring crutches:

1.   With the person in the supine position and wearing shoes, measure the distance from the axillary fold to the shoe plus 2 inches.
2.   Or, measure the distance from the axillary fold to a point 6 to 8 inches away from the person's heel.

The crutch hand grips are adjustable. When the person is standing, the elbows should be slightly bent (approximately 30°) and the wrists slightly hyperextended. The crutches are rubber tipped to prevent slipping.

The person is taught to support himself on the crutches by using his arms and hands. He does not place his weight on the axillary bar. This would cause skin irritation, pressure on nerves in the axillae, poor circulation, and possible paralysis.

Lofstrand crutches (or Canadian crutches) have no axillary bar. Instead, a cuff circles the lower arm to keep the crutches in place.

For good balance, the crutches are placed 4 to 8 inches in front of the feet, and about 4 to 8 inches to the side. This provides a broad base of support. There are four basic crutch-walking gaits:

Two-point   This gait is used if weight-bearing is permitted on both feet. It resembles normal walking. The right crutch and the left foot are placed forward; then the left crutch and right foot follow.

Three-point   This gait is used when only one foot can bear weight. Both crutches and the nonweight-bearing leg move forward and then the weight-bearing foot comes through. The crutches are brought forward immediately and the pattern is repeated.

Four-point   This gait is used when weight is permitted on both feet. Four bases of support are used. The right crutch is placed forward, the left foot forward, the left crutch forward, and then the right foot forward.

Swing-through   This gait is used by the person who can bear weight on one or both feet, and who wants to move about quickly. Both crutches are brought forward and the legs are brought through quickly and placed in front of the crutches.

## PROBLEMS OF IMMOBILITY

When a person maintains a balance between activity and rest, there are few problems. However, recovery from many accidents and illnesses requires that immobility and rest be enforced. When an injured body part is placed at rest, further injury is prevented and tissue repair is encouraged. Lacerations and fractures, for example, are immobilized. If the laceration is on the foot, weight-bearing is discouraged because this delays healing. A fracture is immobilized from the time it is suspected until the bone has healed. A person who has had a heart attack is placed on bed rest, complete or partial. The degree of prescribed bed rest will probably be determined by the extent of injury, the client's personality, and the physician's past experiences with similar clients. Physically maintained bed rest needs to be accompanied by psychological rest. Some persons have a great deal more difficulty than others in adjusting to bed rest. It has been shown, for example, that some persons expend more energy when they are fed than when they feed themselves. In addition, using a bedpan causes more strain than getting out of bed to use a commode. The degree of prescribed rest will be written on the doctor's order sheet and defined by agency policy. The nurse carefully implements, evaluates, and reports the client's response.

When mobility is curtailed, the unused muscles need sufficient exercise to prevent deterioration. Exercise will be prescribed depending upon the health problem. When muscles are immobilized, the process of degeneration begins almost immediately. According to Browen and Hicks (1972), the strength and tone of immobilized muscles (for example, a fractured extremity placed in a cast) may decrease by as much as 5 percent per day in the absence of muscle contractions. The nurse has a responsibility to prevent muscle degeneration. Any person whose mobility is limited requires exercise to the body parts which are not immobilized. It is part of the nurse's role to assess the client's need for exercise, and to provide the required exercises. Isometric exercises (the muscle does not shorten) or isotonic exercises (the muscle shortens but tension on the muscle remains constant; a load is moved) may be prescribed. The client exercises within his energy limits. Fatigue must be avoided. Exercising should occur at regular, prescribed intervals. During the bath and when the person's bed position is being changed are two times when exercise is appropriate, though the client's wishes should determine the time for exercise as much as possible.

Olson (1967) described 3 major musculoskeletal complications of immobility: osteoporosis, contractures, and decubitus ulcers. Prevention and treatment of decubitus ulcers are discussed in the chapter on skin (Ch. 14). Osteoporosis and contractures will be considered here. In osteoporosis, osteoblasts form the osseous matrix, while osteoclasts continuously destroy the matrix through the opposing function of absorbing and removing osseous tissue from the bone.

Since osteoblasts depend upon the stresses and strains of mobility and weight-bearing for proper functioning, normal motor activity is necessary to their function of building up the bone matrix. If there is no activity, as with complete immobility, there is an absence of these daily stresses and strains (Olson, 1967).

Therefore, the process of bone destruction continues without the needed bony build-up. The supply of bone calcium is depleted and there is increased excretion of bone phosphorus and nitrogen, and osteoporosis (porous bone) results. The bones, then, are easily deformed or fractured.

Olson (1967) stressed that nurses need to be aware that decalcification occurs when the person is immobilized, regardless of the amount of calcium ingested. Therefore, the diet should not contain increased calcium because it will not be used. It will only be added to the very large amount being excreted, and may precipitate from the urine as renal calculi or it may be deposited in the muscles or joints.

Weight-bearing, muscle movement, and maintenance of some mobility will prevent or decrease osteoporosis. Placing the person on a tilt table, having him stand or walk if possible, and daily exercises against resistance are important. Encouraging the client to assist in his own care is an appropriate way to provide exercise and mobility.

In contractures, muscle fibers shorten. Maintaining joints in their most functional position, range of motion exercises, and change of position all help prevent contractures. A firm mattress, a bed board, a footboard (placed firmly against the person's feet to keep them at right angles to the legs), and a loose top sheet help keep the body in good alignment. It is important to encourage the client and his family to participate actively in range of motion exercises if the problems of immobility are to be lessened.

## PROMOTION OF REST: PHYSICAL AND PSYCHOLOGICAL MEASURES

Rest may be described as a time of decreased body activity and a resultant refreshed feeling. Rest should follow activity so that the body can recover. The nurse is alert to signs of fatigue in herself and her clients. Fatigue is avoided by resting when the body indicates the need to refresh itself. Most people are aware of measures that are restful for them. Certainly the client himself should be the one to decide what rest measures the nurse can help him implement. These may vary from a quiet walk or a warm bath to a pleasant conversation or a nap.

The amount of rest required varies from person to person, just as the means to obtain rest vary. When rest is medically prescribed, the amount and type of rest and activity permitted are carefully explained to the client and arrangements are made to help him carry out the prescription. He may be on complete bed rest, which may mean that he can do nothing for himself except breathe. Agency policy defines the constraints of each type of bed rest, complete or partial. The client may be allowed up in a chair twice a day or his activity may be permitted as tolerated. The health condition will dictate the degree of activity permitted.

Freedom from anxiety is essential if a person is to obtain rest. Some people suggest that the hospital is not the place to go if you want to rest. When a person is hospitalized, anxiety is often heightened by the unknown. "What will they do to me when I have a thyroid scan?" "What was the result of the test they did this morning?" "Are things going all right at home?" Nurses can lower the client's anxiety by explaining diagnostic procedures and by seeing that test results are made known. Access to family through visiting and telephoning helps lower anxiety. More extensive visiting hours and allowing parents to stay with children are especially helpful. However, sufficient uninterrupted time for rest throughout the day must also be provided. Occasionally it may be necessary to limit visitors or telephone calls. This decision is often left up to the client.

Loud talking, noisy equipment, and the use of the intercom are examples of things that make it difficult for the hospitalized person to rest. The multiple-occupancy room, while often necessary and even desirable, does contribute additional activity and noise, and thereby makes it more difficult for the client to rest.

A warm bath can be provided for the person who finds this restful. A relaxing backrub and clean, neat bedding provide rest. Proper positioning, of course, provides comfort. If a specific drink or snack encourages rest, it is usually available. As quiet an environment as possible should be provided. Dim lights or darkness may be requested, but if the nurse must make frequent checks on the client, he will probably find it acceptable to keep the lights on rather than having them turned on while he is resting or sleeping.

## Relaxation Techniques

Relaxation techniques are growing increasingly popular. The following are suggested for muscle relaxation: rotate the head gently, shrug and relax the shoulders, rotate the arms at the shoulders. This usually helps relieve tension in the neck and upper body.

Controlled abdominal breathing aids relaxation. It is most effective when it is deep, slow, and accompanied by relaxing movements. For example, inhale deeply as you slowly raise your shoulders. Then exhale slowly and consciously relax as you lower your shoulders. Continue the inhaling, contracting a different group of muscles, and exhaling as the body part is relaxed. Do this until all the parts of the body are relaxed.

Hoffman (1977) states that meditation, Yoga, and other relaxation techniques can actually decrease oxygen consumption, respiratory rate, heart rate, blood pressure, and muscle tension. He suggests the following slightly different technique:

1. In a quiet, peaceful environment, assume a comfortable position in which all your muscles can eventually relax.
2. Close your eyes and take a very deep breath.
3. Visualize a peaceful, tranquil scene. Each time you exhale, repeat a word that has special meaning for you.
4. Relax all the muscles of your body beginning with the feet and continuing up to the head.
5. Do this over a 15 to 20 minute period.
6. Now sit normally for several minutes and enjoy the feeling.

## Yoga, Biofeedback, and Meditation

Yoga, biofeedback, and meditation are additional techniques to promote rest and relaxation. Stern and Ray (1977) suggest that, while they are examples of a multitude of techniques, they all suggest a common process. Certain responses are *allowed* to come forth rather than *made* to come forth. For example, you cannot make yourself relax, you can only allow yourself to become relaxed.

**Yoga**   Yoga has been a total way of life for millions of people for over 6,000 years. It teaches that a whole person consists equally of body, mind, and spirit. All three must be fully developed if the person is to reach his full potential.

There are benefits to be gained from practicing the therapeutic postures, the breathing, relaxation, concentration, and meditation exercises of Yoga. Ross (1975) states that all Yoga requires is "a few minutes of your time each day, a few postures to assume, a few correct deep breaths, a little thought, some small silence" (p. 11). She describes complete Yoga breathing:

Seated comfortably in your chosen position, your hands resting on your knees, inhale completely as follows:

1) Inhale into the abdomen by extending the abdominal muscles as far as is comfortably possible.

2) Expand the thoracic cage so that the ribs expand and the chest swells.

3) Raise the clavicles (collar bones) as far as you can without hunching the shoulders.

This is all done in one inhalation, smoothly, progressively, and in this order. Now exhale slowly. Then time control is learned. The exhalations take twice as long as the inhalations. There can be a pause between inhalation and exhalation. Muscle relaxation is accomplished muscle by muscle, starting at the toes and working up to the face.

The Yoga positions are demonstrated in Ross's *The New Manual of Yoga*. Concentration and meditation excercises are also described. The reader who is interested in Yoga as a means of relaxing is referred to the references at the end of the chapter, as well as to many others currently available.

**Transcendental Meditation and Biofeedback**   Stern and Ray (1977) describe transcendental meditation as follows: "You sit for 20 minutes twice a day and say a word which is called a mantra over and over in your mind." They describe biofeedback as having three aspects: techniques for gaining control over one's physiological functioning; a means of developing awareness of one's body and learning which aspects are related to various types of functioning; and a certain attitude in order to gain control over physiological functioning.

In biofeedback, the responsibility for changing one's condition is clearly up to oneself. Stern and Ray believe that if a response can be recorded and fed back to the subject, he can learn to control it. The possible uses of biofeedback are many. Current literature will provide information about biofeedback as therapy for insomnia, pain relief, and other problems.

## SLEEP

Burgess (1978) considers sleep a recurrent healthy state in which the body decreases its response to stimuli. Noback and Demarest (1975) believe that sleep is a state of diminished consciousness in which there is a change in the quality of the brain's reaction to events in the environment. The reticular activating system, which controls the degree of central nervous system activity, controls wakefulness and sleep. This system consists of nerve cells and fibers originating in the brain stem and extending upward through the mesencephalon and thalamus. They are then distributed throughout the cerebral cortex (Nordmark and Rohweder, 1975). Sleep occurs when the reticular activating system is sufficiently depressed by the reduction of stimuli from the cerebral cortex and periphery.

## Sleep Assessment Guide

These questions serve as a guide to the nurse as she assesses the client's sleep habits:

1. How much sleep do you require per night?
2. What time do you usually go to bed? Get up?
3. Do you nap during the day? If so, for how long?
4. How long does it take you to fall asleep?
5. How often do you awaken after you have fallen asleep?
6. Do you need to urinate during the night?

7.  Do you feel rested when you awaken in the morning?

8.  Do you have any bedtime routine? (e.g., beverage, backrub, warm bath)

9.  How many pillows and blankets do you use?

10.  Do you keep a night light on?

11.  What noises usually waken you?

12.  Do you have any sleep problems (e.g., insomnia, sleep walking, talking in your sleep)?

13.  Do you take any medicine to make you sleep?

## Variations in Sleep Requirements

The amount of sleep required varies considerably among individuals. At different life stages, varying amounts of sleep are required. Some guidelines for sleep requirements at various ages follow.

The newborn's sleep is broken into many short periods of heavy and light sleeping distributed throughout 24 hours. During the first week, he averages 16 to 20 hours per day. By 12 to 16 weeks, his sleep is reduced to 14 or 15 hours a day. This pattern continues throughout the first year. Nap times get shorter until the morning nap is eliminated (Meilach, 1972). Murray and Zentner (1975) state that the toddler requires 12 hours sleep at night plus a nap. The pre-schooler requires 9 to 12 hours; the 6-year-old, 11 hours; the 11-year-old, 9 hours. Adolescents and adults of all ages generally require 7 to 9 hours of sleep each day. Sleep needs may be increased by illness, stress, or the lack of motivation to stay awake.

## Stages of Sleep

Sleep is divided into two major categories: rapid eye movement (REM) and nonrapid eye movement (NREM). Physical changes occur as the person becomes drowsy and continue throughout the stages of sleep. Nonrapid eye movement (NREM) sleep is divided into four stages. Drowsiness precedes these stages. The eyes are closed and the body is not moving. Body temperature declines, and the electroencephalogram (EEG) begins to show a regular alpha rhythm of 8 to 12 cycles per second. Respirations and heart beat grow more regular. The person may have fleeting, aimless thoughts. It is a serene and pleasant state. The person may feel that he is floating into sleep. At this stage the person may be easily awakened. Then, consciousness begins to decrease and the person enters Stage I sleep.

In Stage I, body muscles are relaxing, respirations grow more even, and the heart rate becomes slower. Alpha rhythm (regular pattern, low voltage 8–12 cycles per second) is present, but the waves are more uneven and of lower voltage than when the person was drowsy. A noise or a spoken word will awaken the person and he may insist that he was not really asleep.

In Stage II, the EEG traces quick bursts known as spindles (14–16 cycles per second). There are rapid crescendos and decrescendos of waves. The individual is quite sound asleep and relaxed but he is easily awakened. If awakened at this stage, he might say he had been thinking. If undisturbed he soon descends to Stage 3.

When Stage III occurs, large, slow brain waves (high amplitude, about 1 per second) begin to be interspersed with the spindle and irregular rhythm of the earlier stage. His muscles are very relaxed, his breathing even, and his heart rate slower. His blood pressure is falling and his temperature continues to decline. This stage may occur 20 to 30 minutes after falling asleep. It would take a louder noise to awaken the person now.

Stage IV is the stage of deep sleep. It can last from 10 to 20 minutes and it is very difficult to waken a person during this stage. Very slow and high waves (delta; 1-2 cycles/sec) appear on the EEG. The person is completely relaxed and may not move. It is believed that during this stage, growth hormones are released in greater amounts and tissue healing occurs. There is a 10 to 20 percent decrease in blood pressure, respirations, and basal metabolic rate (BMR). The heart rate and temperature are still declining. Respirations are slow and even. Sleep-walking occurs during this stage, as does bedwetting.

During the first few hours of sleep, more time is spent in Stage 4 sleep than in later cycles. It appears that, after the age of 30, the length of Stage 4 sleep begins to decrease.

REM   About 90 minutes after falling asleep the individual begins the ascent from Stage 4 through Stage 3 and 2. Then REM stage begins. The EEG shows an irregular low-voltage wave similar to that in Stage I. There are rapid eye movements, and vivid dreaming occurs. The heart rate, blood pressure, and respirations may fluctuate widely. Adrenal hormones are released in spurts. In males, from infancy through adulthood, penile erections occur during the REM stage. Other muscles are almost totally relaxed. If the person is awakened during REM sleep he will report dreaming, but if he is awakened a few minutes later when he is in another sleep stage he will have forgotten it. He is more difficult to awaken during REM sleep than during any other stage.

Sleep is a succession of repeated cycles, and one full cycle covers 90 to 120 minutes. A normal night's sleep consists of from 4 to 6 cycles. The relative amount of NREM to REM sleep shifts with age. Neonates divide their sleep equally between NREM and REM. By the age of one year, 35 percent of sleep is REM. By 5 years, REM is 20 percent. It rises slightly in the young adult and approximates 25 percent for REM sleep. In the aged, about 13 percent of sleep is REM. The REM period of the first cycle is usually the shortest (5 minutes, or even absent). The later REM periods may last from 30 to 60 minutes. Most REM sleep occurs during the last third of sleep.

## Circadian Rhythm

Humans, like other living things, are cyclic. They experience certain patterns of activity and inactivity which are repeated about the same time in each 24-hour period. This pattern is called circadian rhythm, which means "approximately a day." Sleep and wakefulness are circadian patterns; eating is another example. Body temperature varies rhythmically about a degree or two throughout the day. The highest temperature usually coincides with a person's best hours of wakefulness. The lowest temperature usually occurs in the late hours of sleep. Many biochemical body functions are subject to circadian cycling. The adrenal hormones follow the same rise and fall as the temperature. The concentration of eosinophils in the blood also mirrors the 24-hour cycle.

Circadian rhythms have many implications for health. Individuals can benefit from a greater sensitivity to their own daily rhythms. The study of biological (circadian) rhythms promises to yield important information that can influence timing of medications, treatments, and surgery, for example. The effect of rotating shifts on the worker has a special interest for nurses. The shift from working days to working nights means a shift in the synchronization of the carcadian cycle and an inevitable period when the individual is out of phase. At least a month should be allowed between shifts, or not more than two or three nights at a time, with time between such scheduling to allow resynchronization (Levine, 1969). The case against rotating shifts for nurses was posed as early as 1965 (Mott, 1965). Felton (1976) and others are still reporting the adverse effects of shift rotation. Altering body rhythms may be a serious matter which will eventually lead to illness. Nurses who have some control over their own scheduling apparently choose more frequent shifting, rather than a pattern that would allow synchronization of body rhythms.

## Deviations from Normal Sleep

Sleep deprivation causes a decreased attention span, irritability, nervousness, anxiety, decreased reaction time, and a lowered pain threshold. The greater the sleep deprivation, the more intensified the symptoms become. Altered perceptions can cause confusion, disorientation, or hallucinations.

Sleep deprivation can occur when there is not enough time allowed for sleep, or when sleep is frequently interrupted (especially during Stage 4 or REM). This has implications for clients who may be deprived of sleep because of interruptions for nursing care. Careful planning of care will lessen the need to interrupt sleep. Murray and Zentner (1975) state that a reduced period of sleep is *not* a miniature of a full night's sleep. The person remains mostly in Stage 4 sleep and little necessary REM sleep occurs.

Insomnia   Insomnia is by far the most common of all sleep disturbances. It occurs when people have trouble falling asleep, when they wake during the sleep period, or when they awaken too early in the morning. Insomnia may be caused by some physical conditions, disturbances in body rhythms, or by worry and anxiety. Often being afraid of not being able to sleep can cause insomnia.

Assessing the cause of insomnia and then instituting means to provide relaxation and sleep are important nursing actions. Explaining the variations in sleep requirements or sleep stages may be reassuring and, therefore, help relieve insomnia. For example, the older person can be told he needs less sleep—that may be why he wakens so early in the morning. Usually a person sleeps when he needs to and for as long as necessary, given the right environmental conditions.

If insomnia is caused by the need to get up during the night to urinate, cutting down on the fluids taken several hours before bedtime helps. Avoid eating a heavy meal just before bedtime. If you feel keyed up at bedtime, practice some relaxation exercises. Tossing and turning in bed is not helpful. Getting up for an hour or so is better.

Nurses frequently find that persons believe they have not slept at all when they were observed to be asleep. The depth of sleep may be the reason for their belief. Explaining the depth of sleep during the various sleep stages is reassuring.

As a last resort in insomnia, drugs may be required to ensure sleep. The use of drugs presumably causes some problems. A tolerance to the drug develops and larger doses are required to induce sleep (chemical dependency). Some drugs are known to depress the normal REM stage of sleep (barbiturates, for example). Older persons who are given barbiturates may become confused and excited rather than sleepy because of the depression of that part of the brain—the mesencephalic portion of the reticular activating system—responsible for inhibitory activity (DuGas, 1977).

There is a growing body of nursing research related to sleep. One study by Dittmar and Dulski (1977) attempted to determine a relationship between the early administration of sleep medication to the hospitalized elderly, and its effect on their social behavior and on their ability to perform activities of daily living. They gave the prescribed sleeping medications to 21 subjects at 8 p.m. Their findings indicated these individuals improved in their daily living performance, but showed negative social behavior. The authors suggested that the negative social behavior might indicate a mobilization of energy, a reaction to the environment, and dissatisfaction. They suggest a need to reexamine these behaviors.

**Somnambulism**    The sleep disorder known as sleepwalking (somnambulism) is seen more often in children than in adults. Precautions to prevent injury during sleepwalking are essential (e.g., locks on doors). Sleepwalking occurs during Stages 3 and 4 of sleep. The subject does not usually remember having walked in his sleep. While his eyes may be open, he does not seem to see.

**Enuresis**    Enuresis is involuntary urination, frequently called bedwetting. This disorder is more common in children than adults. It occurs in about 5 to 15 percent of preadolescents and in about 2 percent of adults. Enuresis occurs in Stage 4 sleep in those who are heavy sleepers. Attempts to stop bedwetting include being sure the bladder is empty at bedtime, limiting fluids for several hours before sleep, and use of a drug that lightens sleep.

## Nursing Actions To Promote Sleep

The measures indicated previously to promote rest are, of course, helpful in promoting sleep. Following the individual's routine to induce sleep is important. If he usually watches the 11 P.M. news before he retires, he may not be able to sleep if his TV is turned off at 10P.M. Some people find hot chocolate helps them sleep, while others can sleep after they have had coffee or tea. A dark, quiet room may be important for some people. Others may have difficulty sleeping if it is too quiet or the sounds are unfamiliar. The city dweller who goes camping in the woods and can't sleep is one example of a person reacting to environmental changes.

A comfortable position and freedom from pain are necessary for sleep. The nurse should be available to listen to her clients. Encouraging daytime activity also helps the person sleep at night. When the person is asleep, it is important that he be permitted to remain asleep. Keeping a light on in the room or using a flashlight is more acceptable than turning on a light to check a client. The older person who cannot sleep with a light on may find a flashlight placed beside him a safeguard when he must get up during the night.

Hospital records need to include information about the person's sleep patterns (obtained from the sleep assessment) as well as effective nursing measures to induce sleep.

## SUMMARY

The importance of physical fitness and good body mechanics for the nurse and her clients has been stressed. The musculoskeletal assessment focus was on active range of motion. Nursing actions in assisting a client with changes in mobility included turning and moving as well as use of assistive devices. Techniques for promotion of relaxation were introduced. Nursing actions to promote sleep were presented, as were the stages of sleep and a few common sleep problems.

## LEARNING ACTIVITIES

1. Describe the physiological benefits of exercise on each of the body systems.
2. Identify your own strengths and limitations as they affect your participation in an exercise program.
3. Design for yourself a realistic physical fitness program.
4. Describe the method for stabilizing the pelvis and thereby supporting the back muscles.
5. Assume you have one of the following musculoskeletal injuries. Spend a

day carrying out your usual activities while you have a) your dominant hand in a sling or b) one leg which is not permitted to bear weight.

6. Based on your knowledge of normal musculoskeletal function, assess someone with an abnormality of the musculoskeletal system.

7. Teach a family member how to get a helpless adult out of bed onto a chair.

8. How can you utilize your knowledge of the stages of sleep to implement nursing care?

## REFERENCES AND SUGGESTED READINGS

Bailey, D. A., et al. A current view of Canadian cardiorespiratory fitness. *Canadian Medical Association Journal,* 3 (1974), 24–30.

Brower, Phyllis and Hicks, Dorothy. Maintaining muscle function in patients on bed rest. *American Journal of Nursing,* July, 1972, pp. 1250–1253.

Burgess, Ann Wolbert, 1978. *Nursing: levels of health intervention.* Englewood Cliffs, N.J.: Prentice-Hall.

Cooper, Kenneth H., 1970. *The new aerobics.* New York: Bantam Books.

*Current research on sleep and dreams.* U.S. Department of Health, Education, and Welfare, 1966.

Denlinger, Ken. Rodgers easy winner in blossom. *Washington Post,* April 3, 1978, pp. D-1 and D-7.

Diekelmann, Nancy, 1977. *Primary health care of the well adult.* New York: McGraw-Hill.

Dittmar, Sharon S. and Dulski, Theresa. Early evening administration of sleep medication to the hospitalized aged: a consideration in rehabilitation. *Nursing Research,* 26 (July–August 1977), 299–303.

Downs, Florence S. and Fitzpatrick, Joyce J. Preliminary investigation of the reliability and validity of a tool for the assessment of body position and motor activity. *Nursing Research,* 25 (November–December 1976), 404–408.

DuGas, Beverly, 1977. *Introduction to patient care.* Philadelphia: W. B. Saunders.

Ellis, Janice R. and Nowlis, Elizabeth A., 1977. *Nursing: a human needs approach.* Boston:Houghton Mifflin.

*Essentials of life and health.* New York: Random House, 1972.

Felton, G. Body rhythm effects on rotating work shifts. *Nursing Digest,* 4 (January–February 1976), 29–32.

Foss, G. Body mechanics: use your head and save your back. *Nursing 73,* March, 1973, pp. 25–32.

Friedman, Bonnie and Knight, Katherine. Running for life, health, and pleasure. *American Journal of Nursing,* April, 1978, pp. 602–607.

Gordon, Marjory. Assessing activity tolerance. *American Journal of Nursing,* January, 1976, pp. 72–75.

Guyton, Arthur, 1976. *Textbook of medical physiology.* 5th ed. Philadelphia: W. B. Saunders.

Hoffman, Norman S., 1977. *A new world of health.* New York: McGraw-Hill.

Kavanagh, Terence, 1976. *Heart attack? counter-attack!* Toronto: Van Nostrand Reinhold.

Levine, Myra, 1969. *Introduction to clinical nursing.* Philadelphia: F. A. Davis.

Lewis, LuVerne, 1976. *Fundamental skills in patient care.* Philadelphia: J. B. Lippincott.

Maltz, Stephan; Zellmer, Verne; and Chandler, Harold, 1973. *College health science.* Dubuque, Iowa: Wm. C. Brown.

Meilach, Doria. Your baby's sleep. *Young Mother,* 1972.

Mellor, Bryan. Relaxation therapy. *Nursing Times,* November 11, 1976, 1776–1777.

Michelsen, Dana. Giving a great back rub. *American Journal of Nursing,* July, 1978, pp. 1197–1199.

Miller, Helen M. Physically fit for nursing. *American Journal of Nursing,* March 1970, pp. 520–523.

Mott, Paul. The case against rotating shifts. *Nursing Outlook,* April, 1966, 51–52.

Murray, Ruth and Zentner, Judith, 1975. *Nursing assessment & health promotion through the life span.* Englewood Cliffs, N.J.: Prentice-Hall.

Noback, Charles and Demarest, Robert, 1975. *The human nervous system.* 2nd ed. New York: McGraw-Hill.

Nordmark, Madelyn and Rohweder, Anne, 1975. *Scientific foundations of nursing.* 3rd ed. Philadelphia: J. B. Lippincott.

O'Dell, M. L. Human biorhythmology: implications for nursing practice. *Nursing Forum,* 1975, Vol. 14, No. 1, pp. 43–47.

Olson, Edith V. ed. The hazards of immobility. *American Journal of Nursing,* April, 1967, pp. 788–790.

Pennino, Walter. Aging make run on father time. *Washington Post,* July 2, 1978, p. D-4.

Prior, John and Silberstein, Jack, 1973. *Physical diagnosis.* 4th ed. St. Louis: C. V. Mosby.

Ross, Karen, 1975. *The new manual of Yoga.* New York: ARCO.

Stern, Robert and Ray, William, 1977. *Biofeedback.* Homewood, Ill.: Dow Jones-Irwin.

# 21

# Body Temperature

Introduction
Physiology of Body Temperature Control
Factors Affecting Body Temperature
Measuring Body Temperature
Problems of Hypothermia and Hyperthermia
Applications of Heat and Cold
Summary
Learning Activities
References and Suggested Readings

## Behavioral Objectives

Upon completion of this chapter, the student will be able to:

1. Describe the physiology of temperature control.
2. State specific factors that affect internal body temperature.
3. Decide the method to use for taking a temperature and, after practice, take temperatures by all routes, using both glass-mercury thermometers and electronic thermometers.
4. Explain when hot and cold applications are indicated and, after practice, be able to apply them.
5. Given selected problems of hypothermia and hyperthermia, assess, plan, implement, and evaluate nursing measures to overcome these problems.

## Key Terms

| | | |
|---|---|---|
| antipyretics | heat stroke | radiation |
| aquathermia pads | hydrocollator | sitz bath |
| axilla | hyperthermia | temperature |
| centigrade | hypothalamus | core |
| conduction | hypothermia: induced, | surface |
| convection | accidental; hypothermia | environment |
| evaporation | machines | thermometer |
| Fahrenheit | malignant hyperthermia | glass-mercury |
| frostbite | pyrogens | electronic |
| heat exhaustion | | |

## Introduction

The human body is able to maintain a remarkably constant internal temperature regardless of the temperature in the external environment. Changes in the internal temperature occur when there are problems with the temperature-regulating mechanisms or when disease processes exist.

In this chapter the physiology of body temperature control will be described. Selected problems of hypothermia and hyperthermia will be presented, with emphasis on nursing measures to correct these problems. Determining the proper route for temperature measurement in specific instances, the procedure for taking temperatures, and the need for accurate instruments are stressed. The chapter ends with a discussion of the purposes of hot and cold applications and techniques for their application.

## PHYSIOLOGY OF BODY TEMPERATURE CONTROL

Body temperature represents a balance between the heat produced in the body and the heat lost. Heat is continually produced as a by-product of metabolism. Heat production and loss are regulated in the preoptic and adjacent regions of the hypothalamus. The normal internal body temperature is about 98.6°F (37°C). In health, the internal body temperature seldom varies more than a degree above or below 98.6°F. Even when the environmental temperature ranges between 55° and 140°F, if the humidity is very low, studies have shown that a nude person will maintain a constant body temperature. The surface temperature rises and falls with the temperature of the environment, but the core temperature does not.

Body heat production is influenced by the basal metabolic rate, muscle activity, the effect of thyroxine on cells, the effect of norepinephrine and sympathetic stimulation on cells, and increased temperature of body cells (Guyton, 1976).

Heat is lost from the skin through radiation, conduction, convection, and evaporization. With radiation, body heat is lost in the form of infrared heat rays. If the temperature of the body is greater than the surrounding temperature, more heat is radiated from the body than to it. When the surroundings become warmer than the human body, as in the summer, more radiant heat is transmitted to the body than from it.

In conduction, body heat is lost by direct contact with cooler objects in the environment. Loss of heat by conduction to objects is small, although conduction to air represents a considerable proportion of body heat loss. Conduction of body heat to air is self-limited unless the heated air moves away from the skin so that new, unheated air is brought into contact with the skin. Convection is the movement of heat by air currents. Heat must first be conducted to the air and then carried away by convection currents. Evaporation is the removal of moisture from the body surface by vaporization. Heat is also lost from the body through the lungs, in urine, and feces.

Heat is tranferred from the internal body core to the skin through the flow of blood. A high rate of blood flow allows heat to be conducted efficiently from the internal core to the skin, while reduced blood flow is less efficient. The amount of vasoconstriction in the vessels supplying blood to the skin controls the rate by which heat is conducted to the body surface. The sympathetic centers of the posterior hypothalamus control the dilatation and constriction of the blood vessels in the skin.

Temperature receptors are required for the operation of the feedback mechanisms which operate through the temperature-regulating center in the hypothalamus. Probably the most important temperature receptors are the neurons located in the preoptic area of the hypothalamus. Other receptors include a few cold-sensitive neurons found in different parts of the hypothalamus, the septum, and the reticular substance of the midbrain; skin temperature receptors, and temperature receptors in the spinal cord, abdomen, and possibly other internal structures of the body (Guyton, 1976).

## FACTORS AFFECTING BODY TEMPERATURE

Part of the nurse's assessment is to find out her client's normal body temperature, if it is known to him. Then, his current temperature is measured and compared with his base-line temperature. Keep in mind that various factors, such as the time of day affect body temperature. For persons who are awake during the day and asleep during the night, the lowest body temperature occurs in the early morning hours, and the temperature peaks in the late afternoon and early evening. Thus, if temperatures are to be measured just once a day, late afternoon would be the time that would indicate the most accurate temperature. For persons whose lifestyle requires them to be awake at night and asleep during the day, the low and high temperature points are reversed. The person's wake-sleep pattern is, therefore, an important factor in body temperature measurement.

The menstrual cycle and pregnancy also affect body temperature. There is a slight temperature drop just before ovulation and then a rise during ovulation of .5° to 1.0°F above normal. This rise continues until a day or two before menstruation. During pregnancy, because of the increased metabolic rate, the woman's temperature may be elevated consistently until about the fourth month.

The muscle action during physical exercise generates heat. Exercise may produce some body temperature variation because the temperature regulating mechanisms are not 100 percent efficient. Personal behaviors help control temperature. If we feel cold, we exercise to get warm by moving about, rubbing our hands, jumping up and down. Jogging, for example, generates considerable heat. If the circulation is adequate and the sweat glands are functioning properly, the excess heat produced by this exercise is given off through perspiration and the internal temperature remains constant.

Body temperature is influenced by age. In infants, because of the immaturity of heat-regulating mechanisms, body temperature may show marked fluctuations. Clothing and environmental temperatures are adjusted accordingly to maintain the infant's temperature within the normal range. Nalepka

(1976) stated that the shivering mechanism is absent in premature and other infants during the first month of life. These infants also have little or no subcutaneous fat and therefore little or no insulation. These infants are especially dependent upon others to help maintain their normal body temperature by controlling the environmental temperature and their clothing.

The elderly person tends to have a low body temperature because of circulatory deficiencies, loss of subcutaneous fat, and malfunction of heat-producing mechanisms (such as loss of shivering mechanism). For these reasons, cold weather is not tolerated well by the elderly, and hypothermia may become a problem.

Those who have deficient or absent sweat glands are in serious danger when the environmental temperature is greater than their body temperature. When the temperature of the surroundings is greater than that of the skin, the body gains heat from the surroundings and the only way it can lose the heat is by evaporation. Therefore, since perspiration and evaporation of the perspiration cannot occur, body temperature rises. Environmental conditions may cause some body temperature variations in those with normal sweat glands. When the humidity is high we are extremely uncomfortable. There is truth in the phrase, "It's not the heat, it's the humidity." In high humidity, the sweat that is formed stays on the skin since it cannot evaporate into the air that is already saturated with moisture. Therefore, body temperature may approach or even exceed environmental temperature. Lack of air movement prevents effective evaporation in the same way that it prevents cooling by conduction of heat to the air. Convection currents cause air that is saturated with moisture to move away from the body to be replaced by unsaturated air. This explains the value of fans in hot, humid weather.

Clothing affects body temperature through conduction and convection. Clothing traps air next to the skin and decreases the flow of air currents. Therefore, the rate of heat loss by conduction is decreased. For these reasons, clothing that is layered is more effective in heat conservation than one bulky piece of clothing. When clothing is wet, heat loss is considerable because water is a good conductor of heat.

Certain medications affect body temperature by interfering with the temperature-regulating center. These drugs include the phenothiazines, barbiturates, and alcohol.

The effect of extremes of environmental temperatures and disease processes on body temperature will be discussed in some detail later in the chapter.

## MEASURING BODY TEMPERATURE

Important health care decisions are based on measurements of body temperature: a medication is initiated or terminated; surgery is performed or cancelled; diagnosis is established or not; a client is discharged or retained in a hospital. The clinical thermometer is an assessment tool of almost limitless value in such decision-making. An accurate thermometer correctly used is essential, then, in measuring body temperature.

How accurate are thermometers? Questions about their accuracy are raised periodically (Palmer, 1949; Barber, 1971; Abbey et al., 1978). In a study reported by Abbey et al. (1978), new thermometers, stored but not used thermometers, and used and then stored thermometers were shown to be inaccurate. The inaccuracies ranged from 2 percent in new thermometers to nearly 24 percent in those used and then stored for ten months. It would seem that the department dispensing thermometers has an obligation to test and provide accurate instruments. In any case, if the nurse believes the temperature she gets does not accurately represent her client's body temperature, it is her responsibility to take the temperature again, using a different thermometer.

Many types of thermometers (as well as other temperature-sensing devices) are available today and new ones will, no doubt, continue to be developed. Glass-mercury thermometers, disposable paper thermometers, and electronic thermometers are among those currently available. Directions for taking temperatures vary depending upon the instrument used. The manufacturer's directions should be followed.

The amount of time required for oral, rectal, and axillary temperature placement has been the object of considerable research. At this time, it is generally agreed that accurate readings are obtained with the glass-mercury thermometer when the oral thermometer is kept under the tongue for 8 to 9 minutes; the thermometer kept under the arm for 10 minutes for an axillary temperature; and the rectal thermometer kept in the anus for two minutes. Usually a rectal temperature measures slightly higher than the oral, and the axillary measures about a degree lower.

## Selecting the Method for Taking the Temperature

An oral method is the most convenient when the client is alert, able to hold the thermometer under his tongue safely, and can keep his mouth closed during the time required for an accurate reading. Oral temperatures would not be taken when a person is receiving oxygen, has a naso-gastric tube in place, is a mouth breather, is unconscious, or is a young child. While agency policy frequently indicates the age and conditions at which rectal and axillary temperatures are taken, nursing judgment should be included in the determination of the appropriate method. If the policy states that children over the age of 5 may have oral temperatures taken and those under 5 require rectal temperatures, the nurse might ask the mother how she takes her child's temperature. Usually the nurse can use the same method the mother does. If a rectal temperature is required for the child, the mother might like to take it. The nurse must use her own judgment about asking parents to assist.

Ordinarily, axillary temperatures are taken on infants following an initial rectal temperature to assess the patency of the anus. Routine rectal temperature measurement stimulates rectal elimination, which is not desirable.

## Thermometers

Fahrenheit and Centigrade (Celsius) thermometers are available. Generally, the Fahrenheit thermometer is calibrated to register from 90° to 106°F. The Centigrade scale ranges from 35° to 43.3°C. On the thermometer scale, only the even numbers are printed (e.g. 90, 92, 94). In addition, each long line on the scale indicates a full degree; each short line indicates .2 (2/10) of a degree.

The following formula is used to convert temperatures from Fahrenheit to Centigrade: subtract 32 and multiply by 5/9. To convert from Centigrade to Fahrenheit, multiply by 9/5 and add 32.

**Special Considerations**
Before the nurse takes an oral temperature, she determines when her client last had something to eat or drink. Hot or cold food or fluids, smoking, or gum chewing within 30 minutes before the oral temperature measurement will influence the temperature.

The oral thermometer has a long, slender bulb which provides a greater surface for contact with tissues than that found in the stubby or bulb-shaped mercury tips on the rectal thermometers. While some oral thermometers have stubby tips, thermometers used for oral and rectal temperatures are not interchangeable, for esthetic reasons. Mouth thermometers are used for mouth temperatures and rectal thermometers for rectal temperatures. An oral thermometer is used for measuring an axillary temperature.

Several brands of electronic thermometers are available. They all have separate probes for mouth and rectal temperatures. Ordinarily, the tip of the oral probe is white and the rectal probe red. Plastic disposable tips cover the probe and eliminate the need for cleansing between use. This portable battery-operated thermometer registers the body temperature in 30 seconds or less. A signal (either light or sound) indicates when the temperature should be read. Immediate recording of the temperature is required because the reading is eliminated when the probe is replaced in its slot.

While the only sure way to assess a person's body temperature is to measure it with a thermometer, the following guide provides important additional data.

## Guide for Assessing Body Temperature

Ask the client:
1. Do you know your normal body temperature?
2. Do you know your present body temperature?
3. Do you know of any times when your temperature varies?
4. What is your wake–sleep pattern?
5. For women of child-bearing age: when was your last menstrual period?
6. Do you have trouble tolerating heat or cold?
7. Has anyone in your family had an unexplained problem during surgery?

## Performance Checklist
### Taking an Oral Temperature

1. Wash hands.
2. Select a clean glass-mercury thermometer. If cleansing is done by soaking in a chemical solution, rinse thermometer under cold running water.
3. Read the thermometer by holding it horizontally at eye level and rotating it slowly until the mercury column can be seen.
4. If it registers 96° or higher, grasp the end of the thermometer with the thumb and index finger, and by snapping the wrist, shake the mercury to the lowest marking.
5. Place the thermometer under the tongue in the sublingual pocket (where the tongue and the floor of the mouth are joined by the frenum lingulae). Instruct the person to keep his lips closed.
6. Keep the thermometer in place 8 to 9 minutes.
7. Remove the thermometer and wipe with a tissue from end to mercury bulb (minimizes spread of organisms to cleaner area) using a twisting motion. Dispose of tissue appropriately.
8. Read and record temperature.
9. Place thermometer in designated area for replacement, or cleanse by washing with detergent, cool water, and soaking in designated solution.

*Axillary Temperature*
1. Follow steps 1 through 4 above.
2. If necessary, wipe axilla dry.
3. Place thermometer bulb in axilla and have client position arm across chest.
4. Keep thermometer in place 10 minutes.
5. Follow steps 7 through 9 above.

*Rectal Temperature*

1. Wash hands.
2. Select a rectal thermometer.
3. Read thermometer and shake it down as necessary.
4. Lubricate mercury tip of thermometer to lessen friction.
5. Assist client to a side-lying position and insert thermometer into anus, approximately 1½".
6. *Hold* thermometer in place for 2 minutes.
7. Remove thermometer, clean it, read and record temperature, and return it to designated area.

*Electronic Thermometers*

1. Select the appropriate oral or rectal probe and plug it into the outlet on the thermometer.
2. Attach disposable probe cover.
3. Slide probe slowly into sublingual pocket (oral temperature) or insert probe into anus (rectal).
4. When the body temperature has registered, remove and discard probe cover, record temperature and replace probe in slot.
5. Replace thermometer on storage base.

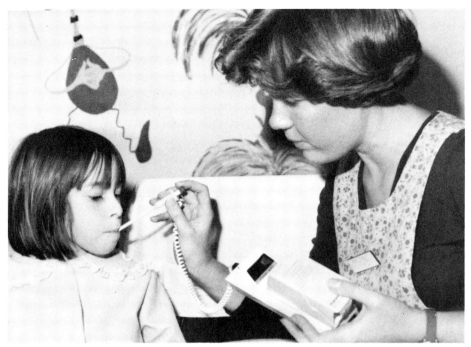

**Figure 21-1.** *Taking a child's temperature orally with an electronic thermometer.* *(Photo by Frank R. Engler, Jr.)*

Do the following:
1. Measure your client's temperature.
2. Take the pulse, blood pressure, and assess the cardiac rhythm (Ch. 15).
3. Check the peripheral circulation by inspecting for color and taking pedal pulses (Ch. 15).
4. Check the intactness of the sense of touch.
5. Are there any broken skin surfaces?
6. Feel the temperature of the skin on the abdomen or between the thighs.
7. See if the skin is pale or flushed.
8. Is there any shivering?
9. How alert is your client?

## PROBLEMS OF HYPOTHERMIA AND HYPERTHERMIA

### Hypothermia

Hypothermia is defined as abnormally low body temperature, typically 95°F (35°C) and below. Low body temperatures can be induced for medical reasons or they can be accidental.

*Induced hypothermia* is useful during surgery when, as a result of the hypothermia, circulation can be stopped for relatively long periods because the oxygen needs of the tissues are greatly reduced. Blood pressure is low and bleeding is minimal. Humans can tolerate body temperatures of 70°-75°F, without permanent ill effects (Ganong, 1977).

*Accidental hypothermia* occurs when there is prolonged exposure to the cold. Individuals of all ages who are exposed to extremely cold temperatures without protection may become victims of accidental hypothermia. The elderly, however, become victims of accidental hypothermia after exposure to relatively mild cold. Half of all victims of accidental hypothermia are elderly. Infants under one year of age are also highly susceptible because of their immature temperature controls.

The most likely candidates for accidental hypothermia are the very old, the poor who are unable to afford adequate heating, and those whose bodies respond abnormally to the cold. The aged with temperature-regulation defects are the most endangered because they cannot shiver and conserve the badly needed body heat.

**Assessment**   The only sure way to detect hypothermia is to take the person's rectal temperature with a special low-reading clinical thermometer (one with a scale that goes below the usual low point of 94°F (34°C). Feel the skin of the abdomen, which in hypothermia is cold to the touch. The person may be confused and may progress to a state of coma if the temperature drops below 90°F (32.2°C). The face may be puffy and pink. There is no pallor or shivering. The pulse is slow and the blood pressure low.

**Nursing Implementation**   General medical opinion is that rewarming of the hypothermic person should take place slowly (Butler and Shalowitz, 1978). The person should be covered with blankets and placed in a warm room (80°F). The blood pressure is monitored and maintained at a steady level. Body temperature (rectal) is monitored frequently. It usually returns to normal within 24 hours (Millard, 1977; Butler and Shalowitz, 1978).

Prevention is an important aspect of nursing in hypothermia. Many old people live in surroundings that are too cold. While the energy crisis has encouraged people to turn down room thermostats, comfortable temperatures must be maintained for the elderly. Comfortable clothing that provides insulation also helps prevent hypothermia. Drugs that affect temperature control should be avoided.

**Frostbite**   Frostbite is a condition of true tissue freezing. Rapid rewarming by thawing in warm water (100–108°F) is recommended (Mills, 1976). The body part should *not* be rubbed with ice or snow. No friction or rubbing of any kind should be used, because of the danger of tissue damage.

## Hyperthermia

Hyperthermia (also called pyrexia or fever) is a body temperature above normal. It may be caused by abnormalities in the brain itself or by toxic substances that affect the temperature-regulating centers. Chemical substances causing an elevation in the heat-regulating center are called *pyrogens*. With this increase in the thermostatic setting, mechanisms to increase body temperature begin to work. Peripheral vasoconstriction decreases heat loss. There is a subjective feeling of chilliness and the skin feels cold. Shivering which may become severe occurs as the body attempts to increase heat production. Then, after increased heat is produced, the peripheral blood vessels dilate and the skin is flushed, hot, and dry.

Increased metabolic rates such as those seen in hyperthyroidism result in elevated body temperature. Decreased heat loss occurs with obesity, dehydration with decreased secretion of sweat, peripheral vasoconstriction, and absence of sweat glands. Damage to the heat-regulating center can occur after head injury (including brain surgery), cerebrovascular accident, or abnormally high body temperatures. Tissue destruction, inflammatory response, and infectious diseases also affect the heat-regulating centers.

**Assessment**   In hyperthermia, the body temperature will be abnormally elevated. The pulse and respirations will be rapid. The skin may appear red, hot and dry, or damp with perspiration. The person will feel either chilly or uncomfortably warm. There may be chills, headache, restlessness, and general malaise (tiredness). The client may suffer delirium or loss of consciousness if the fever remains high. Convulsions occur rather frequently in infants and small children.

**Nursing Implementation**   Nursing measures for the person with hyperthermia are centered around attempts to reduce the amount of heat produced in the body and increase the amount of heat eliminated from the body. Additional nursing measures are aimed at lessening the effect of fever on the body.

To reduce the amount of heat produced, mental and physical rest are encouraged. Bed rest is enforced and physical activities are restricted. Mental rest is more difficult to achieve but it is encouraged when procedures and treatments are explained, needs are anticipated, and assurances are provided. More detail on techniques for providing psychological rest is given in the chapter on activity, rest, and sleep (Ch. 20).

A cool, comfortable room increases heat elimination and encourages rest. Bed clothes should be light. A fan increases air circulation and facilitates removal of body heat when air conditioning is not available.

Antipyretic drugs are given to reduce the fever and thereby prevent damage to the body from excessive body heat. Salicylates are popular antipyretic drugs (Aspirin is a salicylate, Acetylsalicylic acid). The antipyretic effect of the salicylates appears to involve inhibition of the synthesis of prostaglandins. Pyrogens cause generation of Prostaglandin E-like substance in the brain. This effect is inhibited by salicylates (Goodman and Gilman, 1975). Antipyretics may be ordered at regular hours or p.r.n. depending upon the temperature; for example, "give Aspirin gr 10 q 4 h for a temperature above 102°F." In addition, antibiotic drugs are often given (on a regular basis such as q 4 h or q 6 h) to the person whose fever responds to antibiotic therapy.

A sponge bath is useful for rapidly lowering the body temperature. It can be carried out easily in either the home or the hospital. Mothers should be taught the procedure, because young children with high fevers often have convulsions if the temperature is not lowered quickly.

## Special Considerations

Because the body loses heat by conduction to a cooler substance, in this instance from the hot body to the tepid water, by evaporation of the water from the skin surface, and by convection as the air carries the heat away, sponging serves to lower the temperature. Occasionally alcohol sponging is ordered. Then alcohol is substituted for the water or added to the water. Because alcohol evaporates at a lower temperature than water, cooling occurs faster.

---

### Performance Checklist
### Tepid Sponge Bath

1. Take the vital signs.
2. Wash hands.
3. Get a basin of water 85° to 100°F (30° to 38°C), towels, wash cloths, bath blanket, and bottle of rubbing alcohol.
4. Sponge large areas at a time; e.g., one side of leg, arm, chest, and abdomen. Use long strokes.
5. Place wet wash cloths in axillae and groin to assist cooling. Keep them there and replace with fresh, cool ones as needed.
6. Dry the sponged areas by patting gently (rubbing will increase heat production).
7. Gently rub back with rubbing alcohol.
8. Replace clothing.
9. Take vital signs after 20 minutes.
10. Repeat sponging until designated body temperature has been reached (stop before normal temperature is reached because further drop occurs after sponging ends).

---

**Hypothermia Machines**   Hypothermia pads or blankets are used when rapid surface cooling of the body is desired, when it is essential to lower the body temperature quickly, or when artificial cooling must be maintained for a prolonged time period. The hypothermia machine consists of a refrigeration unit with attached pads or blankets. A solution (usually ethyl alcohol and distilled water) maintained at the desired temperature circulates through the tubes contained in the pads or blankets that are in direct contact with the client's skin.

Specific operating instructions will be available with the machine. A temperature probe is inserted into the rectum and the body temperature is

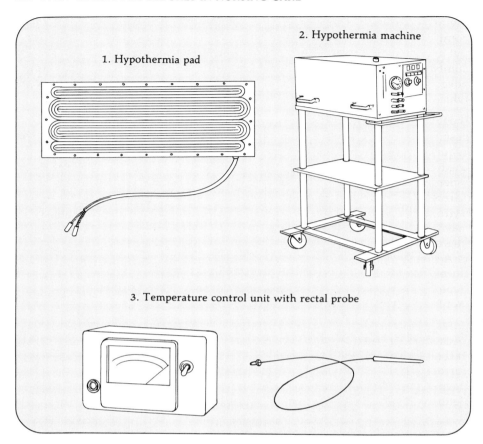

**Figure 21-2.**  *The hypothermia machine consists of: (1) hypothermia pads; (2) a refrigeration unit; and (3) a temperature control unit and a probe for measuring rectal temperature.*

continuously registered. The client's skin is checked at regular intervals for circulatory changes indicated by color, swelling, pain, and numbness. Emotional support is given throughout the time the person remains on the blankets. Shivering must be controlled, if it occurs, by use of medications, or else heat production is increased. The doctor will prescribe the body temperature desired and the length of time the temperature is to be maintained.

## Controlling the Effects of Fever

Comfort measures, hydration, and nutrition lessen the effects of fever on the body.

**Comfort measures**   The person with a fever requires good hygiene because diaphoresis (profuse sweating) frequently accompanies fever. Bathing as needed and assistance in changing clothing and bedding contribute to comfort. The client should be encouraged to use the cotton clothing provided by many agencies rather than the synthetic bed clothes which are less comfortable because they do not absorb perspiration. Good oral hygiene and adequate fluids usually prevent cracks in the corners of the mouth and tongue which otherwise accompany fever.

Hydration   Because of the fluids lost by perspiration and increased respirations, fluids must be replaced. In addition, increased fluid intake is required to help eliminate the waste products from increased metabolism and the toxic substances that may be present. The desired daily intake of fluids for a person with fever is 3,000 ml. If the total amount cannot be taken orally, parenteral fluids will be required. The person is offered oral fluids of his choice (within prescribed parameters). Warm fluids are comforting if the person is having a chill, otherwise the temperature of fluids should be that desired by the client.

A record is kept of all oral and parenteral fluid intake. Urine output is measured and the amount of sweat estimated. This estimate can be made by reporting how often gown and bedding need to be changed as well as whether or not the clothing is damp or soaking wet.

Nutrition   Contrary to popular belief, we should not "starve a fever." Because the metabolic rate is increased with fever, both proteins and carbohydrates are required in the diet. Proteins are needed to aid in tissue formation and carbohydrate to supply energy. The person with a fever should have his weight checked regularly. His dietary intake should be evaluated to determine whether or not he is eating the foods prescribed for him.

Reporting   Close observation of a person's vital signs is important. An elevated temperature is significant and should be reported promptly. Accuracy of temperature measurement is assumed and has been discussed in some detail previously. The frequency of temperature measurement will vary with the health problem.

## Heat Exhaustion and Heat Stroke

In heat exhaustion, the client's temperature is about normal—a little above or a little below. Skin is cool and moist and the client is usually conscious. Heat exhaustion and heat prostration—progressive lassitude (weakness and exhaustion) and inability to work—are followed by severe headache, vomiting, tachycardia, and hypotension. Water depletion and hypovolemia are accompanied by hemoconcentration, hypernatremia, and hyperchloremia associated with concentrated urine. The treatment is rehydration and rest (O'Donnell and Clowes, 1974).

In heat stroke, the person's temperature is very high, between 105.8°F and 108°F. The outlook is bleak for the person whose temperature reaches 108°F. The skin is hot, dry, and red. Sweating has ceased and thermal energy is stored when sweating is blocked. As a result the person is hyperthermic. He is usually severely confused or comatose. Hypotension occurs in about half the persons with heat stroke.

Fatigue, lack of physical conditioning, failure of acclimatization, increased heat and humidity, and obesity predispose to heat stroke. Teaching measures for prevention of heat stroke, then, include counseling to take it easy in a climate warmer than the accustomed one. For example, playing tennis in 95°F accompanied by relatively high humidity is risky if one is not used to this activity and climate.

When the diagnosis of heat stroke has been made, the first goal is rapid reduction of temperature. This may be accomplished by putting the client in an ice bath. To counteract the peripheral vasoconstriction caused by the ice bath, the skin is massaged during the bath to promote circulation to the skin. The client is removed from the bath when his temperature reaches 102°F. In young people with heat stroke (and most of those studied with heat stroke were young) who receive the proper treatment, neurological and circulatory symptoms are usually corrected within six hours (*Emergency Medicine*, 1976).

**Malignant Hyperthermia**  Malignant hyperthermia is an unexplained fever occurring during anesthesia when certain anesthetic agents such as halothane, succinylcholine, or methoxyflurane are used. While the etiology of this problem is not known, it is believed to be a part of a generalized human stress syndrome. Therefore, the hyperthermia may be a reaction to stress and not necessarily to the anesthetics. There seems to be a familial incidence. For this reason it is important to take a thorough family history, looking for multiple drug allergies, unexplained surgical deaths in family members, or a history of muscle weakness and associated diseases. Preoperative stress should be minimized. Careful monitoring during surgery, while it will not prevent the problem, will allow prompt detection and treatment of the problem should it occur (Zelechowski, 1977).

## APPLICATION OF HEAT AND COLD

Heat and cold are applied frequently in both the home and the hospital; in the hospital setting, a doctor's order is ordinarily required before heat or cold is applied.

### Heat

Heat is used to relieve pain, reduce swelling, congestion and inflammation, to relieve muscle spasm, to provide comfort, to decrease the blood supply in other areas of the body, and to raise the body temperature. Heat causes dilatation of blood vessels, and thereby increases the supply of blood to the area. The dilated blood vessels carry away toxins and excess tissue fluid, thereby reducing swelling and congestion. Reduced swelling decreases pressure on nerve endings and relieves pain. Because heat increases the blood supply to the injured part, healing is promoted. Heat stimulates metabolism and the temperature rises. It also causes redness in the area of heat application.

Prolonged exposure to heat can damage tissues. Special care is required when heat is applied to the very young and the very old who do not tolerate heat well. In addition, persons who have circulatory disorders, are debilitated, have decreased or absent response to pain, or are unconscious require special consideration in application of heat.

Heat applications can be either local or general; either moist or dry. A local application is one that is applied to a specific part of the body; a general application is one applied to the entire body.

### Special Considerations

Dry heat is applied with a hot water bottle, heating pad, or heat lamp. Hot water bottles are generally not applied to a person who has decreased or absent sensation. The skin will tolerate greater temperatures if the heat is dry than if it is moist, because water is a good conductor of heat and air is not.

---

**Performance Checklist**
**Applying a Hot Water Bottle**

1. Fill the hot water bottle 1/2 to 2/3 full of water, 115–125°F.
2. Place the bottle on a flat surface and expel the air.
3. Tightly close the hot water bottle.
4. Wipe the bottle dry.
5. Cover hot water bottle with pillow case (or other cover) to slow heat transmission, lessen danger of burning, and provide comfortable, soft surface.
6. Place hot water bottle on designated area.
7. If treatment is to continue, refill hot water bottle as water cools.
8. Observe skin for redness, heat, swelling, pain, circulation. Chart observations.

---

**Disposable Hot Packs**   Disposable hot packs are prefilled plastic packages containing an exact amount of interacting ingredients which, when activated (by striking or squeezing), produce a sustained temperature of 101°-114°F. The manufacturer's directions for use and length of time heat is maintained (usually 20-60 minutes) should be read carefully. The pack is applied directly to the designated area (no cover is required).

**Electric Heating Pads**   While many agencies do not permit the use of electric heating pads, they are commonly used in the home. Safety requires that the heating mechanism be in proper working condition, that the pads not be used in or near water, that they be covered, and that the control button be placed on "low." The skin is checked for redness, pain, and circulation during the pad's use. If the pad causes pain, it is removed.

Heat Lamp    A 60-watt bulb placed in a lamp 18 to 22 inches away from the body provides a safe amount of heat by radiation. The lamp is secured so that it maintains the correct distance and does not fall. The lamp is kept on for the length of time ordered (usually 10 to 15 minutes).

Aquathermia Pad    The aquamatic K pad is made up of an electric control unit and a container of distilled water which is heated and circulated through the unit and the pad. The temperature is set at 105°F, the pad is covered with sheeting or a bath towel, and the pad applied to the designated area. Throughout the treatment, the skin is assessed for swelling, redness, circulation, pain, and numbness.

Moist Heat    Baths, soaks, and compresses are the usual modes for application of moist heat. Baths and soaks are used to apply moist heat to the entire body or to a specific part. The usual water temperature is 105° to 110°F, and it should be carefully tested for safety reasons. Higher temperatures may cause tissue damage. Length of time for treatment varies, but a tub bath is usually 10 to 30 minutes long and a sitz bath 15 minutes. A sitz bath is one in which warm or hot water is placed in a tub (or basin) and the client sits with the pelvis in the water. Special tubs and basins are more appropriate than regular bath tubs for this purpose because the pelvis, but not the legs and feet, should be in the water. Sitz baths are used for relief of pain, to encourage voiding by producing relaxation, and to promote healing. The water temperature varies depending upon the purpose of the bath. If the purpose is to provide heat: 110° to 115°F for 15 minutes; for cleansing to promote healing 94° to 98°F. During the bath the person is assessed for weakness, faintness, and any other changes that might result from circulatory shifts.

Warm Compresses    Warm compresses may be either sterile or not. Sterile compresses are applied to an open wound. Then a sterile basin with sterile solution is heated to 105°-110°F. The compresses are wrung out using forceps and applied to the body part as indicated. For insulation, a waterproof cloth is used to cover the sterile dressings. Unless otherwise indicated the compresses are changed every 5 minutes for 15 to 20 minutes. When compresses are applied to intact skin, they need not be sterile.

Commercially prepared moist sterile compresses are available. They are heated in the package in the unit provided and applied as any sterile dressing is applied.

Hot Packs    Hot packs are used to cover large body areas and are applied as hot as they can be tolerated without burning the skin. Hot towels are often used for this purpose. The hydrocollator is an appliance that steams special hot packs. Plastic sheeting is placed under the part to be treated. The pack is removed from the water with forceps and placed where indicated. It is then covered with a towel. Because the packs are heavy, it is fatiguing if they are placed on top of the body part. If possible, they should be placed under the part. Proper body alignment is maintained during all the treatments.

# Cold

Cold applications cause vasoconstriction with reduced blood flow to the skin; therefore, the skin becomes pale, mottled, cool to the touch, and numb. Whether the application is cold or warm, temperature tolerance varies with the individual, the part of the body to which it is applied, the area of application, and the length of time it is applied. For example, the eyelid is thinner and more sensitive to ice than the thick sole of the foot.

Cold applications are used to provide topical anesthesia (placing an ice bag on the injection site before giving the injection, for example), to prevent edema (after bruises, sprains, and strains), to lessen hemorrhage, to reduce inflammation, decrease metabolism, and to lower body temperature.

The temperature for cold applications should be prescribed as either tepid, cool, cold, or ice. As with hot applications, cold applications are either local or general, moist or dry.

Dry Cold   An ice cap, collar, or disposable pack is used to provide dry cold. An ice cap or collar is filled with crushed ice, air expelled from the container, and sealed. Any water on the outside is wiped off, the container is covered with a special cover, a wash cloth or towel, and the container is applied to the area indicated. A disposable pack contains interacting ingredients which, when activated, create a temperature ranging from 50° to 80°F. The cold action lasts from 30 minutes to 4 hours, depending upon the product used. The manufacturer's directions should be followed. Usually no cloth cover is required and the pack is applied directly to the designated area. The skin is inspected throughout the treatment for signs of circulatory change. Continued mottling or pain necessitates removal of the application.

Moist Cold   The use of tepid sponges and ice baths was discussed in the previous section under hyperthermia. Cold compresses and ice packs will be discussed here.

Cold Compresses   Usually gauze pads, wash cloths, or towels are used for cold compresses. They are soaked in a basin of ice chips plus a small amount of water. The compresses are wrung out and applied to the area indicated.

Ice Packs   Ice packs may be applied to the entire body to lower the temperature or hyperthermia pads may be used. The skin is covered with a cloth before ice packs are applied to a large surface. Then an additional layer of cloth covers the ice pack to slow the melting.

Ice packs or compresses stay cold for different time lengths depending on the environmental temperature and the person's temperature. Fifteen to 20 minutes is the approximate length of time the packs remain cold. Often the client will be able to tell the nurse when the pack or compress needs to be changed if he is not able to change it himself. The skin is inspected for changes.

## SUMMARY

Body temperature represents a balance between the heat produced in the body and the heat lost. Heat regulation takes place in the hypothalamus. Heat is lost from the skin by radiation, conduction, convection, and evaporation.

Many factors affect body temperature, including body rhythms, menstrual cycle, muscle action, age, deficient sweat glands, environmental conditions, and medications. Because many health decisions are based on body temperature readings, accuracy in temperature-taking is essential.

Problems of hyperthermia and hypothermia require nursing assessment, planning, implementation, and frequent evaluation. Applications of heat and cold are part of this treatment. Whether the application is cold or warm, temperature tolerance varies with the individual and the part of the body to which it is applied. Length of time of the application, size of application, and whether it is moist or dry affect tolerance.

## LEARNING ACTIVITIES

1. Given the age and health state of an imaginary client, decide which route to use for measuring the body temperature.
2. You suspect a client is hypothermic. What do you include in your nursing assessment?
3. Describe nursing measures for the person who is hyperthermic.
4. Describe the physiology of temperature control.
5. Explain the body's physiological response to heat; to cold.
6. State two health problems that require the application of heat; of cold.

## REFERENCES AND SUGGESTED READINGS

Abbey, June C., et al.   How long is that thermometer accurate? *American Journal of Nursing,* August, 1978, pp. 1375–1376.

Barber, C. R.   The calibration of thermometers.   London: National Physical Laboratory Department of Trade and Industry, 1971.

Butler, Robert N. and Shalowitz, Ann.   A winter hazard for the old: accidental hypothermia. *Journal of Nursing Care,* 11 (March 1978), 16–17.

Davis-Sharts, Jean.   Mechanisms and manifestations of fever. *American Journal of Nursing,* November, 1978, pp. 1874–1877.

DuGas, Beverly, 1977. *Introduction to patient care.* Philadelphia: W. B. Saunders.

Felton, Cynthia.   Hypoxemia and oral temperatures. *American Journal of Nursing,* January, 1978, pp. 56–57.

Fuerst, Elinor; Wolff, LuVerne; and Weitzel, Marlene, 1974. *Fundamentals of nursing.* 5th ed. Philadelphia: J. B. Lippincott.

Ganong, W. F., 1977. *Review of medical physiology.* 8th ed. Los Altos, Cal.: Lange Medical Publications.

Goodman, Louis and Gilman, Alfred, 1975. *The pharmacological basis of therapeutics.* 5th ed. New York: Macmillan.

Guyton, Arthur, 1976. *Textbook of medical physiology.* 5th ed. Philadelphia: W. B. Saunders.

Leddy, Susan. Sleep and phase shifting of biological rhythm. *International Journal of Nursing Studies,* Vol. 14, No. 1 (1977, Pergamon Press), 137–150.

Millard, P. H. Hypothermia in the elderly. *Nursing Mirror,* 145 (November 3, 1977), 23–25.

Mills, William J. Out in the cold. *Emergency Medicine,* 8 (January 1976), 135–147.

Nalepka, Claire. Understanding thermoregulation in newborns. *Journal of Obstetric, Gynecological, and Neonatological Nursing,* 5, (November/December, 1976), 17–19.

O'Donnell, T. and Clowes, G. Heat stroke and heat exhaustion. *New England Journal of Medicine,* 291 (September 12, 1974), 564–566.

Palmer, D. H. A check on acceptability of clinical thermometers. *Hospitals,* 23 (May, 1949), 87–88.

Some new light on heat. *Emergency Medicine,* 8 (July, 1976), 107–109.

Wood, Lucile, 1975. *Nursing Skills for Allied Health Services, Vols. 2 and 3.* Philadelphia: W. B. Saunders.

Zelechowski, Gina. Hidden killer: malignant hyperthermia. *Nursing 77,* September, 1977, p. 35.

# 22

# The Sensory System and Pain

## Behavioral Objectives

Upon completion of this chapter, the student will be able to:

1. Assess a client's sensory status.
2. Describe ways to prevent sensory alterations.
3. Implement and evaluate nursing actions for persons with sensory alterations.
4. Describe safety measures for a person with perceptual distortion.
5. Assess a client's level of consciousness.
6. Assess the person in pain; include the psychological aspects as well as the physiological.
7. Compare the gate control theory with the specificity theory and indicate pain relief measures based on each theory.
8. Discuss the validity of the belief that culture affects the pain experience.
9. Implement and evaluate nursing measures to prevent and relieve pain.

## Key Terms

| | | |
|---|---|---|
| acuity | coma | corneal-scleral junction |
| affect | confusion | delerium |
| alertness | conjunctiva | disoriented |
| analgesic | consciousness, levels of | dorsal column stimulator |
| cognition | cordotomy | gate-control theory |

| | | |
|---|---|---|
| hallucinations | perception | sensory deprivation, |
| Harrington rod | perceptual distortion | deficit, overload |
| hemorrhoids | perceptual disturbance | sensory disturbances |
| ischemia | placebo | sensory system, status |
| oriented | placebo effect | Snellen eye chart |
| pain | reticular activating | special care unit |
| pain reaction | system | specificity theory |
| pain threshold | scoliosis | stupor |
| pallor | sensory alterations | trigeminal neuralgia |
| pattern theory | | visceral |

## Introduction

An intact sensory system is necessary if we are to interpret our environment
accurately. The title *The Miracle Worker*, a play about the teaching-learning
experiences of Helen Keller, who was deaf and blind, and her teacher, suggests
the difficulty involved when two of the major senses are impaired. Somewhat
differently, a person who has had a cerebrovascular accident (a stroke) may
not feel the heat of his soup or taste its saltiness. So the danger of burning his
mouth and overloading his body with salt are hazards resulting from damage
to the sensory system. If the sense of smell is temporarily impaired, as in the
case of a head cold, the appetite is depressed. However, the nurse who has an
extremely efficient sense of smell may find, in many instances, that it helps
her to make certain important nursing assessments.

A sensory status assessment guide and a guide to assess the level of
consciousness are presented. Nursing actions for the client with sensory
alterations, including safety measures for the person with sensory distortion,
are stressed. While care of the newly deaf or blind person will not be included,
measures to assist the deaf or blind person who enters the health-care system
for another reason are included. Special interventions in the care of the elderly
person with sight and hearing problems are presented.

## SENSORY FUNCTION

The senses include hearing, sight, taste, smell, touch, position, and organic
sensations by which we maintain contact with the environment (Chodil and
Williams, 1970). In 1974, Bolin stated that "the exact mechanism through
which we receive and organize patterns of stimulation is not known, but there
is increasing evidence that the reticular activating system (RAS) plays an
important role in the efficient processing of stimuli and the resulting
behavior." The RAS "controls the overall degrees of central nervous system
activity, including control of wakefulness and sleep, and control of at least part
of our ability to direct attention toward specific areas of our conscious minds"

(Guyton, 1976). An altered sensory environment, therefore, upsets the balance of function of the RAS.

The level of sensory stimulation necessary for well-being differs from person to person. If the environment can be manipulated to increase or decrease sensory input as necessary, a balance will be maintained and sensory alterations—deprivation or overload—will be avoided.

## Sensory Alterations

While authors use different terms to describe sensory alterations, the following terms will be used as defined: *sensory deprivation* is a reduction in the amount and intensity of sensory input; *sensory overload* is a condition of highly intense stimulation that is not patterned (Bolin, 1974). Alterations in the sensory environment may result in changes in affect, cognition, and perception. *Perceptual distortions*, such as seeing dots before the eyes, hearing strange sounds, or having the sensation of floating may occur. An incorrect interpretation of sensory input is considered a perceptual distortion.

## ASSESSING SENSORY STATUS

Appropriate parts of the following guide may be used to assess a client for a sensory deficit or alteration.

1.  Is there a known sensory deficit? Hearing, sight problems? If so, does he hear better in one ear; see better in one eye?
2.  If there is a deficit, what is his reaction to it?
3.  Does he use any corrective device such as glasses or hearing aid?
4.  What is his usual level of sensory input? For example, from what environment does he come? Does he live alone or with others? What are his usual daily activities?
5.  Does he appear restless, bored, irritable, anxious, or fearful?
6.  Does he appear indifferent to people or events affecting him?
7.  Do *you* (the nurse) have trouble getting or keeping his attention?
8.  Is he oriented to time, place, and person?
9.  Does he experience any perceptual distortions?

## Physical Assessment

The beginning student will find several techniques important in her assessment of sight and hearing. They include the following screening test for visual acuity:

The client is asked to cover first one eye and then the other with a piece of opaque paper while he reads any print available.

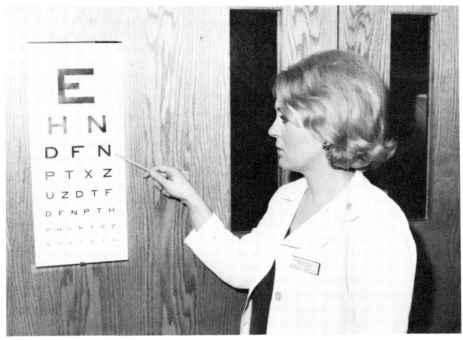

**Figure 22-1.** *The nurse checks the client's visual acuity by having him read the letters on the Snellen eye chart. (Photo by Frank R. Engler, Jr.)*

The Snellen eye chart produces more precise information about vision and is usually available. If the client ordinarily wears corrective lenses for distance, he should wear them during this part of the assessment. He stands 20 feet from the chart and reads the smallest line of print he can. Each eye is tested separately; an opaque eye cover as previously described is used. The smallest line of print from which he can accurately read more than half the figures is identified. The visual acuity level is printed at the right side of each line. The client's acuity is assessed and recorded as a fraction, e.g., 20/30. The numerator indicates the distance the person was standing from the chart and the denominator the distance at which the normal eye could read the line on the chart. The larger the denominator, the worse the vision (Bates, 1974).

## Removal of Foreign Body from Eye

For visual examination of the eye if a foreign body is suspected, the upper lid must be everted. Then the client is encouraged to try to relax his eye while he looks down. The nurse grasps the upper lashes and gently pulling them down, places an applicator stick about a half inch above the lid's margin. The lid everts when the upper lid is pushed down. Throughout the procedure, the client must continue to look down. The conjunctiva is inspected. When the foreign body has been identified and removed by gently touching an applicator tip to it, the upper lashes are gently pulled forward; the client is instructed to look up, and the eyelid will return to its normal position.

## Removal of Contact Lenses

It is important for nurses, especially those in an emergency room, to know how to remove contact lenses from the eyes of those persons who are unable to do so for themselves. In 1976, an estimated 10 million persons in the U.S. wore contact lenses (Gould, 1976). This number has probably increased.

The cornea is oxygenated primarily through the exchange of gases in the atmosphere and tears. During sleep, the metabolic rate of the cornea decreases and there is enough oxygen in the blood to maintain health.

When eyes are closed for a prolonged time period, contact lenses must be removed. The metabolic rate of the cornea increases in contact lens wearers and if the eyes are closed for long periods, and there is a lens in place, damage to the cornea occurs. The amount of damage is directly related to the length of time the lens has been in place and the extent of the interference with tissue metabolism. Should corneal damage occur, it will usually affect the epithelial layer, which is the most regenerative. Damage is seldom permanent.

The proper technique for lens removal follows. The lens is identified by its size: the hard lens is always smaller than the cornea; the soft lens extends beyond the corneal-scleral junction. To remove a hard lens, a thumb or finger is placed on the upper eyelid, at the margin, and the lid is raised. A thumb or finger of the other hand is placed at the margin of the lower lid and the lid is lowered. The lids are brought together slowly and the lens is trapped between the upper and lower lid margins. If the lens has moved off center, it is recentered before removal is attempted.

The soft lens should move as the lids are manipulated. If the lens does not move easily, saline solution should be dropped on the cornea. Then the upper lid is pulled up and the lens pinched with the fingers of the other hand and removed.

If a contact lens suction cup is available, it can be used to remove a hard lens, but not a soft lens. The lenses are stored after removal in a marked container (left lens; right lens) filled with either saline or distilled water.

A medic-alert bracelet is valuable in alerting others that contact lenses are in place; a wallet identification card is an alternative safety alert.

## PREVENTING SENSORY ALTERATIONS

Preventing sensory alterations includes protecting the person from acquiring sensory deficits, as well as protecting him from sensory deprivation or overload.

Visual screening, teaching, and vigilance will prevent some sight problems. Unfortunately, medical therapy has resulted in some serious vision problems (for example, retrolental fibroplasia from excessive use of oxygen in the

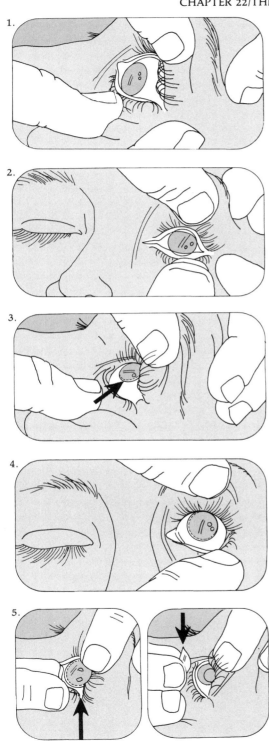

**Figure 22-2.** *Removing hard and soft contact lenses: (1) Place a thumb or finger on the upper eyelid margin and raise the lid; place a thumb or finger of the other hand on the lower eyelid margin and lower the lid. (2) As the lids are brought together, the lens is trapped between the margins of the upper and lower eyelids. (3) The soft lens can be identified by its size—it usually extends 1 to 4 mm. beyond the corneal-scleral junction. (4) The soft lens should move as the lids are manipulated. If it does not, moisten the lens with saline solution to prevent damage to the cornea. (5) Pull the upper lid up with a finger or thumb of one hand and pinch the lens with the fingers of the other hand for removal.*

treatment of premature infants). Keeping sharp objects and especially dangerous toys away from children will protect their sight as well as that of their playmates. Prompt treatment of eye infections will help prevent damage. Early visual screening will identify the child who needs corrective lenses. A child who holds a book close to his face to read, who sits close to the television set, who doesn't see a friend across the street, who can't read what is on the blackboard, is in need of visual screening. Parents who have not picked up the clues that a child has a visual deficit have been stunned to hear their child, fitted with corrective lenses, say he had no idea how pretty the flowers in their yard were.

Childhood deafness can result from maternal rubella, meningitis, prematurity, hereditary factors, and blood factors (Carty, 1972). About one-third to one-half of deafness is of unknown origin. In so far as the conditions known to cause deafness can be prevented, the possibility of preventing hearing deficits exists. An ear problem is often indicated when the young child tugs persistently at his ear. Upon examination, the ear may be found to be tender and warm to the touch. Prompt medical care helps prevent hearing difficulties resulting from ear infections. Children should be protected from putting objects in their ears. Careful nose blowing is important in preventing ear infections. Pressure in the nostrils should be kept equal as the nose is blown. Parents need to be reminded that this simple process has to be taught to their children—one seldom thinks about the fact that a child does not known how to blow his nose. Ears should be protected from high intensity sounds, such as industrial noises and loud music. Any change in a person's hearing acuity indicates the need for prompt medical intervention.

Sensory deprivation and overload can be prevented more easily when the client's usual level of sensory input is known. A person who lives alone, is retired, and does not seek social contacts probably has less sensory stimulation than a person who has a job and shares a household with others. The nurse should try to maintain a level and quality of sensory input similar to the client's accustomed level. For example, some people find certain sounds unacceptable. It is important to think of this, when hospital roommates are assigned. Age and cultural differences can cause a sensory overload in the person who has to listen to a radio station not to his liking, even if the volume is normal and the time exposure minimal.

Sensory overload in hospitalized clients may be prevented by limiting the number of people with whom the client is required to interact. Nursing students, medical students, interns, residents, staff doctors, staff nurses, auxiliary personnel, other health team members—the list of persons going in and out of a hospital room in the course of a day seems endless.

Sensory deprivation may be encountered by the active client who has had a heart attack and is on bed rest with no visitors and no phone calls permitted. Possible deprivation can be identified by knowledge of his lifestyle. Other stimuli can be increased, such as radio, television, or hobbies within the client's range of interests and the required medical regime. Knowledge that the nurse comes in to check frequently and that she will come when called decreases the problem. The use of intercoms as they relate to overload, deprivation, or distortion seems to be a fertile field for study. Further discussion of nursing interventions related to sensory alterations will follow.

## NURSING ACTIONS FOR PERSONS WITH SENSORY ALTERATIONS

After the sensory problem has been identified, nursing actions are planned. First, let us consider nursing for the person with a known sensory deficit who seeks health care for a problem unrelated to his deficit. This discussion is limited to the person who is blind or deaf or who has a sight or hearing problem as a result of prior disease or accident or of aging; problems of the newly blind or deaf person or those with other sensory deficits will not be considered in this text.

### Deafness

The person who cannot hear is forced to perceive his environment through his remaining senses. He has abilities; he has also learned to live with his disability. He can become an active partner in the plan for his care. The nurse must learn how he communicates. In a study in 1972, Carty reported that nurses usually communicate with their deaf clients through verbal language because they believe the deaf read lips very well. The second most common method of communication is the written note. Carty states that nurses who believe they are communicating effectively with their deaf patients by speech and written note are not being very realistic. Very few deaf persons are competent lip readers. It has been found that even under ideal conditions (proximity of speaker, good lighting, absence of distracting features such as a mustache or dental deformities), only 20 to 30 percent of the spoken words were comprehended (Furfey and Harte, 1968). In addition, persons who were deaf before the development of language could read at approximately the fourth-grade level (Furth, 1966). For such clients, understanding notes is difficult.

Nurses seldom felt it was necessary to seek an interpreter for their deaf clients. Yet for their clients who spoke only a foreign language, an interpreter would be obtained. While not all deaf persons understand sign language, it is a valuable tool for the nurse to have. Because the deaf have such difficulty expressing themselves and understanding others, they may tend to withdraw. They may become suspicious because they miss and misinterpret so much sensory input. Carty (1972) found that a smiling, friendly staff member may be viewed by the deaf client as one who is making fun of him. Perceptual distortion may be caused by the visual overload of several persons around the deaf person's bedside—each one doing something different and each one talking. The deaf person may become anxious or suspicious because he doesn't know if he is being talked to or about.

In caring for the deaf, it would seem that important nursing actions include the use of an interpreter (family members or others), and the prevention of visual overload in the environment. Without the use of an interpreter, nurses may honestly believe they have met their client's needs when, in fact, they have not.

## Blindness

One nursing author has suggested the importance of anticipating the needs of the person with a sensory impairment—especially the blind or the deaf. But it is important to recognize that this may be, for some people, an inappropriate assumption. All clients should be approached, as much as possible, as individuals, and this rule applies certainly to the blind and deaf.

When a blind person enters a hospital or health agency, however, the new environment should be described in detail. The nurse should then help him arrange his personal belongings if he wants help, and should not rearrange them without his knowledge. It is important to show him where the call light, the telephone, the bathroom, etc., are located. These actions acknowledge and encourage independence in a new environment and help prevent accidents.

The blind person has learned to adapt to his loss of sight. The nurse must determine his abilities and preferences regarding his care. For example, does he want to know where the food is located on his tray? An effective method of locating the food is to describe the plate as the face of a clock; the meat is at 6:30, the potatoes at 12, and so forth. Mummah (1976) points out the importance of talking to blind persons before touching them to avoid startling them. Any procedure, no matter how simple, should be described before the nurse begins to implement it. The blind person should be greeted by name; and in groups, each person to whom the nurse is speaking should be identified by name. It is important for the blind client to know when the nurse is leaving his presence and when she plans to return.

Mummah (1976) describes a staff education program that illustrates the care of the blind. When a nursing instructor in rubber-soled shoes placed a food tray in front of a blindfolded student, the student screamed and jumped. Then the teacher started to wash another student's face with a wet washcloth without explaining what she was doing. The students were soon telling the instructor that she should explain what she was doing. These suggestions should prove useful in helping a client who is blind.

## The Aged with Sight or Hearing Problems

Decreased visual acuity makes one less able to interpret visual stimuli accurately, whether one is old or young.

During the normal aging process, a number of physical changes occur that make a person susceptible to perceptual distortion or that reduce their sensory perceptions. Changes in sight may cause either of these sensory problems. Elderly clients should be encouraged to wear their glasses. If age or illness has created a change in their vision, they should be assisted in having their lenses changed. If a client wears glasses but comes to the health-care agency without them, the nurse should arrange to have them brought in. The client should be helped to keep his glasses clean. If the glasses are speckled with dirt, they have lost their efficiency. A little soap and water will clean the lenses. They can be dried with a soft cloth.

Older people need more light for satisfactory vision than younger people. Snyder (1978) states that 3 times as much light is needed by the elderly as by the 20-year-old. Snyder also reports that eliminating the glare from lights increases the older person's attention span.

Nursing assessment should identify the older person with a hearing deficit. If the client ordinarily uses a hearing aid, he should be encouraged to wear it. The nurse may be responsible for checking the proper functioning of the aid. She should know how to change the batteries and help the client keep the aid dry.

Snyder (1978) offers the following suggestions when caring for the elderly who are hard of hearing: one should *lower* rather than elevate the voice pitch, because the elderly have difficulty hearing sounds in the higher frequency range. One should come to eye level to speak and direct the voice to the older person's ear, standing close to him when speaking—a "hand-shake's distance away" (p. 46). Competing noises should be eliminated. Some older people and, indeed, all partially deaf people have difficulty understanding speech when there are background noises such as radio, TV, background conversations, etc. Snyder believes that "compensation for audiological impairment is one-sided; the responsibility rests with the speaker to make adjustments; there is little the older person can do."

## NURSING INTERVENTIONS RELATED TO SENSORY DEPRIVATION AND OVERLOAD

Nursing interventions attempt to prevent sensory deprivation. For persons with sensory deprivation, the goal is restoration of adequate sensory stimulation and normal perception. The signs of sensory deprivation are: restlessness, irritability, boredom, inactivity, slowness of thought and disturbances in thought processes, daydreaming, increased sleeping, anxiety, panic, or hallucinations.

The effects of sensory deprivation occur rapidly; the recovery from deprivation also comes quickly. Downs (1974) found that normal, healthy persons who were subjected to social isolation for only 2¾ hours experienced distorted sensory perceptions. When sensory input was increased, recovery was rapid.

The following suggestions for nursing intervention are meant to be individualized according to the client's particular needs. Evaluation of their effectiveness is essential, since  research in this area is limited.

A changing environment with adequate sensory stimulation is provided. If the client is confined to bed, the bed might be placed so that he can see out of the window or the door. There is occasionally a problem in hospitals because the adjustable beds are expected to be kept in the low position. If this keeps the client from seeing out of the window, arrangements can be made to overcome this obstacle if the client wishes. Anyone who can move about, either independently or not, is encouraged to go from one area to another. Even the person on bed rest can usually be placed on a stretcher and taken to a porch, a lounge, or the dining room. A person confined to his home can be encouraged to move from room to room. A novel by Graham Green, *Travels with My Aunt*, describes the pleasure one man obtained as he moved each week to a different room in his house. His purpose, of course, was somewhat different from the need to prevent sensory deprivation in the hospitalized client, but in both cases, change of environment adds sensory stimuli. In a similar manner, changing the environment of the multiple-handicapped person from an institution or private home to that of a camp in a beautifully wooded park provides distinct, though unmeasured, behavior changes.

A telephone, radio, television, reading material, games, and letter writing equipment are all helpful in increasing sensory stimulation. A clock in the room or a watch on the client's wrist helps orient a person to time. This seems obvious, but it is an often overlooked way to add sensory input. A calendar also helps with orientation. Without a calendar, many of us would not know the date. Newspapers enable the person who wants this information to know what is happening in the world.

While the importance of the nurse's presence to the sensory deprived person has been mentioned before, it cannot be over-stressed. By her presence she serves as a source of sensory input. She listens, talks, and uses touch as a means of communication with her client. She remembers to explain what she is doing no matter how routine the procedure. She encourages the client to participate in planning and carrying out his own care as a means to stimulate his senses.

Stimulation should be aimed at as many different senses as possible. The sights, sounds, smells, body positions, and textures should vary. A familiar food from home helps vary the available tastes and consistencies of food.

To stimulate smell, incense can be provided for those who like it. The nurse may choose to wear a light scent. She can help the person who likes to see things grow plant seeds in a garden or in a pot on the window sill. A bowl of fish or an aquarium provides changing movement and color. The value of a pet in increasing sensory stimulation for the handicapped and mentally retarded has been documented.

## Social Contact

Prevention of social isolation is an important nursing goal. Family and friends are a great help in this respect. Whenever possible, visiting should be encouraged throughout the day. In addition, groups of clients can eat together, play games, and do range of motion exercises together. Volunteers make valuable visitors for the client who is alone. Other community resources are often available to help the person who needs more sensory input (e.g., senior citizens groups, hot lines, dial-a-prayer).

Social isolation is a risk for persons in private rooms. Those in prescribed isolation because of their illness are especially prone to suffer sensory deprivation. Whether the client is a child or an adult, it seems that being in isolation limits even the interaction between client and nurse, to say nothing of visitors. Nurses may think it is too much trouble to put on gown and mask, and wash the hands unless they are required to give a medication or treatment to the person in isolation. In these cases, there also is the possible perceptual distortion when all the client sees is the eyes of the gowned, masked worker.

The measures used for lessening sensory deprivation should be evaluated. Have the signs and symptoms of deprivation lessened or disappeared? If they have, the efforts have been successful. Because what works for one person may not work for another, it takes a creative, imaginative nurse to find a way to lessen sensory deprivation.

## Sensory Overload

All of us have experienced, or are aware of, sensory overload. Meetings seem interminable, the phone rings constantly, interruptions seem inevitable. The staff nurse, the student who shares a house, or the faculty member probably all have learned how to bring sensory input back into balance. Some time alone in the library, a walk, or a weekend in the country where there is no phone, newspaper, or radio may be ways to restore balance. Given the opportunity, most persons can solve their own sensory overload problems. But not everyone has the opportunity. The clients in the intensive care units, clinic waiting areas, or semiprivate rooms are almost trapped in the stimuli of their environment. Although all sensory receptors adapt either partially or totally, continued or excessive stimulation of the senses causes fatigue or irritability.

The bright lights, the strange machinery, the alarms, the numbers of people, the amount of talking that goes on, and the total unfamiliarity of special care units, have all been studied as sources of sensory overload. People who are ill are especially vulnerable to sensory overload. They need rest so that the body can repair and restore itself. It is important for the nurse to plan needed care so that there are uninterrupted times for rest and sleep. This is one way that environmental stimuli are reduced. Special care units are being designed so that the very ill are placed in private rooms. This decreases noise from personnel and equipment. Some agencies arrange for equipment to be kept outside the unit, when possible, and the leads attached to the client (such as electrocardiograph leads) to be removed as soon as possible to provide for more mobility. Decreasing noise, lights, smells are ways to decrease stimuli. Explaining all the treatments as well as why certain equipment is needed helps prevent perceptual distortion.

## Sensory Disturbance

Sensory disturbance can be exhibited as a change in perception, cognition, or affect. This can occur in the client who suffers from deprivation or from overload. The nurse's goal is to assist the client to overcome this disturbance. Unless the client is completely oriented, she must assume responsibility for his safety.

A person suffering a sensory disturbance may not feel free to share his experience for fear he may not be believed or that the nurse or doctor may think there is "something wrong with him." It helps some persons to relate their experiences to another. The client needs to be assured that sensory disturbances are usually transitory and not unusual. A perceptual or thought disturbance can occur without disorientation. Downs (1974) believes sensory disturbances are probably far more widespread than has been suspected.

The nurse calls a client by name every time she comes into his presence. She tells him where he is and why; she keeps him as mobile as possible. Clocks, calendars, and familiar articles from home such as photographs provide orientation. All information should be communicated in nontechnical language. The measures used to help a client maintain a sensory balance can be used here.

Occasionally, for safety of the client or staff, physical restraint may be required. Sometimes raised bed rails are sufficient to protect the restless or confused person. If, however, the person attempts to crawl over the bed rails or remove needed tubes or dressings, protective restraints may be required. A physician's written order is required because of the legal restrictions against restraint. Restraints are available that permit movement—sitting, turning, but prevent falling. Restraints are applied so that they are neither too loose nor too tight. Padding is required around ankles or wrists to prevent irritation. The client still needs to have his position changed at regular intervals and restraints temporarily removed while the nurse is in attendance. The clients' families are often upset by the use of restraints. A careful explanation of the reason for their use is necessary.

## ALTERATIONS IN CONSCIOUSNESS

Any loss or decrease in level of consciousness makes orientation difficult or impossible. The levels of consciousness are described in various ways. This makes it essential for the nurse to describe the client's behavior rather than to label him as in a stupor or a coma.

The three terms often used to designate levels of consciousness are alertness, stupor, and coma. the person who is *alert* is in full possession of his senses. The person in a *stupor* appears unconscious but can be aroused sufficiently to respond to commands. Reflexes are usually present. The person in a *coma* is unconscious and cannot be aroused even by powerful stimuli. His reflexes are usually abnormal or absent.

The *oriented* person recognizes time, place, or persons. The *disoriented* person does not recognize time, place, or persons. *Confusion* may be manifested by lack of attention, mental slowness, incoherent thinking, or distorted perception of the environment. *Delirium* is a state of disturbed awareness resulting in confusion, agitation, and hallucinations.

## Assessing Level of Consciousness

1. Does the client know who he is, where he is, and what day and time it is?
2. Does he respond readily and accurately to stimuli?
3. Does he respond to but misinterpret environmental stimuli?
4. Does he appear unconscious but can be aroused? Are reflexes present?
5. Is he unconscious and unable to be aroused even by powerful stimuli?

The nurse is totally responsible for any client who is not completely conscious and oriented. Frequent observations and provisions for safety are essential. External stimuli are reduced; this includes limiting the number of personnel taking part in his care.

The nurse talks to the person who appears unconscious. Many persons have reported, upon regaining consciousness, the value of hearing someone talking to them. Wisser (1978) reports a conversation with a man who had been a patient of hers months before. When she asked him if he remembered her (he was unconscious the entire time she cared for him and talked to him) he said, "'Yes. God, I remember your voice. It was the only way I knew I was alive and not dead. You were the first one who told me what the hell had happened. I was scared to death, but then I'd hear your voice, and I knew I would be all right.'"

## PAIN

Pain is one of the most frequently encountered health-care problems. What pain is, how to prevent it, and measures to relieve it will be discussed here, including whether or not culture influences pain. Health professionals' beliefs about pain will be presented as they are described in the literature.

Pain is a personal problem. When we are in pain, no one else knows how it feels. When the client is in pain, only he knows how it feels. Nurses have been heard to say, "How can you need pain medication? You only had a hysterectomy and that was two days ago." Many persons experience pain two days after removal of the uterus. This example is cited not to indicate that medication for pain is the only cure for pain—far from it. Many nursing measures help the person in pain to be more comfortable and, therefore, require less pain medication. It is hoped, however, that the nurse will not permit her own beliefs about pain to interfere with her nursing interventions when a person says he has pain.

The pain of a sunburn, of a finger burned against an oven rack, of a twisted ankle, of sorrow, or of rejection, are familiar to most of us. Psychological pain may require somewhat different interventions than physiological pain, but it causes no less suffering. Pain and suffering are among the most frequent problems the nurse encounters. What then is pain? What is suffering? Does pain have a purpose? Pain is usually meant to protect the body when tissues are either damaged or threatened with damage. Pain, for example, causes the person to remove his finger from the hot oven to prevent further damage. But pain does not always indicate threat of tissue damage. For example, phantom pain which is perceived in a body part that is no longer present (after amputation, for example) does not warn of tissue damage.

## Pain Defined

There are as many definitions of pain as there are persons asked to define it. Many dictionaries describe it as a feeling of distress, suffering, or agony caused by stimulation of specialized nerve endings. A broader definition states that pain refers to distressing experiences on either a physical or emotional level. When the health professional focuses on the *person* having pain, "pain is whatever the experiencing person says it is and exists whenever he says it does" (McCaffery, 1972).

What is suffering? It is the response to pain. It is the state of anguish of one who bears pain, injury, or loss (Copp, 1974).

If nurses are to implement plans to relieve pain, it is important to understand why the person feels pain and why he responds to it as he does.

## Pain Threshold and Reaction

Pain threshold is defined as "the lowest intensity of stimulus that will excite the sensation of pain when the stimulus is applied for a prolonged period of time" (Guyton, 1976). Guyton also believes that thresholds for pain do not differ significantly from person to person or in the same person at different times. The issue of whether or not pain thresholds vary is controversial. It seems that everyone agrees, however, that the reaction to pain differs remarkably among individuals. Anguish, anxiety, crying, depression, and other signs vary considerably from person to person. McCaffery sums it up in the following sentence: "At any rate it is doubtful that the uniformity of the pain perception threshold, if it does exist, has any relationship with the pain experience of patients" (1972).

## Theories of Pain

Several theories have been proposed: the specificity theory, the pattern theory and, most recently, gate-control theory. The traditional view of pain is based on the *specificity theory*. Specific pain receptors in the body tissues send pain signals by way of afferent pain fibers to the postero-lateral portion of the spinal cord where two actions occur. 1) Some impulses are relayed to the motor fibers of the reflex arc so that the involved muscles respond immediately. 2) Other impulses in the spinal cord cross over to the opposite side and ascend to the thalamus where pain is perceived. Then the activated cerebral cortex interprets the impulses in relation to location and intensity of pain, etc. The cortex initiates descending nerve impulses (efferent fibers) that result in autonomic, skeletal muscle, and psychic responses (Siegele, 1974). Melzack (1975) believes this theory "assumes that the amount of pain is proportional to the intensity of stimulation, and that the location of the stimulus determines the location of the pain." This theory has been challenged because it does not adequately explain some clinical phenomena such as pain persistence after nerve tracts have been destroyed.

The *pattern theory* actually includes several different theories. In general, all of them have in common "the concept that patterning of the nerve impulses generated by receptors forms the basis of a code that provides the information that there is pain" (McCaffery, 1972).

In 1965, Melzack and Wall proposed the more comprehensive *gate-control theory*. While it is still controversial, it is gaining increasing support. The theory suggests that the transmission of pain signals a dynamic process—not a fixed, unchanging one. This dynamic process "stems from a series of gatelike mechanisms in the pain-signaling system. If a gate can be closed, full analgesia follows because pain signals from injured tissues cannot reach the brain" (Melzack, 1975).

Impulses in the sensory nerve fibers can open or close the gates. Activity in large afferent fibers tends to close gates and lessen pain; small afferent fiber activity tends to open gates and increase pain. The gates can also be opened or closed by activity in the fibers descending from the brain stem reticular formation. Fibers from the cortex can also either open or close the gates (Melzack, 1975).

Because the cerebral cortex is the center for memory, attention, anxiety, and interpretative function, the individual's present and past experiences have an effect on the gate-control system. The gate-control theory explains why comparable stimuli will be felt as pain by one person and not by another. It explains the persistence of pain following the severing of nerve pathways, the effectiveness of acupuncture, and the effectiveness of the dorsal column stimulator to lessen chronic pain. Gramse (1978), in writing about the effect of the dorsal column stimulator, stated that the "stimulation of larger myelinated peripheral fibers or their extensions into the dorsal column will inhibit, at the first spinal synapse, activity produced by stimulation of the small fibers that carry pain impulses."

## Types of Pain

In theory, there are three types of pain: pricking, burning, and aching. Delta type A fibers are involved in *pricking-type pain* (e.g., a needle prick, a knife cut, a widespread area of irritation). Type C fibers are involved in *burning* (when the skin is burned) and *aching* pains (deep pains—not on the body surface) (Guyton, 1976).

When a person is asked to describe his pain, he may use terms such as: feels like a knot, a twinge, gnawing, stabbing, stinging, vise-like, throbbing, cramping, shooting, cutting, knife-like, sharp, dull, burning, sore, numb, ache, discomfort.

Another classification of pain describes it as superficial, deep (visceral), or referred. *Superficial pain* occurs when the cutaneous receptors are stimulated. *Deep pain* is usually dull and aching and arises from the muscles, viscera, or periosteum. It is usually more diffuse and more persistent and more difficult to locate precisely. *Referred pain* is usually from a viscera. It is pain felt in a part of the body distant from the actual lesion. A classic example of referred pain is that which radiates down the left arm when the person has a heart attack (myocardial infarction).

Pain is described as mild, moderate, or severe. But because these terms are interpreted differently by different people, a description of the pain is best when it is recorded exactly as the client describes it.

## Stimuli Resulting in Pain

Mechanical, thermal, chemical, and electrical agents stimulate the pain receptors in the skin and superficial organs to cause pain. The reaction to pain is different when it is unfamiliar. Similar pain in the future will be modified by a first experience. For example, anxiety may be less; self-blame or guilt may be greater.

Sunburn is an example of pain caused by a thermal agent. Diaper rash, an acid burn, results from a chemical stimulant, while a static electric charge is an example of an electrical stimulus causing pain. A sustained muscle contraction (e.g., a charley horse) and ischemia (decreased blood flow to a part) also stimulate pain receptors. The pain of ischemia occurs when the legs are crossed for even a brief time or when one is required to sit still for a long period without being able to move.

Pain receptors differ from all the other sense organs; they do not adapt to continuous stimulation. This nonadaptability is protective because the stimulus warning of possible or real tissue damage continues to be transmitted. Persons who cannot feel pain are in danger. They have no warning when they must shift position as a part becomes ischemic, for example, or when thermal injuries occur because the temperature of the bath was not identified as being too hot.

## Assessment of Pain

McCaffery (1972) sees assessment itself as a form of nursing intervention. While she talks to the person about the pain, the nurse is showing concern, reducing her client's isolation by her presence, and lessening anxiety by helping him focus his attention.

The following guide includes important aspects to be investigated when the client has pain. The nurse must ask questions to determine the source of the pain.

1. Where is the pain? Can you point to it?
2. What does it feel like?
3. How much does it hurt?
4. How and when did the pain start? What seems to bring it on? How long does it last?
5. What do you do to relieve the pain?
6. What do you think is causing it?
7. Is there anything else you can tell me about the pain?

How is the person responding physiologically to the pain? The blood pressure, pulse, respiration, skin moisture, color, pupil dilatation, muscle tension, alertness, and gastro-intestinal motility should be assessed. With superficial pain, the body prepares for flight or fight with increased blood pressure, pulse, and respirations, perspiration, pallor, pupil dilatation, increased muscle tension, general mental alertness (this may take the form of restlessness), and a decrease in gastro-intestinal motility. With severe deep or visceral pain, the blood pressure may drop, the pulse may decrease, and weakness and nausea may occur. There is an increased blood flow to the internal organs.

How much does the client move his body? Does he move slowly, carefully, or not at all? Does he strike out or grasp your hand? Does he "splint" the part that hurts? Is he trembling or pacing the floor? How does he respond psychologically?

1. What does he say about the pain, for example, its intensity?
2. Is he able to talk about the pain or does he only moan?
3. What is his facial expression? Does he wince, frown, grimace, or show general body tension?
4. Is he withdrawn? Does he turn his face to the wall to shut out everything but the pain itself?
5. Can his anxiety be assessed?

What is his emotional status? It has been shown that anxiety greatly increases the reaction to pain. Is the person generally anxious or does the pain make him anxious? Location of the pain influences anxiety. For example, the belief that one's sight has been damaged is very frightening. Pain near the heart raises anxiety. Fear of pain modifies behavior. A person with trigeminal neuralgia will protect his face. He will not want to be washed, touched, or shaved. He will be afraid to chew, brush his teeth, or talk very long.

What does the client see as the purpose of the pain? Does the child or adult interpret it as punishment? Is the pain seen as a means to an end? Some religious persons see suffering as a means of achieving Heaven. Older adults may be accustomed to accept pain as a part of the human condition, as a sacrifice, or as a test. While no studies have been identified that examine the influence of religion on pain and suffering, there would seem to be a relationship.

## Effects of Culture on Pain

What health professionals believe about the pain experience has an effect on their pain-relieving interventions. The nurse who thinks medication is not necessary for pain relief 2 days after a hysterectomy may have difficulty understanding a woman who can find no relief without it.

Some people believe that persons from ethnic backgrounds different from their own respond in different ways to pain. For example, people of Asian origin are said to be stoic. Are they? Davitz, et al. (1976) asked nurses in Japan, Taiwan, Thailand, Korea, Puerto Rico, and the United States to indicate the degree of physical pain and psychological distress they thought each in a group of simulated patients was suffering. Japanese and Korean nurses believed that the patients suffered a relatively high degree of physical pain and psychological suffering. American and Puerto Rican nurses thought that the same patients suffered a relatively low degree of pain.

Whether the persons of one culture suffer more than those of another is not the point of such a study. However, when the nurses think there is a difference in the experience of physical pain and psychological distress (and these did) between one cultural group and another, this belief may affect their responses to requests for pain relief. The person experiencing the pain should be the center of concern, and when he says he has pain, regardless of his cultural group, he must be believed.

In a famous study reported in 1969, Zborowski identified some differences in response to pain among patients of Old American (Anglo-Saxons), Jewish, Irish, and Italian descent. "The clinical impressions of medical practitioners that patients of Jewish and Italian origin tend to be more emotional while experiencing and expressing pain than the Anglo-Saxon—the Old American—was confirmed" (p. 239).

The Old American and the Irish subjects tended to de-emphasize their pain and to report it unemotionally. The Jewish and the Old American subjects were more precise in describing their pain. The Irish and the Old American said they preferred to hide their pain and the Jewish and Italian preferred to show it. These subjects cried, complained, were demanding, and stated that they could not tolerate pain. The Jewish subjects most frequently expressed anxiety and worry. Pain was the reason they sought hospitalization. They wanted to understand the meaning of their pain and showed less confidence in the doctor than the other patients did. The Old American and the Irish placed all their trust and confidence in the doctor.

This study also examined the level of education of the subjects. There were differences in only two areas: the less educated seemed to worry more and the more educated had more confidence in surgery than the others.

## Age and Sex as Related to Pain

Some nurses also believe that the response to pain varies with the age and sex of the client. For example, infants and children are expected to cry when they have pain. Aging persons are accepted when they react emotionally. Women, whatever their age, are permitted to react emotionally to pain. Adult males may not be.

It seems more valuable to eliminate the stereotypic beliefs about responses to pain and focus on the person experiencing the pain. Then the client's needs can be met in ways that are acceptable to him whatever his age, sex, or cultural background.

## NURSING INTERVENTIONS FOR THE PERSON IN PAIN

The goal of complete or temporary pain relief is planned together by the nurse and client. If there are several choices for pain relief, the client should choose. Because loss of control is a major concern of the person in pain, every attempt is made to keep the client in control.

## Understanding the Cause of Pain

Anxiety is decreased if the person understands the cause of the pain and the reason it occurs. If a certain procedure, for example, is painful, the client in most cases should be told, though not too far in advance. There are some people who really do not want to know in advance about painful procedures. Of course, this wish is respected. The nurse will need to know the client's wishes and also what procedures are painful. This is somewhat difficult because of the subjectivity of pain. Many nursing students consider receiving an injection very painful, while their clients may not find them especially unpleasant. One nurse refused consent for a liver biopsy because of her notion of the pain associated with it. Another nurse described her feelings after having a Harrington rod inserted in her spine for correction of a scoliosis. She wrote: "In no way could I have foreseen how intense the pain would be, but I'd have given anything if someone had said to me the night before the operation: 'you're going to experience pain like you've never felt before, but we'll be here to help you'" (Cady, 1976).

The person in pain must have permission to react to it in whatever manner works best for him. Also the privacy, if it is needed (when for example, screaming or swearing is what helps), must be provided.

It was suggested earlier that assessment itself helps serve as a nursing intervention in the pain experience, because the nurse is present—the person in pain is not alone. The nurse listens. She also talks with the person about the experience. She offers support—maybe by holding the client's hand during a painful procedure. Support can also come from family and friends, auxiliary personnel, and other health-team members.

## Removing the Source of the Pain

If the source of pain can be removed, this is an effective means of intervention. If there is a speck of dirt in the eye, the pain is relieved when it is removed. If the baby's wet diaper is causing pain, removing it and cleansing the skin is the action necessary. Is an abdominal binder too tight? Loosening and readjusting it will relieve the discomfort. Is a distended bladder causing pain? Offering the bedpan may help. In some instances the cause of the pain must be removed surgically (e.g., gall stones). Drugs are also frequently given to reduce inflammation, swelling, spasm, and thereby relieve the pain.

While comfort measures such as a cold, wet washcloth on the forehead, a warm bath, a massage, or a snack may or may not provide physiological relief, they provide the caring which relieves the psychological distress.

## Preventing Pain

Pain can be prevented if the pain receptors are prevented from reacting. A cloth over the eyes may protect them from light and prevent a headache. Cream on the skin protects it from diaper rash or sunburn. A scarf protects the skin from exposure to air and prevents the pain of trigeminal neuralgia. Aspirin may decrease the sensitivity of pain receptors. A topical anesthetic agent relieves the pain of sunburn or hemorrhoids. If pain is a warning of tissue damage, as it often is, medical care is needed to identify the cause of the pain.

Some interventions work by interrupting the pain impulse somewhere along its pathway. Spinal anesthetics work in this fashion. Cordotomy (severing the nerve) for intractable pain is another attempt at pain relief. Dorsal column stimulation, previously mentioned, is effected by a battery device to block pain impulses to the spinal cord in severe, chronic pain when other methods have failed. An internal electrode is surgically implanted. When the person activates the buzzer, a buzzing sensation is felt instead of pain. Dorsal column stimulation is based on the concept that stimulation of large fibers will inhibit activity of the small fibers that carry pain impulses.

## Decreasing Pain Perception

Analgesics are the drugs of choice for pain relief. They act on the nervous system by interfering with the transmission of pain stimuli or by altering pain perception at the cerebral level. Analgesics are classified as narcotic or strong analgesics (such as morphine), and nonnarcotic analgesics such as aspirin. Narcotic analgesics relieve pain by altering the emotional response to pain.

Those who receive morphine for pain say that the pain is still present but it does not concern them. Analgesics are best given before the pain becomes severe. Repeated frequent administration of narcotic analgesics eventually leads to tolerance; the medication requirements are high and pain relief inadequate. While narcotics should not be given when nonnarcotics will provide pain relief, avoiding the use of narcotics should not be carried to an extreme (Drakontides, 1974). Concern about addiction should not keep one from providing the relief afforded by narcotic analgesics in the illnesses and injuries for which they are without equal. Postoperative patients and those who are terminally ill, for example, should not be deprived of the necessary analgesics. Especially in terminal illnesses, persons who are assured that they will receive their medication for pain, stay in control as they live out their lives.

Historically, the control of p.r.n. (as necessary) analgesics has been given to the nurse. We should attempt to refocus this practice so the client is in control. When an analgesic has been prescribed every four hours p.r.n. and the client needs it after three and a half hours, a medical re-evaluation seems to be required. The nonnarcotic analgesics are used to relieve mild or moderate pain. They are usually administered orally and seldom cause addiction. Aspirin and Tylenol are frequently used nonnarcotic analgesics.

The pain interpretation can be modified by the nurse-client relationship. When the client has confidence and trust in the health professional, pain appears to be less (the placebo effect). When a drug is given it can be accompanied by a statement such as, "I think this will help." This increases the client's confidence and helps relieve pain.

The interventions for pain relief should be evaluated at regular intervals. When the nurse has given a medication, she tells the client she will be back in 30 minutes to see how the medication is working. When she returns she will determine if her client is comfortable, asleep, or not at all relieved by the intervention. If the pain has not decreased, then the process must begin again to discover a different intervention for pain relief. Since the original assessment identified the ways the client handled pain in the past, these same interventions can be put into practice once more. In addition, any method to encourage relaxation and provide rest will modify the pain experience. The person who is fatigued has more pain than the one who is rested and relaxed.

Distraction lessens pain. In the hospital, clients have been observed laughing and talking with their visitors, apparently not experiencing pain. When the visitors left, these persons needed something for pain relief. The visitors had served as a distraction from the pain. In a similar manner, taped music, radio, or television distract from pain. Any activity that proved useful in the past should be tried over again. Cady (1976) reported that she wrote letters to her pain. This was a distraction and, therefore, useful. Night time is a bad time for the person with pain possibly because there are fewer distractions.

Touching the client sometimes helps relieve pain: rubbing the back, holding the hand, or holding a baby are familiar examples.

## SUMMARY

Sensory disturbances are probably fairly widespread. Maintaining environmental stimuli at a level that can be accurately processed will reduce sensory disturbances. Careful assessment will help identify the problems so that they can be relieved. Careful evaluation of nursing interventions is required because of the limited clinical nursing research in this area.

The person's pain experience requires careful assessment, intervention, and evaluation focusing on the individual with his own unique response to pain. The nurse who tries to understand the one who is suffering has made a most important contribution to the relief of pain.

## LEARNING ACTIVITIES

1.  Assess someone in pain. Use the guide presented in the chapter.
2.  Compare the gate-control theory with the specificity theory.
3.  Using the research findings cited in the chapter as a basis, discuss the effects of culture on the pain experience.
4.  Describe nursing measures to relieve the pain of a client two days after abdominal surgery.
5.  Assess a person's sensory status.
6.  Describe nursing measures for a person with a) a hearing or b) a sight deficit who comes to the hospital for an unrelated problem.
7.  Explain how you would attempt to prevent sensory deprivation in a bedridden middle-aged man with a heart attack.

## REFERENCES AND SUGGESTED READINGS

Bates, Barbara, 1974. *A guide to physical examination.* Philadelphia: J. B. Lippincott.

Bolin, Rose. Sensory deprivation: an overview. *Nursing Forum,* Vol. 13, No. 3, (1974), 241–259.

Boore, Jennifer. Old people and sensory deprivation. *Nursing Times,* November 10, 1977, pp. 1754–1755.

Brown, Marie S. The Gordons needed all the help they could get. *Nursing 77,* October, 1977, pp. 40–43.

Burgess, Ann W., 1978. *Nursing: levels of health intervention.* Englewood Cliffs, N.J.: Prentice-Hall.

Cady, Jane. Dear pain. *American Journal of Nursing,* June, 1976, pp. 960–961.

Carty, Rita. Patients who cannot hear. *Nursing Forum,* Vol. 11, No. 3, (1972), 290–299.

Chodil, Judith and Williams, Barbara. The concept of sensory deprivation. *Nursing Clinics of North America*, Vol. 5, No. 3 (1970), 453–465.

Copp, Laurel. The spectrum of suffering. *American Journal of Nursing*, March, 1974, pp. 491–495.

Davitz, Lois; Sameshima, Yasuko; and Davitz, Joel. Suffering as viewed in six different cultures. *American Journal of Nursing*, August, 1976, pp. 1296–1297.

Downs, Florence. Bed rest and sensory disturbances. *American Journal of Nursing*, March, 1974, pp. 434–438.

Drakontides, Anna. Drugs to treat pain. *American Journal of Nursing*, March, 1974, pp. 508–513.

DuGas, Beverly, 1977. *Introduction to patient care.* Philadelphia: W. B. Saunders.

Feeley, Ellen M. and Reid, Elizabeth. Roommates: to have or have not. *American Journal of Nursing*, January, 1973, pp. 104–107.

Fuerst, Elinor; Wolff, LuVerne; and Weitzel, Marlene, 1974. *Fundamentals of nursing.* 5th ed. Philadelphia: J. B. Lippincott.

Furfey, Paul and Harte, Thomas. Interaction of deaf and hearing in Baltimore City, Maryland. *The Catholic University of America, Studies from the Bureau of Solid Research*, No. 4, December, 1968, p. vvi.

Furth, Hans S., 1966. *Thinking without language.* New York: The Free Press.

Gould, H. How to remove contact lenses from comatose patients. *American Journal of Nursing*, September, 1976, pp. 1483–1485.

Gramse, Carol. Dorsal column stimulation. *American Journal of Nursing*, June, 1978, pp. 1022–1025.

Greene, Graham, 1970. *Travels with my aunt.* New York: Viking.

Guyton, Arthur, 1976. *Textbook of medical physiology.* 5th ed. Philadelphia: W. B. Saunders.

Kiersnowski, Cynthia; Martsolf, Donna; and O'Brien, Patricia. Miss Greene thought we were torturing her. *Nursing 76*, September, 1976, pp. 58–60.

McCaffery, Margo, 1972. *Nursing management of the patient with pain.* Philadelphia: J. B. Lippincott.

Melzack, Ronald. Shutting the gate on pain. *Science Year, 1975*, Field Enterprises Educational Corporation, Chicago, pp. 56–57.

Mummah, Hazel. Fingers to see. *American Journal of Nursing*, October, 1976, pp. 1608–1610.

Shelby, Jane. Sensory deprivation. *Image*, June, 1978, pp. 49–55.

Shiery, S. Insight into the delicate art of eye care. *Nursing 75*, June, 1975, pp. 50–56.

Siegele, Dorothy. The gate control theory. *American Journal of Nursing*, March, 1974, pp. 498–502.

Snyder, Lorraine. Environmental changes for socialization. *Journal of Nursing Administration*, January, 1978, pp. 44–49.

Storlie, Frances. Pointers for assessing pain. *Nursing 78*, May, 1978, pp. 37–39.

Wisser, Susan.   When the walls listened. *American Journal of Nursing*, June, 1978, pp. 1016–1017.

Zborowski, Mark, 1969.   *People in pain.*   San Francisco: Jossey-Bass.

Zubek, John P., 1969.   *Sensory deprivation: fifteen years of research.* Century Psychology Series, New York: Appleton-Century-Crofts.

**5**

# Professional Nursing and Health Care

# Nursing Trends Past and Present
## Current Health Care Concerns

Part 5 discusses nursing as a profession within the health care field. Historical perspectives of the development of the nursing profession are used to help the student focus on the present and future of nursing within the health care system.

# 23

# Nursing: Past, Present, and Future

## Behavioral Objectives

Upon completion of this chapter, the student will be able to:

1. Describe current concepts and definitions of nursing.
2. Identify historical influences on nursing as a profession.
3. Describe professional organization in nursing.
4. Describe current issues in nursing education, practice, and research.
5. Identify criteria necessary for a profession, and apply these criteria to nursing.
6. Describe the American Nurses Association Code of Ethics.
7. Define nursing practice.
8. Describe selected factors in society that have an impact on the future of nursing.

## Key Terms

American Nurses Association (ANA)
certification
clinical nurse specialist (CNS)
code of ethics for nurses

licensure
National League for Nursing (NLN)
National Student Nurse Association (NSNA)
Nurse Practice Acts

nursing practice
nurse practitioner
professional nursing
Sigma Theta Tau
standards of nursing practice

## Introduction

The past century has seen the evolution of nursing from an activity to a profession. Nursing activities, those human actions which assist in the care of others, are performed in all societies by various members with assorted talents. Nursing as a profession is a new phenomenon in a historical sense, having been developed in recent times. This chapter will discuss nursing as it is understood today in light of its past. The three basic areas of education, practice, and research are considered, as well as basic professional responsibilities and future directions of nursing.

## CURRENT CONCEPTS AND DEFINITIONS OF NURSING

Nursing is not viewed in isolation. It is an integral part of the total system of health care. In order to better view its relationship to the total health-care system, it is necessary to understand the concept of nursing—what it is, and what it is not. This conceptualization is not merely an academic consideration. It is a foundation on which an individual builds her nursing practice.

An important factor that today's nurse needs to consider is that whatever her personal concept of nursing is or may become, she will practice in a changing world. While being aware of the importance of having an individual philosophical foundation and concept for nursing, the nurse will need to be prepared to adapt her nursing concept to everchanging practice situations.

In attempting to develop an individual concept of nursing, consider some of the common images of nursing. The consumer of nursing services, who is not a health professional, may have an image of nursing that does not coincide with the definitions of the profession. The word "nurse" stimulates an image response in many minds that includes such commonalities as someone who carries out doctor's orders and "does" something such as giving an injection. There is a further image, usually based on experience, that is a value judgment. Some perceive nurses as warm, helpful, and caring. Others describe nurses as cold, unemotional, and mechanical. Very few people, when asked to give their impressions of nursing, will describe what the professional responsibilities of the nurse are. They will usually describe specific impressions of a person (a woman), performing an action (related to physical care of the sick), on a patient (an individual), in a given place (a hospital).

While these common images reflect a part of what nursing is, they fail to include an expanding number of variations in practice and performance that exist in nursing today. The nurse (man or woman) shares nursing expertise in many areas, including techniques of physical assessment, interpersonal skills, co-ordination of care, consultation with other health professionals, administration, education, and research. The nurse may work with an individual of any age, in any setting. She may work with an individual, or the main focus of her efforts may be with a family, a group, a community or a large organization.

Nursing literature of the past few decades reflects the views of many within the profession. Virginia Henderson (1964) stated that:

The unique function of the nurse is to assist the individual, sick or well, in the performance of those activities contributing to health or its recovery (or to peaceful death) that he would perform unaided if he had the necessary strength, will or knowledge. And to do this in such a way as to help him gain independence as rapidly as possible.

Orem (1971) further defined nursing as assisting man in his self-care. She described nursing as a service that has as its special concern "man's need for self-care action and the provision and management of it on a continuous basis in order to sustain life and health, recover from disease or injury, and cope with their effects." Orem saw nursing as a service to the family and the community as well as to the individual.

Ida Jean Orlando (1961) described nursing as helping the patient meet his needs, and this description of nursing emphasized the nurse–patient relationship as a key to nursing care. Ernestine Wiedenbách (1964) described nursing as a deliberative action with some components similar to those mentioned above.

Myra Levine (1969) described nursing as "human interaction" and stressed the importance of adaptation between the patient and his environment. Martha Rogers (1970) saw nursing possessing scientific knowledge that could be utilized in a social context—interacting with man's environment.

These are a few of the many nursing writers who have described their images of nursing. In developing a personal concept of nursing today, it is important to understand the past on which our present state of the profession is built.

## HISTORICAL PERSPECTIVES OF NURSING

It is reasonable to assume that many of the activities performed by nurses today have been accomplished by various people since the beginning of human society. History records these activities in varying detail within cultures. Midwives and wet-nurses ministered to the needs of maternal and infant populations. Priests and priestesses reigned over health customs in some of the earliest civilizations. Early Egyptian history records diagnoses and treatments of many diseases. Ancient Babylonians gathered in the market place to share their illnesses with those designated to treat them. The early Jews practiced preventive nutrition and community health with their laws of eating and sanitation. The Greeks in early times expanded the practices of the Egyptians. Hippocrates of Greece attempted to teach with science rather than magic and the oath of Hippocrates remains a tradition in medicine to the present time.

Religion has long been a factor in the cultural experience of sickness and health. Ancient gods and their mortal representatives presided over the powers of life and death. Judaism and later Christianity considered the care of the sick and dependent as a high priority and the men and women involved in the delivery of this care were awarded status within the community. The Moslem culture developed many hospitals which carried on practices similar to early Greek medicine. The history of even the smallest of primitive tribes is replete with examples of concern for the health of its people, including many examples of medicine men and spiritual healers.

In the nineteenth century nursing as an occupation declined. Religious altruism of earlier years no longer permeated the culture of western Europe. The status of women who worked in nursing had shifted and reflected nursing as a job which had long hours, poor pay, and was done by those in society with little education and few other options.

The mid-nineteenth century witnessed many efforts for rights of women. Education, job opportunities, and the right to vote were matters of feminine concern in both the U.S. and Europe. Nursing—predominantly a female activity at that time—reflected a general upgrading of its women employees. Professional nursing as it exists in the U.S. today had its formal beginnings with the work of Florence Nightingale (1820–1910) in England. Miss Nightingale was a lady of wealth, education, and social standing. Her far-reaching vision realized the need for adequate training for those who cared for the sick. She recommended that candidates for nurses' training come with preparation in broad fields of education and culture.

The group of nurses which Florence Nightingale took to the Crimea to nurse the soldiers in the war (1854), cared for families and concentrated on efforts to make the community a healthier environment for its members. The American poet Longfellow left a vignette of Florence Nightingale in American literature with his description of her and her nursing in "Lady of the Lamp."

During the latter part of the nineteenth century, nursing in the U.S. began its attempts to establish training schools. Most of these schools were financially supported and administered by physicians. The schools were affiliated with hospitals and the apprentice method of training was used.

The American Civil War resulted in many deaths and casualties in both the North and the South. It is known that a large number of these losses were due to the poor conditions under which the wounded were treated as well as the poor environment in which the soldiers lived, travelled, and fought. Florence Nightingale was a consultant to American health care providers during the Civil War and her influence in nursing thought was substantive. Dorothea Dix rallied the first Army Nurse Corps to serve during the Civil War. Their efforts did not substantially stem the influence of disease and infection. The need for more and better trained nurses was apparent. During the postwar years, Clara Barton established the Red Cross society here in America. This was part of the international Red Cross with its headquarters in Geneva, Switzerland. It provided nurses for service in disasters, including wars.

The latter part of the nineteenth century saw schools of nursing begin to increase in the U.S. A number of competent and committed women guided the nursing profession here in its early days. In keeping with the guidelines suggested by Florence Nightingale, these schools began as educational enterprises, separate in administration from hospitals. Economic pressures placed priority on nursing service over nursing education as time went on. The interaction between the hospital's need for the services of student nurses and the student's need for educational experiences created a tension that lingered long after nursing education became recognized as a prerequisite to practice.

Schools of nursing developed in different locations. The first of these was at the New England Hospital for Women and Children in Boston in 1872. In the following year, nursing schools were also opened at Bellevue Hospital in New York, New Haven Hospital in Connecticut, and Massachusetts General Hospital in Boston. There were 35 hospital training schools in the U.S. in 1890. Two decades later there were 1,129 schools.

Linda Richards (1841–1930) is remembered for her leadership in education in the Boston Schools of Nursing. Isabel Hampton Robb made numerous contributions to the development of nursing as a profession, including her role in founding the American Nurses Association and the American Journal of Nursing. She also guided the progress of the School of Nursing at Johns Hopkins in Baltimore. Her successor there was M. Adelaide Nutting (1858–1948) who later accepted a position at Columbia University, becoming the first known professor of nursing. Miss Nutting's contributions extended into many nursing organizations, including the International Council of Nurses.

Although the training of nurses occurred in hospitals, graduate nurses for the most part practiced as private duty nurses in homes. Hospital staffing was accomplished by student nurses. One notable exception to this trend of practice was the beginning of community health nursing. Lillian Wald (1876–1940), a graduate of New York Hospital School of Nursing, helped develop the Henry Street Settlement in New York City. Here, social needs as well as health concerns of the community were focused upon. Miss Wald was the first president of the National Organization for Public Health Nursing and was the first nurse to be elected to the Hall of Fame for Great Americans. Another famous founder in the field of public health nursing was Mary Sewell Gardner (1871–1961). She worked with Lillian Wald in founding the Organization for Public Health Nursing and was a pioneer in writing and publication in this field.

Annie W. Goodrich (1866–1954) brought her knowledge as a nurse educator to influence nursing education. She was a leading force in the shift from apprentice-type training to professional education. She was appointed first dean of the newly developed Army School of Nursing in 1918—established to prepare nurses to serve in the military service.

## PROFESSIONAL ORGANIZATIONS IN NURSING

The evolution of nursing as a profession is reflected in the formation of professional organizations. Professional organizations have a responsibility both to their members and to the public. Criteria for a profession and professional responsibilities will be discussed in more detail later in this chapter.

Organization of nurses in the U.S. began with the formation of alumnae groups from nursing schools. As the number of nursing schools mushroomed at the turn of the century, and the focus of organizations expanded to include professional goals, alumnae organizations became inadequate. The American Nurses Association blossomed from the seeds of the alumnae organizations and continued to grow as a professional organization. Its original purposes had included improving standards of nursing education, establishing an ethical code, and uniting nurses as a group. These purposes have been maintained and expanded. The present ANA code of ethics is well-defined and this organization continues to develop and monitor standards of practice for professional nursing.

Concern for the educational process in nursing was reflected in the formation of organizations to monitor nursing schools and help with curriculum development. The American Society of Superintendents of Training Schools for Nurses began in 1893 and became the National League of Nursing Education in 1912. The same year, the National Organization for Public Health Nursing was formed to organize and standardize nurses engaged in public health nursing. Membership in this organization was open not only to nurses, but also to others working in public health.

After World War II, the nursing profession began a restructuring of its professional organizations. The six main organizations existing at that time were: the American Nurses Association (ANA), the National League of Nursing Education (NLNE), the National Organization for Public Health Nursing (NOPHN), the National Association of Colored Graduate Nurses (NACGN), the American Association of Industrial Nurses (AAIN), and the Association of Collegiate Schools of Nursing (ACSN). The AAIN opted to remain a separate organization. The NACGN ceased its activity since by 1951 all ANA constituent organizations admitted registered nurses to membership with no color discrimination.

The ANA continued to be the official professional organization of nursing with membership open only to registered nurses. The remaining three organizations mentioned (NLNE, NOPHN, and ACSN) consolidated their functions into the National League for Nursing in 1952. The ANA and the NLN are presently the largest nursing organizations. While different in function and structure, they complement each other and work together for the profession of nursing and for the public who utilize that profession. Both the ANA and the NLN have a national membership and constituent chapters within each state. The two organizations have joint committees in areas where concerns are overlapping.

The ANA sets standards for nursing practice and education. It is the official voice of nurses in legislative matters, represents U.S. nurses in community organizations including the International Council of Nurses, promotes professional development, and works to promote the general and economic welfare of nurses. It also stimulates and promotes research and publication.

The NLN attempts to identify society's need for nursing and plans programs to help meet those needs especially in regard to comprehensive health care. The NLN, which has both agency and individual memberships, includes not only nurses but also allied health professions, community members, and health and educational institutions. It strives to improve nursing services and educational programs in communities with accreditation services, testing, consultation, research, and publications.

A third important organization within nursing is the National Student Nurse Association (NSNA). Originally established in 1953 with some assistance from the ANA and NLN, this group became legally incorporated in 1958 as an autonomous nonprofit organization. It is administered and supported by nursing students and voices their concerns. NSNA policies and programs are voted by a house of delegates, consisting of elected members from state student nurse associations. The group publishes *Imprint* as its official journal. Some of NSNA's activities include recruitment, workshops, activities on health and nursing legislation, and interdisciplinary contact with students in other health-related fields such as medicine, pharmacy, and dentistry. Membership in NSNA is available to any student in a state-approved nursing program that leads to registered nurse licensure.

The national honor society of nursing in the U.S. is Sigma Theta Tau, Inc. The purposes of this society include recognition of superior achievement and development of leadership, fostering high professional standards, encouraging creativity in work, supporting research, and strengthening commitment to the ideals and purposes of nursing. Membership is derived from selected students and faculty in NLN accredited programs at the baccalaureate or higher degree levels, and selected leaders in nursing practice. Sigma Theta Tau publishes its activities in *Image*.

## NURSING EDUCATION

Florence Nightingale had originally envisioned autonomy for nursing education. In the U.S., as in England, this goal could seldom be implemented for economic reasons. Since nursing schools for the most part were financially supported by hospitals, the ultimate control of nursing education also rested with the hospital administration.

Gradually, baccalaureate programs were developed in nursing as the need to offer nursing education in an educational setting was recognized. The first baccalaureate program was begun at the University of Minnesota in 1909. Since that time, the number of baccalaureate programs in the U.S. has continued to grow. During the 1950s, with the rise of the community college as an educational resource, a third type of nursing program developed—the associate degree program in nursing. The graduate of this program is identified as a technical nurse with preparation that is appropriate to a technical level of nursing function under the direction of a professional nurse or physician.

In 1948, the Carnegie Corporation supported a study of nursing education which was directed by Esther Lucile Brown. This report recommended that "professional" nurses be graduates of accredited professional schools. It further recommended that nursing schools be university-affiliated and responsible for their own budgets. Since that time there has been increasing support for nursing education to be associated with educational institutions. The number of hospital diploma programs has decreased dramatically. Most remaining diploma programs have arrangements with nearby colleges for teaching of basic sciences and other courses supportive to their curricula. This allows the diploma student to earn transferable college credits for her learning. The ANA has proposed a position that the baccalaureate degree be the basic educational preparation for entry into practice for all professional nurses by 1985.

Practical/vocational nursing is another level of nursing education. Graduates of these programs take examinations to be Licensed Practical Nurses (LPNs). These programs are usually 12 to 18 months in length and are found in hospitals, vocational schools, and community colleges. LPN education emphasizes technical nursing skills and direct patient care, usually in hospitals and nursing homes. The graduate is prepared to function under the direction of a professional nurse or a physician.

Postbaccalaureate and graduate nursing education is sought by growing numbers of nurses. Some baccalaureate-prepared nurses seek postbaccalaureate training in a specific clinical area and thus work toward becoming skilled practitioners. Others seek academic routes to higher education via master's and doctoral degree programs. There is considerable variety in the quality and scope of graduate programs available to nurses today.

## Continuing Education

Continuing education is a concept currently being implemented in nursing as in other health professions. The overall need for continuing education in light of a growing body of knowledge and skills in health fields is generally agreed upon within the nursing profession. However, there is not general agreement regarding what criteria constitute valid continuing education for an individual in practice, where this education can best be offered, and whether it should be a mandatory requirement for renewal of licenses. A wide variety of continuing education opportunities are available. Hospitals and other health agencies offer courses and workshops as part of inservice programs. Schools of nursing and departments of continuing education within universities and community colleges offer programs and continuing-education credits. Although the idea of continuing education is widespread, it may be a number of years before there is a consensus within the profession on related issues.

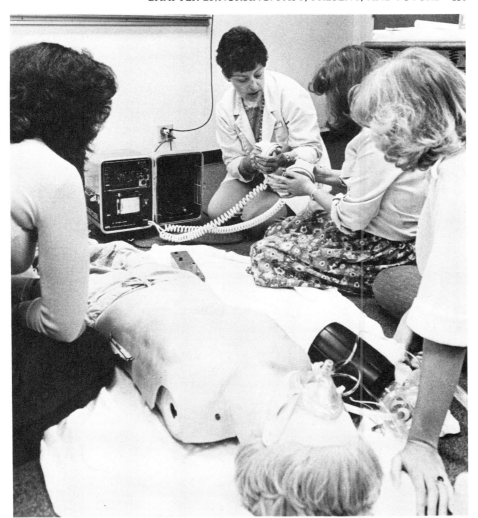

**Figure 23-1.** *In-service training in the use of defibrillator. (Photo by Jose Mercado/News and Publications Service, Stanford University)*

Career mobility in nursing is a matter of concern to many, but especially to those who begin their nursing education in a diploma or associate degree program and then wish to progress along the educational continuum of baccalaureate and higher degrees. The Open Curriculum Concept which allows flexibility in achieving learning objectives, and assesses previous learning for relevance to present goals, is supported by the NLN and facilitates upward mobility.

Use of many aspects of educational technology is evident in current nursing education. Individualized planning, programmed instruction, media centers, and instructional designs with criterion-referenced objectives are seen. The entire field of nursing education is in an exciting period of expansion and growth as it attempts to keep in rhythm with the rapid changes both in our society and in the fields of health care and education.

## NURSING PRACTICE

Nursing is a practice discipline and the profession thus assumes responsibility for development and implementation of standards of practice. The need for close communication and cooperation between nursing service and nursing education in promoting standards of practice is evident. According to the International Council of Nurses, the nurse promotes health, prevents illness, restores health, and alleviates suffering. Within this broad definition of nursing practice, there is much room for the variety of practice situations that exist today. The nurse gives care to clients, protects the client's environment, teaches the client, helps carry out treatments for illness, and helps coordinate the many factors within the health care system to assure the best available care. The "client" may refer to an individual or may be a family, group, or community.

Nursing was originally practiced fairly independently in the U.S. with graduate nurses working outside of hospital settings in public health and private homes as well as occupational settings. The economic stresses of the 1930s lowered these job opportunities and motivated many graduate nurses to accept lower salaried positions in hospitals as dependent workers subject to the policies of hospital administration. Concurrent with the concerns of women in other types of employment, there has been the concern of nurses with both economic security and job satisfaction. In search of these, nurses have explored expanded roles—some of these similar to nursing as it was practiced prior to the migration of nurses to hospitals, and some that reflect new dimensions of health care.

The primary care nurse is seen giving initial and comprehensive nursing care to a client and/or family, including coordination of care with other health professionals. Frequently, this nurse may be a nurse practitioner with advanced skills in physical assessment within specialized clinical areas.

The clinical nurse specialist is another practice-based nursing role, similar in some ways to the primary care nurse, but including educational preparation at the master's level. The Clinical Nurse Specialist can function as a teacher, consultant, researcher, change agent, or therapist and practitioner.

Nursing practice today includes components of dependence, interdependence, and independence. The nurse is in a dependent role when she is performing actions that implement orders prescribed by another such as a physician. She is in an interdependent role when working with the physician and other health professionals to coordinate a comprehensive plan of care. The nurse functions in an independent role when she assumes the primary responsibility for nursing diagnosis and care of a client. The scope of nursing—practice and services which the nurse can offer as an independent practitioner—is defined by the Nurse Practice Acts of each individual state. Some states are more liberal in their interpretation of what constitutes nursing practice than others. Another area that may be vague regarding interpretation of nursing practice is in financial reimbursement for nursing services. At this time, insurance companies vary rates for direct payment of practitioners in the health field and nursing rates are among the lowest. As an integral part of a large system of health care delivery, the nurse needs to continue to adapt her practice to changing health needs without lowering the professional standards.

The general standards for nursing practice in any setting have been developed by the ANA. They include the following criteria:

1. The collection of data on the health status of the client is systematic and continuous. The data are accessible, recorded, and communicated.
2. Nursing diagnoses are derived from health status data.
3. Nursing care plan includes goals from data in nursing diagnosis.
4. Nursing care plan includes priorities and the prescribed nursing measures to achieve goals.
5. Nursing actions provide for client participation in health promotion, maintenance, and restoration.
6. Nursing actions assist the client to maximize his health capabilities.
7. Client progress toward goal achievement is determined by the client and the nurse.
8. Client progress or lack of progress toward goal achievement directs reassessment, reordering of priorities, new goal-setting, and revision of the nursing care plan.

## NURSING RESEARCH

Nursing research is essential to the development of knowledge and theory within the profession. Florence Nightingale gave nursing a research orientation in her systematic data-gathering and the utilization of these data to make needed reforms. It was not until the 1930s that the value of nursing research was emphasized by U.S. leaders in the profession. The focus of nursing research at that time was primarily on nurses and their image. Research was often done by social scientists rather than nurses. Gradually, as nursing programs developed within university settings, there was impetus for research by faculty and students. The publication *Nursing Research* began in 1952 and became a written vehicle for dissemination of findings of research in nursing. Federal funding of nursing research projects aided progress in this field although this source of funding fluctuates with various political and economic changes within the government. The past 25 years have seen a major focus in research on nursing education. There has recently been an increasing interest in nursing research related to clinical practice. Expanding

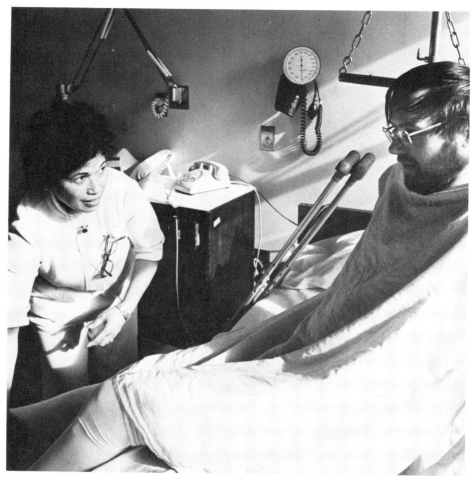

**Figure 23-2.** *Nursing actions assist the client to maximize his health capabilities. (Photo by Jose Mercado/News and Publications service, Stanford University)*

roles in nursing practice, development of criteria for evaluating quality of patient care, specific clinical practice areas, and utilization of scientific principles in nursing practice are all topics of current interest in nursing research. Interdisciplinary research with other allied health groups and collaborative studies of nurses in various clinical areas and settings are also being done.

The need for close communications among researchers, educators, administrators, and practitioners is obvious if nursing research is to reflect the reality as well as the theoretical basis of the profession. Circulation of research results, and the utilization of findings for improvement of patient care and health-care delivery needs to be a concern of every nurse regardless of where she practices.

# PROFESSIONAL AND LEGAL RESPONSIBILITIES IN NURSING

Criteria for a profession have been delineated by many competent sources. One of the earliest descriptions was that of Dr. Abraham Flexner in 1915. He identified the following characteristics as essential to a profession:

1. Involvement of essentially intellectual operations accompanied by large individual responsibility.
2. Learned in nature with members constantly resorting to the laboratory and seminar for a fresh supply of facts.
3. Practical in aims, not merely academic and theoretical.
4. Possessing a technique capable of communication through a highly specialized educational discipline.
5. Self-organized, with activities, duties, and responsibilities which engage participants and develop group consciousness.
6. Responsible to public interest and increasingly concerned with the achievement of social aims.

In applying these criteria to nursing, it is evident that only in recent years have some of the characteristics of a profession been identifiable. The intellectual operations of the profession begin in basic nursing educational programs which include components of general education as well as professional subjects. Individual responsibility in nursing begins after graduation from a school of nursing. The nurse is tested for knowledge at a minimum level via the State Board Test Pool Examinations prior to licensure. Licensure in nursing in the U.S. is done within each state. Students who have graduated from state accredited nursing programs are recommended by their school as qualified to take the examinations. Licensure in other states can be accomplished by endorsement. The nurse applies for endorsement by giving evidence of licensure in the state in which Board Examinations were taken. It is the individual's responsibility to maintain a current license to practice as required by the State Board of Nursing in a given state.

Nursing draws its learning from physical, behavioral, and social sciences as well as from professional knowledge. The profession seeks continuing development of new knowledge and theory appropriate to the changing world. This goal is reflected in the emphasis on continuing education in nursing. In some states continuing education credits are required for annual renewal of licensure. This is an effort to assure a continuing updating of knowledge among professional nurses.

The practical aim of nursing is evidenced in nursing practice. In addition to licensure, the practice of nursing is guided by the Nurse Practice Acts which are developed in each state. These attempt to define nursing practice and identify minimum standards necessary for nursing practice in that state. Certification, which is a fairly recent program within the ANA, is a further effort within the nursing profession to describe levels of practice above the minimum or licensure level. The certification process gives recognition to nurses who have achieved advanced standing in a given practice area.

Nursing has a technique able to be communicated by a specialized educational system. Earlier discussion of nursing education describes the evolution of this system up to the present.

Nursing is a self-organized profession with activities and responsibilities which develop group consciousness among participants. The professional organizations in nursing assume responsibility for group consciousness as well as for standards of practice, peer review and political awareness.

Responsibility to the public is governed by a code of ethics—The Code for Nurses—which the ANA adopted in 1950. This code includes the following ethical responsibilities of the nurse:

1. Provision of services with respect for human dignity and individual uniqueness regardless of social or economic status, personal attributes, or the health problem.
2. Safeguarding of the client's right to privacy and protection of confidential information.
3. Safeguarding the client and the public if health and safety are affected by the incompetent, unethical, or illegal practice of any person.
4. Assuming responsibility and accountability for individual nursing judgment and actions.
5. Maintaining competence in nursing.
6. Using informed judgment with individual competence as criteria in seeking consultation, accepting responsibilities, and delegating nursing activities to others.
7. Participating in activities that contribute to ongoing development of the profession's body of knowledge.
8. Participating in professional efforts to implement and improve standards of nursing.
9. Participating in professional efforts to establish and maintain conditions of employment conducive to high quality nursing care.
10. Participating in professional efforts to protect the public from misinformation and misrepresentation and to maintain the integrity of nursing.
11. Collaborating with members of health professions and others in promoting community and national efforts to meet public health needs.

In addition to professional considerations, the nurse needs to be aware of legal responsibilities, including the scope of nursing practice as defined by law in the state where she is practicing. The suggested ANA definition of nursing practice was set forth in 1955:

The practice of professional nursing means the performance for compensation of any act in the observation, care, and counsel of the ill, injured, or infirm, or in the maintenance of health or prevention of illness of others, or in the supervision and teaching of other personnel, or the administration of medications and treatments prescribed by a licensed physician or dentist; requiring substantial specialized judgment and skill and based on knowledge and application of the principles of biological, physical, and social sciences. The foregoing shall not be deemed to include acts of diagnosis or prescription of therapeutic or corrective measures.

Expanding roles in nursing have been covered by an addition to the above statement made in 1970 which refers to additional acts that may be performed under emergency or special conditions. Each nurse in practice is responsible for malpractice insurance and liability. The nurse must be aware of the many facets of law that are of concern to the health fields, such as patient's rights, negligence, accident reporting, informed consent, Good Samaritan laws, privacy, drug legislation, and wills. Many agencies have legal counsel available but the responsibility to seek answers when questions arise, and to act in accordance with the law is ultimately the responsibility of the individual nurse.

## NURSING IN THE FUTURE

There are many present realities to be considered in anticipating and planning for the future of nursing. The students who enter nursing today bring with them a variety of educational and life experiences. People with degrees and experience in other fields are choosing nursing for many reasons such as job availability and a desire to work within the health care system. Women who are raising children are beginning and completing their nursing education and preparing to combine home and career responsibilities. The rising divorce rate has forced many women to deal with the realities of self support and the support of children. Nursing offers these and other women who seek job security a wide variety of career options. Men are increasing their percentage in the profession which has long been predominantly female. All of these factors increase the human resources from which nursing can draw. Nursing needs to be prepared to develop this potential and help define its utilization in health care delivery.

New roles will continue to evolve in keeping with societal changes. Expansion of existing roles in some areas, and the deletion of roles no longer needed, can be expected. Nurse clinicians in all areas will have the responsibility of ongoing definition of their role as it fits with others involved in health related services. Nursing careers in government, military, and industrial agencies offer many opportunities. Aerospace nursing will continue to emerge as society expands its boundaries into the universe.

Self-care and client participation in nursing and health care are increasingly expected by both consumers and providers of health care. Prevention and wellness continue as high priorities in nursing. Treatments for illness often requires sophisticated scientific knowledge for optimum results. The implementation of treatment requires the support system of caring, continuity and coordination that nursing can provide. Utilization of auxiliary nursing personnel and technicians needs to be continually evaluated for maximum utility of the abilities of all. The assumption of widespread participation in health care assumes a foundational knowledge of prevention and health behaviors. The nurse is one of many involved in this process of health education to consumers.

Legislation will have considerable impact on the future of nursing. The outcome of the struggle for the Equal Rights Amendment will have important implications to many members of the nursing profession. Resolution of issues relative to National Health Insurance will influence delivery of nursing services. A matter of special importance to nurses seeking roles in independent practice is that of direct payment for nursing services. At the present time nurses are paid poorly in relation to other health professionals for services that are reimbursed by health insurance. The ANA is presently working to encourage nurses to seek, and insurers to provide, a fair share of the economic enforcers available to providers of independent professional services.

Nursing needs to continue to develop and maintain its standards, adapt to societal needs and develop its own vision. The future depends on planning ahead realistically while maintaining sound professional practices on which the future can be built.

## SUMMARY

The image of nursing and nurses has evolved historically. Nursing as a profession is a fairly recent concept which reflects this evolution. The last century has witnessed many changes in nursing education and practice. The focus of nursing education has shifted from that of learning only skills to provide services under the direction of other professionals, to learning to be responsible for the knowledge base as well as the skills needed to practice nursing as a profession. Nursing education is now primarily offered in institutions of higher education. Professional nursing organizations provide structure and support in areas of education, practice and research.

Nursing practice has developed within the limits of existing state laws. Expanded roles of nurses continue to emerge in an attempt to meet changing and increasing health care needs of society. Professional and legal issues relevant to nursing are an ongoing challenge. The future of nursing is intertwined with many aspects of society such as legislation, economics, and health care delivery.

## LEARNING ACTIVITIES

1. Begin to keep an informal, written record of your image of a nurse and nursing as a profession. Update this at regular intervals, adding changes in your perceptions and the reasons for these.

2. Interview several people who are not family members or health professionals, and ask what their image of a nurse and nursing is. Compare your results with your classmates and try to obtain a composite picture of opinions gathered.

3. Write to the state where you plan to eventually practice nursing and request the nurse practice act for that state and the licensing procedures.

4. Attend at least one meeting of a local chapter of the National Student Nurse Association.

5. Visit a nursing program that is different from yours and compare differences as they may relate to the graduates of each program and eventual functioning in nursing.

6. Interview at least one nurse who is practicing in an expanded nursing role in a clinical area of your choice.

7. Read at least two articles relative to nursing research and describe how these will help you in your study of nursing.

## REFERENCES AND SUGGESTED READINGS

American Nurses Association. *Bylaws.*   Kansas City, Mo., 1970.

———— . *Code for Nurses with interpretive statements.*   Kansas City, Mo., 1976.

———— . *Standards of nursing practice.*   Kansas City, Mo., 1973.

Brown, Esther Lucile, 1948.   *Nursing for the future.*   New York: Russell Sage Foundation.

Bullough, Bonnie, 1975.   *The law and the expanding nursing role.*   New York: Appleton-Century-Crofts.

Creighton, Helen, 1975.   *Law every nurse should know.* 3rd ed.   Philadelphia: W. B. Saunders.

*Ethical concepts applied to nursing 1973.* International Council of Nurses News Release, No. 6, September, 1975.

Gortner, Susan R. and Nahm, Helen.   An overview of nursing research in the United States. *Nursing Research,* 26 (Jan.–Feb., 1977) 10–30.

Griffin, Gerald J. and Griffin, Joanne King, 1973.   *History and trends of professional nursing.*   St. Louis: C. V. Mosby.

Flexner, Abraham.   Is social work a profession? Proceedings of the National Conference of Charities and Correction, 1915, pp. 578–581.

Hall, Virginia C., 1975.   *Statutory regulation of the scope of nursing.*   Chicago: The National Joint Practice Commission.

Henderson, Virginia, 1966.   *The nature of nursing.*   New York: Macmillan.

————.   The nature of nursing. *American Journal of Nursing,* August, 1964, pp. 62–68.

Kelly, Lucie Young, 1975.   *Dimensions of professional nursing.* 3rd ed.   New York: Macmillan.

————. Nursing practice acts. *American Journal of Nursing,* July, 1974, p. 1310.

National League for Nursing. *Bylaws.*   New York, 1973.

————.   *The open curriculum in nursing education.*   New York: The Association, 1970.

National Student Nurses' Association. *Bylaws.*   New York, 1972.

Orem, Dorothea E., 1971.   *Nursing: concepts of practice.*   New York: McGraw-Hill.

Orlando, Ida Jean, 1961.   *The dynamic nurse–patient relationship.*   New York: Putnam.

Rogers, Martha, 1970.   *An introduction to the theoretical basis of nursing.*   Philadelphia: F. A. Davis.

Rowland, Howard S., ed., 1978.   *The nurse's almanac.*   Germantown, Maryland: Aspen Systems Corporation.

Wiedinbach, Ernestine E., 1964.   *Clinical nursing: a helping art.*   New York: Springer Publishing.

# 24

# Current Health Care Concerns

Introduction
Types of Health Care
Delivery of Health Care
Funding of Health Care
Chronic Illness
Attitudes Toward Health Care
Consumer Participation in Health Care
Summary
Learning Activities
References and Suggested Readings

## Behavioral Objectives

Upon completion of this chapter, the student will be able to:

1. Describe the focus of emergency care, acute care, and ambulatory care.
2. Compare the functions of official and voluntary health agencies.
3. Discuss sources of funding for health care.
4. Identify common chronic illnesses that interfere with wellness.
5. Discuss current philosophies toward health care, including holistic health care and self-care.
6. Describe the importance of individual behavior as it relates to health.

## Key Terms

acute care
ambulatory care
chronic illness
consumerism
emergency care
enabling factors
health maintenance
  organization (HMO)

high-level wellness
holistic health
official agency
Medicaid
Medicare
national health insurance
  (NHI)

predisposing factors
reinforcing factors
self-care
stress-related illness
third-party payment
voluntary agency
workman's compensation

## Introduction

The accelerated rate of social change that characterizes our society often makes that which was recently seen as new seem obsolete. Yet even amidst constant change, there are human concerns which remain relatively constant. Health is one of these.

This chapter will discuss current types of health care and the agencies and financial arrangements which support these. Chronic illness and the relationship of stress and illness will be briefly described, as well as some of the emerging attitudes toward health and individual participation in health care.

## TYPES OF HEALTH CARE

Health care, as it is presently organized, can be described under the three general categories of emergency care, acute care, and ambulatory care.

### Emergency Care

Organized emergency care was traditionally given in the Emergency Room (ER) of hospitals. Use of the hospital ER for nonemergencies, limitations in available equipment and personnel, and the need for outreach emergency facilities were among the major problems in providing emergency care. The U.S. Congress, in 1973, passed the Emergency Medical Services Systems (EMSS) Act and committed federal funds for the development of better emergency services in the community. The EMSS Act identified the following essential components for an emergency medical services system:

1. Personnel (available on a 24-hour basis).
2. Training (clinical training and continuing education for personnel).
3. Communications (including a central system and control center to join personnel, facilities, and equipment).
4. Transportation (ground, air, and water vehicles with trained operators).
5. Facilities (easily accessible and coordinated with other health-care facilities).
6. Access (appropriate transportation, including ability to handle in-transit care, to specialized medical care units such as intensive care units, burn centers, spinal cord centers, and detoxification centers).
7. Effective utilization (of personnel, facilities, and equipment in cooperation with other public safety agencies).
8. Policy-making (including consumer participation).
9. Payment for service (needed services to be provided to all, regardless of ability to pay).
10. Transfer (of patients to follow-up care and physical, psychiatric, and vocational rehabilitation).

11. Record-keeping (standardized record of patient treatment, consistent with records in other nearby care facilities).
12. Public education (including methods of self-help and first aid).
13. Review (periodic, comprehensive, and independent review and evaluation of services).
14. Disaster capacity (plan to provide services for mass casualties, natural disasters, or national emergencies).
15. Reciprocal services (agreements to exchange services with neighboring facilities).

This encouragement and financial support for emergency care has resulted in greater awareness on the part of all concerned regarding the importance of a total backup system for emergency care. Trauma centers have been developed and the use of helicopters for speedy transportation has increased the number of successful attempts at lifesaving, particularly for victims of car accidents, one of our leading causes of death in younger age groups.

## Acute Care

Acute or episodic care is usually given in hospital settings. Hospitals are classified on the basis of their clinical focus, such as general or orthopedic; or

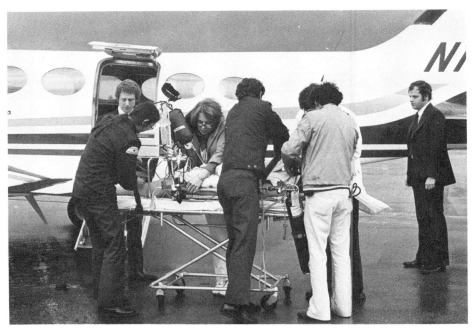

**Figure 24-1.** *Trauma centers increase the number of successful attempts at lifesaving after accidents. (Photo by Laura Hofstadter/News and Publications Service, Stanford University)*

on the basis of control, such as federal, state, or private. Hospitals offer a large variety of services depending on their size, goals, and resources. One of the main problems of hospitals today is the ever-rising cost of inpatient care. Lack of comprehensive planning by geographic area has resulted in a surplus of hospital beds in selected clinical services and geographic locations, while shortages exist in other clinical specialties and locations. Utilization of high-cost hospital services paid for by health insurance, when lower-cost outpatient services and home care could be equally effective, is an issue currently being examined by insurance companies and consumers.

## Ambulatory Care

Ambulatory care is ongoing health care given outside of hospitals and acute care facilities. This type of health care is offered through private practice, community clinics, and the outpatient departments of hospitals. The majority of health care given today is in ambulatory settings. One of its major problems is fragmentation. Specialization of services has increased client accessibility to more expert care providers, but the client may need assistance in navigating through the often confusing maze of multiple health services.

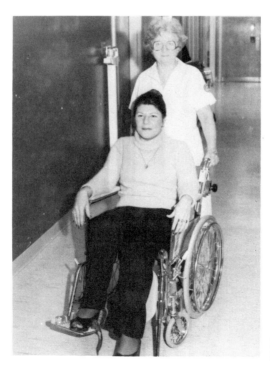

**Figure 24-2.** *Ambulatory health care. (Photo by Frank R. Engler, Jr.)*

## DELIVERY OF HEALTH CARE

Health care delivery systems include private and group practice and health agencies. Health care agencies are described as official or voluntary. An official health agency is tax supported, assumes responsibility for the health of all citizens within its jurisdiction, and is governed by laws. A voluntary agency is supported by funds and donations, usually focuses on a particular health problem such as heart disease or cancer, and is governed by a group of private citizens, often volunteers, with a paid support staff. Both types of agencies exist on local, state, and national levels. There are also official agencies on an international level, such as the World Health Organization (WHO), which functions under the framework of the United Nations; the International Development Agency (IDA), which supplies economic and technical assistance to nations; and the Peace Corps, which provides volunteers to assist with living conditions and health in underdeveloped countries.

Official health departments began in this country on a state level with laws designed to prevent the importation of disease from one state to another. The three major areas of responsibility for health departments are: promotion of personal and community health, maintenance of a healthful environment, and attack on disease and disability (Smolensky, 1977).

The federal agency concerned with health began in 1912 when the Public Health Marine Hospital Service was reorganized and the U.S. Public Health Service was formed. In 1953, the Public Health Service, along with Social and Rehabilitation Services, Social Security Administration, and the Office of Education, were organized to form the Department of Health, Education, and Welfare (HEW). In 1979, this department was split into the Department of Education and the Department of Health and Human Services.

This Federal agency assists the state health departments with grants for initiating new health services, especially those through the Children's Bureau. The Public Health Service is composed of the following divisions:

Food and Drug Administration
National Institutes of Health
Alcohol, Drug Abuse and Mental Health Administration
Health Services Administration
Health Resources Administration
Center for Disease Control

Local health departments are supported by local taxes with some financial aid from the state level. The official agencies attempt to provide leadership to the community and to encourage the community to accept responsibility for its health.

Functions of voluntary health agencies have been described as (Gunn and Platt, 1945):

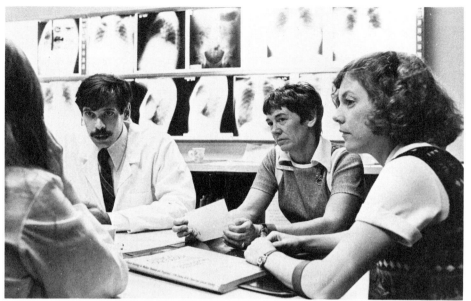

**Figure 24-3.** *An interdisciplinary health-care team at work.* *(Photo by Jose Mercado/News and Publications Service, Stanford University)*

1. Pioneering or exploring with new ways to deal with health problems.
2. Demonstration of practical methods to improve public health.
3. Health education.
4. Supplementation of activities of the official health department.
5. Guarding of citizen interest in health.
6. Promotion of health legislation.
7. Group planning and coordination.
8. Development of well-rounded community health programs.

Associations such as the Heart Association, Cancer Society, and Lung Association can be excellent community resources for both health-care consumers and health-care providers. It is important to the community that these agencies work cooperatively with official agencies.

In addition to official and voluntary agencies, health care is delivered through private practice and health maintenance organizations (HMOs). The best known private practitioner is the physician. Many physicians are now practicing in group practice. This may be with other physicians, or the group may be interdisciplinary and include other health professionals, such as psychologists, clinical nurse specialists, social workers or nutritionists.

HMOs are a growing form of organized health care services. They are a prepaid group practice, where subscribers pay an agreed-upon sum for comprehensive health services, including preventive services. Physicians and other health professionals are salaried. This concept of health care provides economic reward for wellness.

## FUNDING OF HEALTH CARE

Funding of health care is an increasing concern given the reality of spiralling costs. At the present time, apart from prepaid plans, costs are paid in three ways: fee-for-service, third-party payment, and government financing. The fee-for-service or direct consumer payment can be a financial catastrophe to middle- and low-income families in the event of serious illness. To protect themselves against such a situation, many people purchase various forms of health insurance, which assures that a third party—the insurance company—will pay for at least a portion of their health care. Such insurance is financed by premiums. Individuals, employers, or both, assume responsibility for premium payments. Although this type of insurance helps, it does not usually cover payment for preventive health services, is insufficient coverage for catastrophic illness, and is not available to all people.

Government financing of health care has been provided through workman's compensation, Medicare, and Medicaid. Workman's compensation is regulated by state laws which require that employers assume financial responsibility for injuries incurred by an employee while on the job. Medicare assures a health insurance for the aged under the Social Security Act of 1965. Medicaid, created by the same act, is a program within each state designed to help pay costs for health care of the medically indigent and the poor. The federal government assists states in financing Medicaid programs, and sets some of the standards for eligibility and benefits.

Existing health coverage does not meet the needs of many Americans today and adequate health care for all is not available for financial reasons. There is growing pressure for some type of National Health Insurance (NHI) that would alleviate this situation and, despite objections from those who prefer the traditional health-care systems, it seems likely that some form of NHI will be approved by Congress in the near future. This would likely increase the demand for ambulatory care services, including nursing.

## CHRONIC ILLNESS

One of the main threats to optimum health in our society is chronic illness. Chronic illness is defined as any impairment or deviation from normal that has one or more of the following characteristics: is permanent; leaves residual disability; is caused by nonreversible pathological alteration; requires special training of the client for rehabilitation; or may be expected to require a long period of supervision, observation, or care (Commission on Chronic Illness, 1957). Among the common chronic illnesses, especially among the elderly, are heart conditions, kidney disease, arthritis, back and spinal problems, mental illness, hypertension, diabetes, and emphysema. Persons with chronic disease often require long-term nursing supervision. As with other health-related variables, the major factor in treatment of chronic illness is the individual's willingness to promote his or her own health and to seek care early when illness occurs. When a person is disabled by chronic disease, it is important to plan for appropriate rehabilitation to assist him in achieving as much normalcy as possible within the limitations of his disease.

There is an obvious relationship between the changing pace of life today and the increase in stress-related illness. It has been estimated that over 50 percent of hospitalizations are caused or aggravated by stress factors. The relationship of stress to major diseases, including chronic illness, is well-known. There are a number of ways to cope with stress and reduce its effects on health. Relaxation and stress-reduction classes are available in many communities. Some of the individual behaviors that can alleviate stress include avoidance of situations that produce stress when possible and maintenance of activities and relationships that provide satisfaction and working out of negative feelings, such as anger, which add to stress.

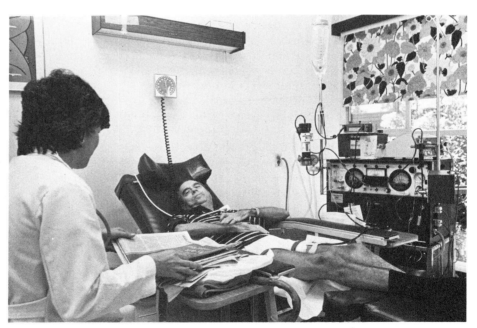

**Figure 24-4.** *A nurse assisting with hemodialysis of a patient with chronic kidney disease. (Photo by Jose Mercado/News and Publications Service, Stanford University)*

## ATTITUDES TOWARD HEALTH CARE

Health care in the United States has been crisis-oriented in the past. People sought out the physician when they were sick and the initial questioning dealt with symptoms of illness. Available services were for illness care.

The World Health Organization definition of health states that health is "a state of complete physical, mental, and social well-being and not merely the absence of disease or infirmity." This definition reflected a shift of emphasis toward wellness. Dunn (1961) introduced the concept of high-level wellness which considered wellness and illness as two ends of a continuum and focused on the interrelationships between health and environment in achieving the highest possible level of wellness.

Recent years have witnessed the emergence of the concept of holistic health care, which sees all persons as "whole beings whose individual psycho-physio-cultural-spiritual relationships with the environment directly affect their state of health." (Smolensky, 1977). Internal, as well as external, factors that influence behaviors are assessed to determine individual health needs. Traditions from ancient, as well as modern, cultures of both the East and West are respected. The individual is expected to modify his own lifestyle according to his unique needs.

Prevention has become a recognized value among health care providers and consumers. Immunizations have contributed to impressive results in the prevention of infectious diseases. This was the result of research, health care practice, and acceptance by the public. Unfortunately, efforts to prevent today's leading causes of death in the United States have been less successful. Research indicates that the major preventive measures in heart disease, cancer, and stroke are changes in individual lifestyles. Diet, exercise, nonsmoking, and stress management are key factors in preventing heart disease. Yet a majority of persons remain unwilling or unable to adapt their lifestyles to habits that promote health rather than illness.

Early diagnosis of cancer through diagnostic check-ups and self-examinations can significantly lower the mortality from that disease. Early detection and control of hypertension can lessen the risk of occurrence and severity of strokes. Yet many people postpone or avoid these preventive measures.

In a society which values the right of individual choice, it must be remembered that this includes the choice of illness over health. Efforts to encourage prevention must take into account that the needed individual behavorial changes cannot be forced or legislated. Education about health, where appropriate, is the responsibility of all health-care providers. The appropriateness of education in any given situation needs to be clearly analyzed. Those factors that respond to behavioral change are valid targets for health education. Nonbehavioral factors that contribute to illness, such as heredity, cannot be influenced by health education.

Green (1979) has described the health education process as including an education diagnosis. Such a diagnosis includes predisposing, enabling, and reinforcing factors, which contribute to behavioral problems affecting health. Predisposing factors include the person's knowledge, perceptions, values, and attitudes. Enabling factors are those which allow the individual to take needed actions and may include skills, availability, and accessibility of resources, and referrals. Reinforcing factors are those which are provided by others, such as the supportive attitudes and behaviors of health professionals, peers, family members, and employers. By considering all of these factors in diagnosing educational needs, the health care professional attempting to encourage prevention through education can avoid placing her energy where the return is minimal. An example of this would be in the area of smoking. Increase in knowledge about the effects of smoking has not changed the habits of many since the predisposing factors include the value judgment that smoking is pleasurable to a given individual. Reinforcing or enabling factors, such as referral to a Smoke Enders group or learning of alternative pleasures, would be a more appropriate focus of health education, as would the reinforcing factors of approval or disapproval of others.

## CONSUMER PARTICIPATION IN HEALTH CARE

Consumerism is a well known concept in most fields of human service, including health care. Increasingly well informed consumers assert their rights to participate through unions, news media, and elected legislators. In relation to their health, consumers claim their right to be participants in planning for their health care and to have their individual decisions respected. They further expect explicit information about factors relative to their health care, and the right to equal health care regardless of their individual differences.

The American Hospital Association, in recognition of consumer rights, has adopted a "Patient's Bill of Rights," which describes the rights of the hospital patient in the following areas:

1. Care which is respectful.
2. Understandable information from his physician regarding his diagnosis, treatment, and prognosis.
3. Needed information for informed consent for any procedure or treatment, prior to its being initiated.
4. Option to refuse treatment as allowed legally, and to be informed of the consequences of refusing treatment.
5. Privacy in relation to his medical care.
6. Confidentiality in relation to all communications and records relevant to his care.
7. Reasonable response to his requests for service.

8.  Information regarding the hospital's relationship with other health agencies and educational institutions as these may relate to his care.

9.  Information regarding the hospital's intent to engage in human experimentation that would involve him.

10. Reasonable continuity of care.

11. Information regarding hospital charges even if he is not paying the bill directly.

12. Information about hospital rules and regulations which are applicable to him.

Consumerism has been a powerful force in shaping the delivery of health-care services. Despite the intervening processes of politics and professionalism, the consumer holds the key to the economic survival of any service system provided he assumes that responsibility and learns how to best wield his power within the total system involved.

Another area in which clients are increasingly demonstrating their participation in their own health care is in the growing interest in health activation. Courses for health activation, the involvement of the individual in health matters, are given for adults in the community, and for school children within the school system. These encourage individual responsibility, teach skills in managing common illnesses and injuries, increase awareness of wellness and identify available health-care resources.

Orem (1971) described a framework for nursing that focuses on self-care and includes many of the implications of holistic health care. The nursing student will find it exciting to note that nursing reflects the momentum of society and that in collaboration with other health care professionals, the nurse can contribute to the efforts of each individual to develop his maximum and unique potential.

## SUMMARY

Health care today can be described in three major categories: emergency care, acute care, and ambulatory care. Health care is delivered through private practice, official and voluntary health agencies, and health maintenance organizations. Funding of health care is accomplished by fee-for-service, health insurance plans, prepaid subscription to a group, and government financing.

One of the major health-related problems in our society is chronic illness. Unmanagable stress is a known barrier to maintaining health and preventing illness. Individual behaviors that promote health rather than illness are important to the control of health problems. Health education relative to behavioral changes needs to include an analysis of all factors related to health, not merely lack of information.

Participation in planning for self-care and assumption of responsibility for health are increasingly evident in the behaviors of health care consumers. As one of the professional providers of health care, the nurse needs to keep an open mind about health-care practices. She must be prepared to offer appropriate support and suggestions to clients with various levels of knowledge and motivation, and to be aware of the large range of values toward health that exist in our society.

## LEARNING ACTIVITIES

1.  Give examples of situations where the appropriate type of health care would be:
    a.  emergency care
    b.  acute care
    c.  ambulatory care
2.  Describe the function of one official health agency with which you are familiar and contrast this with the functioning of a voluntary agency of your choice.
3.  Explain the difference between Medicare and Medicaid.
4.  What behavioral changes would you suggest to a client who was having difficulty managing the stress in his life?
5.  Describe some of the factors that must be considered in diagnosing the health educational needs of a client.

## REFERENCES AND SUGGESTED READINGS

Bill of rights for patients. *Nursing Outlook,* 21 (February, 1973), 82.

Commission on Chronic Illness. *Chronic illness in the United States: I, prevention of chronic illness.* Cambridge, Mass.: Harvard U. Press, 1957.

Division of Emergency Medical Services, Public Health Services. *What is an emergency medical services system?* Washington, D.C.: U.S. Department of Health, Education, and Welfare, 1975.

Dunn, H., 1961. *High-level wellness.* Virginia: R. W. Beatty, Ltd.

Green, L. W., et al., 1979. *Health education planning.* Palo Alto, Cal.: Mayfield.

Gunn, S. M. and Platt, P. S., 1945. *Voluntary agencies: an interpretive study.* New York: Ronald.

Orem, D., 1971. *Nursing: concepts of practice.* New York: McGraw-Hill.

Smolensky, J., 1977. *Principles of community health.* 4th ed. Philadelphia: W. B. Saunders.

Somers, Anne R., ed., 1976. *Promoting health.* Germantown: Aspen Systems.

*Trends affecting U.S. health care system.* Germantown: Aspen Systems. For U.S. Department of Health, Education, and Welfare, October, 1975.

# Glossary

Glossary

A

**abduction**   movement of a limb *away from* the midline.

**abortion, induced**   interference with pregnancy after conception has occurred by removing the premature fetus from the uterus.

**abortion, spontaneous (miscarriage)**   the unaided expulsion of the premature fetus by the uterus.

**abrasion**   a wound that results from scraping off the outer skin layer.

**absorption**   taking up of liquids and other substances into body fluids and tissues.

**accessory muscles of inspiration**   the sternocleidomastoid, upper trapezius, intercostal, and abdominal muscles.

**accommodation**   the ongoing, adjusting process of adapting one's own internal experience to the external environmental demands.

**acid–base balance**   ratio of carbonic acid to base bicarbonate of 1:20 in body fluids; maintenance of normal balance between acidity and alkalinity.

**acidosis**   a condition resulting from an accumulation of acid or depletion of alkaline reserve (bicarbonate) in body fluids.

**active range of motion**   joint movement that can be performed by the individual without assistance.

**active transport**   movement of substances across cell membranes, usually against a concentration gradient.

**acuity**   acuteness or clarity.

**acute care**   care given in hospitals on an inpatient basis; episodic care.

**adaptation**   alteration or modification of behavior in response to stress.

**additives**   coloring agents, artificial sweeteners, antioxidants, and preservatives added to foods.

**adduction**   movement of a limb *toward* the midline.

**adenosine triphosphate (ATP)**   a compound containing three phosphoric acids.

**adipocytes**   fat cells.

**affect**   apparent emotional response: expression of emotions or feelings, or lack of expression of emotions or feelings.

**albuminurea**   the presence of albumin in the urine.

**alertness**   full possession of one's senses.

**alignment**   relationship of body parts to each other.

**alkalosis**   condition resulting from accumulation of base or loss of acid without comparable loss of base; decrease in H+ (hydrogen ion) in concentration.

481

**allergy** an abnormal reaction to a normally harmless substance.

**alopecia** baldness, loss of hair.

**alpha rhythm** regular pattern on EEG with low voltage, 8–12 cycles/second.

**alveoli** tiny sacs in the lung, composed of a thin elastic tissue wall containing capillaries and epithelial cells through which gases can diffuse.

**ambulatory care** health care given in nonresidential settings to persons living in the community.

**ampule** a small sealed glass container holding medication for injection.

**analgesic** medication that acts on the nervous system by interfering with the transmission of pain stimuli or by altering pain perception at the cerebral level.

**analysis** the method of studying the nature of a thing or process and determining its essential features.

**anemia** a deficiency of either quality or quantity of blood.

**anions** ions with a negative charge.

**anorexia** a loss of appetite or lack of interest in food.

**Antabuse** trade name for a preparation of disulfiram used in treatment of alcoholism.

**anticipatory grief** preparation for the loss of a loved one or object.

**anticoagulant** a drug given to prevent abnormal blood clotting.

**anticonvulsant** a medication used to suppress convulsions.

**antidiabetic** a medication used to control diabetes.

**antidiuretic hormone** a secretion of the pituitary gland that directly affects the body's conservation of water.

**antigroup functions** roles of group members who use the group to achieve solely individual aims.

**antihistamine** a drug used to counteract the effects of histamine.

**antihypertensive** an agent that prevents or relieves high blood pressure.

**antioxidant** a substance that inhibits oxidation of other compounds.

**antipyretic** a drug given to reduce body fever.

**antiseptic** any substance that inhibits the growth of bacteria.

**anuria** decreased urine secretion (100 ml or less in 24 hr).

**anxiety** a feeling of dread, fear, forboding, worry or uneasiness; experienced by all people at one time or another. Usually a response to stress.

**apical–radial pulse** simultaneous measuring of pulse at radius and cardiac apex.

**apnea** absence of respiration.

**apocrine glands** modified sweat glands which respond to emotional stimuli.

**appetite** generally pleasant sensations making one aware of the desire for food.

**aquathermia pad** rubber or plastic pad filled with circulating fluid that is either cooled or heated.

**arrhythmia** variation in the normal rhythm of the heartbeat.

**arterial blood gases (ABG)** measurement of the partial pressure of oxygen and carbon dioxide in the arterial blood ($PO_2$ and $PCO_2$). Normal $PO_2$: 80–100 mm Hg; normal $PCO_2$: 35–45 mm Hg.

**asepsis** freedom from infection or infectious material.

**aseptic technique** measures used to prevent the spread of infectious material.

**aspiration** breathing mucus or vomitus into respiratory tract.

**aspirating** pulling back on the plunger of the syringe after needle has been inserted.

**assessment** a continuous and deliberate gathering of data to assist in identification of the client's present and potential strengths.

**assimilation** to incorporate things, people, ideas, customs, and tastes into the self.

**atherosclerosis** hardening of walls of arteries.

**attitude** a position taken regarding values and beliefs.

**autoeroticism** self-arousal of sexually stimulating sensations.

**autonomy** ability to gain control over one's independence.

**axilla** armpit.

## B

**barbiturates** compound derived from barbituric acid used to induce sedation or sleep.

**bargaining** the third stage of the grieving/dying process. The individual tries to "buy" extra time, usually in a spiritual way.

**barrier technique** technique of medical asepsis used when a pathogen is known or suspected to be present. Usually includes gowns, gloves, and mask.

**basic diets** those frequently used for specific health problems, e.g., clear liquid, full liquid, soft, bland.

**basic human needs** Maslow's theory that man has certain needs to be satisfied if he is to reach his maximum level of wellness.

**beliefs** convictions, accepted opinions, trust.

**bereavement** the direct result of a loss: to be deprived of the lost person or object.

**biofeedback** a physiological response, recorded and fed back to the subject, so that he can learn to control it.

**biopsy** removal of tissue for microscopic examination.

**birth control pill** an oral medication that achieves physiological contraception by altering the female hormones so as to suppress the production of ova.

**blended family** parents, and the children of former marriages as well as those of the present marriage.

**blood pH** see pH

**body mechanics** use of musculoskeletal system. Good body mechanics: effective use of musculoskeletal system.

**bradycardia** abnormally slow heart rate, usually less than 60 beats per minute.

**bradypnea** slow rate of respiration.

**breath sounds** the sounds of air taken in or expelled from the lungs.

**bronchi** large passages carrying air to and within the lungs.

**bronchioles** small channels formed as bronchi divide. Carry air into the bronchopulmonary segments.

**bronchitis** inflammation of bronchi.

**bronchoscopy** an examination of the bronchial tree with a lighted instrument (bronchoscope) passed through the anesthetized pharynx.

**buccal** referring to the cheek; inner surface of cheek.

## C

**calculi** stones; small hard masses formed in hollow organs of the body or their passages.

**calisthenics** systematic exercise for attaining strength.

**calorie** the amount of heat required to raise the temperature of one gram of water one degree Celsius.

**cannula** a small tube-like instrument inserted into body orifice; e.g., nasal cannula.

**canthus** the angular junction of the eyelids at either corner of the eye.

**capsule**  a medication enclosed in a gelatinous container; a soluble container for medicine.

**carbohydrate**  a compound of carbon, hydrogen, and oxygen—important source of energy.

**carcinogen**  substance that causes cancer.

**cardiac catheterization**  passage of a tube into the heart chambers. Blood samples are taken to determine the amount of oxygen, the hematocrit, and the pressures of blood within the heart.

**carotid sinuses**  dilated portions of the carotid artery where it bifurcates into internal and external carotid arteries.

**caring**  helping another to be, the process of helping another person to grow and actualize him or her self.

**carrier**  a person free of symptoms who harbors a disease or pathogenic agent.

**cathartic**  an agent that promotes defecation.

**catheter**  a tubular instrument used for draining or injecting fluids through a body passage.

**cations**  ions with a positive charge.

**celibacy**  abstention from sexual relations.

**Celsius**  centigrade; temperature scale on which water freezes at 0° and boils at 100°.

**center of gravity**  the point where mass is centered.

**centigrade (thermometer)**  having one hundred gradations, as the Celsius thermometer.

**certification**  a mechanism for validating the quality of a practitioner's competence in a specialized area at a level higher than licensure.

**chemoreceptors**  special cells or organs that respond to changes in the chemical composition of the blood and other body fluids.

**Cheyne-Stokes**  respirations occurring in cycles: first the breathing is very deep, then it gradually decreases in depth and the respirations cease for a brief period.

**chest p-t (physical therapy)**  tapping and rapid to-and-fro movements on chest to loosen mucus secretions (percussion and vibration).

**CHO**  carbohydrate.

**cholesterol**  a sterol; blood cholesterol level. Normal: 250 mg or less.

**chronic illness**  any impairment or deviation from normal that has one or more of the following characteristics: is permanent; leaves residual disability; requires special rehabilitation training; may require a long period of supervision, observance or care.

**circadian rhythm**  repetition of certain phenomena at about the same time each day.

**Circ-O-lectric bed**  electric turning frames by which a person can be placed prone, supine, or upright at the touch of a button.

**clean technique**  a technique that reduces the number of disease-producing microorganisms.

**clean wound**  wound free of pathogens.

**climacteric**  change of life: physical and psychological changes that occur in males and females due to hormonal changes during middle age.

**cognitive development/cognition**  the mental processes involved in the acquisition and utilization of knowledge.

**colostomy**  an opening made from the colon through the abdominal skin surface for the purpose of emptying the bowels.

**coma**  condition in which person is unconscious and cannot be aroused even by powerful stimuli. Reflexes are usually abnormal or absent.

**commode, bedside** a portable toilet.

**communal family** more than two adults unrelated by blood or law, living in a group.

**communication** the transmission of ideas, thoughts, experiences and feelings through verbal and nonverbal means of expression.

**community** an aggregate of people who live in a defined location and share common values and beliefs; people and the relationships that emerge among them as they develop and use in common, agencies, institutions, and the physical environment.

**community health center** nonresidential health care facility.

**compensation** behavior used to make up for a handicap or limitation.

**compress** gauze pad, often 4 × 3″ or 4 × 4″, for use in covering or applying medication to small area.

**concavity** a depression; a hollowed-out surface.

**condom** a rubber sheath which is stretched over the erect penis prior to sexual intercourse to prevent deposit of sperm in the vagina.

**conduction** heat loss e.g. body heat, through direct contact with cooler objects in environment.

**confusion** state of disturbed orientation manifested by lack of attention, mental slowness, incoherent thinking, or distorted perception of the environment.

**congruence** in communication, state achieved when verbal and nonverbal messages share a common meaning.

**conjunctiva** the delicate membrane lining the eyelids and covering the eyeball.

**conjunctival sac** space formed in lower eyelid when lid is pulled down and away from eyeball.

**consciousness** responsiveness of the mind to impressions made by the senses.

**constipation** passage of hard, dry stools, usually with abnormal delay in passage.

**consumerism** emphasis on consumers' right to participate in planning their health care, with respect for individual decisions.

**contagious disease** a disease readily transmitted by direct or indirect contact.

**contaminated wound** wound containing pathogenic microorganisms.

**contamination** soiling; making something unclean or unsterile.

**contraception** use of various mechanical or chemical methods to prevent fertilization of the ovum by the sperm or implantation of the fertilized ovum and thus to avoid pregnancy.

**contracture** abnormal shortening of muscle tissue.

**contusion** injury to tissues (e.g., bruising) with skin surface remaining intact.

**convection** the transfer of heat by moving air currents.

**convexity** rounded surface - elevated.

**cordotomy (chordotomy)** surgical division of a nerve tract of the spinal cord.

**corneal–scleral junction** point where cornea and sclera intersect.

**costal breathing** use of ribs in breathing—more shallow than diaphragmatic breathing. See also **diaphragmatic breathing**.

**CPR (cardiopulmonary resuscitation)** the basic life support measures of cardiac massage and mouth-to-mouth (or mouth-to-nose) respiration.

**crisis** a temporary situation that requires the reorganization of a person's psychological structure and behavior.

**critical periods** in Erikson's theory of stages of development, the specified amount of time wherein each stage must be mastered.

**culture** a universal experience within a particular society or group; a designated group's values, attitudes, and beliefs; a complex that utilizes the heritage of the people to maintain stability.

**cyanosis**  a bluish tinge to the skin and mucous membranes that is frequently associated with oxygen deprivation.

## D

**decubitus ulcer**  skin breakdown in areas of pressure caused by interference with circulation.

**debridement**  removal of foreign matter and devitalized tissue from a wound; action may be either surgical or enzymatic.

**defecation**  process of eliminating feces from the large intestine.

**defense mechanism**  an adaptation to stress; a psychic activity used to make an unwanted feeling or impulse disappear.

**dehydration**  condition resulting from undue loss of water from body tissue.

**delirium**  a state of disturbed awareness marked by confusion, agitation, and hallucinations.

**delta waves**  very slow and high waves (1–2 cycles per second) on the EEG.

**deltoid**  the muscle that abducts the arm; an inverted triangle that forms a cap on the shoulder.

**denial**  the first stage of the grieving/dying process in which the person refuses to accept the loss or impending loss.

**dental plaque**  material deposited on the surface of the teeth.

**depression**  a common adaptation to stress; characterized by a sense of futility and a loss of self-confidence.

**dermis**  the true skin or corium.

**development**  the orderly and irreversible stages that every person (organism) goes through from conception to death.

**developmental stages**  the sequence of characteristic stages beginning with family formation and continuing through the life of the family to its dissolution.

**dialysis**  a process used in persons with defective renal function to remove from the blood (hemodialysis) or other body fluid those elements normally excreted in the urine. See also **peritoneal dialysis.**

**diaphoresis**  profuse perspiration.

**diaphragm**  1. a small rubber bowl-shaped cap inserted into the vaginal canal to cover the cervix and prevent sperm from entering the uterus. 2. the strong, dome-shaped muscle separating the chest and abdominal cavities.

**diaphragmatic breathing**  that respiration performed mainly by the diaphragm.

**diarrhea**  rapid movement of watery feces through the large intestine.

**diastolic pressure**  the cessation or muffling of sound as cuff pressure and pressure in artery at rest equalize.

**diffusion**  the movement and intermingling of molecules in liquids or gases from higher concentrations to lesser concentrations.

**digestion**  breaking down of food into substances that can be absorbed and used by tissues.

**disinfectant**  a chemical cleaning agent used to kill most pathogenic organisms; does not kill spores and some resistant strains of bacteria.

**disorientation**  failure to recognize time, place, or persons.

**displacement**  the shifting of a feeling or emotion from one object or person to another.

**distention**  stretched-out with matter (gas, etc.); enlargement of abdomen, often caused by gas or liquid.

**diuresis**  excessive secretion of urine; often meant as indication of increased kidney function.

**dorsal**  back surface.

**dorsal column stimulator**  a battery-operated device that blocks pain impulses to the spinal cord. Used in severe, chronic pain when other methods have failed.

**dorsiflexion**  bending a part backward.

**dressing**  compress or bandage applied to an external wound.

**drop factor**  number of drops per ml in intravenous infusion set being used (manufacturers give this information on IV packages).

**drug**  medicinal substance.

**dyspnea**  the state of respiration when a person believes he is having difficulty breathing.

**dysuria**  painful urination.

## E

**ecchymosis**  bruise; escape of blood into the tissues.

**eccrine glands**  glands in the skin that function in heat regulation by evaporation and also in excretion of waste products.

**ecology**  the scientific study of the interrelations of living organisms and their environment.

**edema**  excessive fluid accumulation in intercellular spaces.

**edema, pitting**  sign of the presence of edema: indentation of the thumb remains when thumb is pressed into the soft, puffy tissue.

**edentulous**  without teeth.

**effleurage**  smooth, long stroke used in back massage: hands move firmly up the spine and lightly down the sides.

**egocentrism**  regarding the world from the starting place of one's self; regarding the self as the center of all things.

**electrocardiogram (ECG or EKG)**  a record of the heart's electrical potential.

**electroencephalogram (EEG)**  a tracing of the electric impulses of the brain.

**electrolytes**  substances whose molecules split into ions when placed in water.

**emergency care**  immediate health care designed to deal with trauma and disasters in an effective, speedy manner on a twenty-four-hour basis.

**emesis**  vomitus.

**empathy**  the ability to put one's self inside another person and experience what he is experiencing, without losing objectivity.

**enabling factors**  factors that allow the individual to take needed actions, which may include skills, availability and accessibility of resources, and referrals.

**endurance**  ability to withstand physical stress, based on development of an adequate oxygen transport system.

**enema**  introduction of fluid into rectum.

**entry portal**  the way in which a pathogenic agent enters a reservoir.

**enuresis**  bed-wetting.

**environment**  the aggregate of surrounding things, conditions, and influences, especially as affecting the existence or development of someone or something.

**eosinophils**  medium-sized leukocytes.

**epidermis**  outermost skin layer.

**epigenetic principle**  Erikson's theory that the ego does not have all capabilities at birth and that each part of the ego has a specific time for development; energy is focused on a specific part at any given developmental stage.

**episiotomy**  incision into perineum often performed during second stage of labor to avoid lacerations during delivery.

**erythema**  redness caused by capillary engorgement in lower skin layers.

**ethnic**  referring to the origins or characteristics of a given population.

**evaluation**  continuous process of checking the effect of nursing actions; the fourth stage of the nursing process.

**evaporation**  loss of moisture from the body surface through vaporization.

**eversion**  a turning outward.

**excoriation**  superficial skin loss such as that caused by scratching or chafing.

**excretion**  any of several means by which the body disposes of waste products.

**extended care facility**  a residential facility for long-term nursing care.

**extended family**  nuclear family (parents and children) plus other relatives.

**extension**  straightening; increasing the angle formed by two adjoining parts.

**external respiration**  the absorption of oxygen and removal of carbon dioxide from the body as a whole.

**extracellular fluid**  body water found outside of body cells.

**exudate**  material that has escaped from blood vessels and been deposited in or on tissues.

F

**Fahrenheit (thermometer)**  a thermometer on which freezing point of $H_2O$ is 32° and the boiling point is 212°.

**family**  a unit of interacting personalities consisting of two or more persons.

**family developmental task**  growth responsibilities that a family needs to accomplish at a given stage in its development.

**family function**  the activities the family performs to meet the physical, psychological, and social needs of its members and its responsibilities to the community.

**family health tasks**  family functions that relate to health and illness, such as recognition of interruptions in health, seeking of health care, maintaining an environment conducive to health.

**family planning**  planned reproduction, for purposes both of limitation of births and for assisting couples with difficulty producing children to overcome their problems.

**family structure**  the varied types of families as defined by composition: nuclear, extended, single-parent, blended, communal and living together.

**fatigue**  tiredness, often without apparent cause.

**feces**  stool; excrement; body waste eliminated from intestinal tract.

**fertility**  the ability to produce offspring; one's power to reproduce.

**fiber (dietary)**  that part of plant material which is not digested and is excreted in feces; bulk.

**filtration**  passage through a filter that prevents passage of certain molecules.

**fistula**  an abnormal tubelike passage within body tissue.

**flatus**  gas or air in stomach or intestine.

**flexion**  bending; reducing the angle formed by two adjoining parts.

**fluid volume deficit**  a deficit of both water and electrolytes in approximately the same proportion as they exist in the normal extracellular fluid.

**fluid volume excess**  an excess of both water and electrolytes.

**fluoride**  a chemical salt containing fluorine often added to drinking water.

**fluoroscopy**  visual examination of deep structures of body by means of X-rays that project images of bones and organs on a screen.

**foot drop**  a deformity in which the foot assumes plantar flexion.

**foreskin**  the loose fold of skin covering the glans penis.

**formal group structure**  well defined including delineation of membership, rights and responsibilities of members and the visible relationship of members to each other.

**Fowler's position**  head of bed rolled up to a ninety degree angle.

**fracture pan**  smaller, flatter bed pan used when person has difficulty using a regular bedpan.

**free clinics**  nonresidential health care facilities staffed by volunteers, with no charge to clients.

**frequency**  in relation to voidings, abnormally short intervals between voiding.

**frostbite**  condition of true tissue freezing.

## G

**gastric decompression**  return to normal pressure in stomach after a period of increased pressure.

**gastrointestinal tract**  portion of digestive tract from stomach to anus.

**gastrostomy**  an opening into the stomach; often used for insertion of a feeding tube.

**gatch**  jointed back rest and/or knee rest by which a person can be raised and maintained in a sitting position.

**gate-control theory**  theory that transmission of pain signals stems from a series of gatelike mechanisms. If a gate can be closed, pain signals from injured tissues cannot reach the brain.

**gavage**  tube-feeding; insertion of a liquid diet into a tube which has been passed into the stomach through the nose or mouth.

**generic**  pertaining to the distinctive chemical composition of a drug.

**glans**  the cap-shaped tip of an organ: glans penis; glans clitoris.

**glomerulonephritis**  inflammation of glomeruli of kidney.

**gluteus maximus**  the large muscle located on the dorsal aspect of the ilium, sacrum, and coccyx that extends the thigh.

**gluteus medius**  the muscle that abducts and rotates the thigh medially.

**glycogen**  the chief carbohydrate storage material in animals.

**glycosuria**  excess sugar in the urine.

**grain (gr)**  a unit of weight in the apothecaries' system equivalent to 64.8 mg.

**gravity**  the force of attraction between two objects.

**grief**  the emotion felt as the result of the deprivation due to loss.

**group**  a collection or assemblage of persons or things that are related in some way.

**group consensus**  decision-making process whereby a compromise decision is reached with which all members are comfortable.

**group function**  the ways in which a group accomplishes tasks and meets maintenance needs of its members.

**group leadership**  a process which moves a group toward its goals. May be shared by group members or centered in one specific person.

**group norms**  expected behaviors for members of the group.

**group structure**  the internal organization and arrangement of relationships that exist within a group.

**growth** an increase in size, differentiation of structure, and alteration of form of the living organism.

## H

**hallucination** a sensory impression with no basis in external stimulation.

**Harrington rod** apparatus used in corrective spinal surgery, specifically in scoliosis correction.

**Health Maintenance Organization (HMO)** organized health care services consisting of prepaid group practice; subscribers pay an agreed-upon sum for comprehensive health services including preventive services.

**heart structures** four chambers: right and left ventricle; right and left atrium; valves, arteries and veins, protective sac (pericardium).

**heat exhaustion** a disorder resulting from overexposure to heat or sun.

**heat stroke** condition in which temperature is very high (105.8° F and above); no sweating occurs.

**Heimlich maneuver** procedure to prevent asphyxiation from choking: rescuer presses the fist upward into the victim's epigastrium which elevates the diaphragm, compresses the lungs, and increases the pressure within the tracheobronchial tree which forces an occluding object out through the trachea.

**hematocrit** the quantity of cells in the blood. Normal: 41–48%.

**hematoma** a mass of coagulated blood in a tissue or cavity: e.g., bruise, black eye.

**hematuria** presence of blood in the urine.

**hemodialysis** see **dialysis.**

**hemoglobin** the oxygen-carrying pigment of the blood. Normal: 14–16 g/100 ml.

**hemorrhage** escape of blood from a ruptured vessel.

**hemorrhoid** enlarged vein inside or just outside the anus.

**Hering-Breuer reflex** the reflex that limits inspiration and expiration.

**heterosexual** referring to both sexes; having sexual feelings for a person or persons of the opposite sex.

**high-level wellness** a view that considers wellness and illness as two ends of a continuum and focuses on the interrelationships between health and environment to achieve the highest possible level of wellness.

**Hochstetter's site** ventrogluteal site for intramuscular injection.

**holistic health** a view of all persons as whole beings whose individual psycho–physio–cultural–spiritual relationships with the environment directly affect their state of health.

**homeostasis** uniformity, stability in normal body states.

**homosexual** having sexual attraction toward, or sexual activity with, persons of the same sex.

**host** an animal or plant that harbors and provides sustenance for another organism.

**Hoyer lift** a mechanical device for moving a person from flat to upright position.

**hunger** unpleasant sensations resulting from prolonged food deprivation.

**hydrocollator** an appliance that steams specially provided hot packs.

**hygiene** personal practices of bathing, skin care, and grooming that enhance one's physical attractiveness, comfort, and health.

**hyperalimentation** a method of providing essential nutrients intravenously.

**hyperemia** excessive blood in a part.

**hyperextension** increasing the angle between two parts so that it is greater than the normal range.

**hyperthermia**  pyrexia; fever; a body temperature above normal.

**hypertonic**  having an osmotic pressure greater than that of the solution with which it is compared.

**hypothalamus**  a portion of the brain thought to contain the body's temperature-regulating mechanism.

**hypothermia**  abnormal low body temperature (95° F or below). *Induced* hypothermia is brought about to lower metabolism during surgery. *Accidental* hypothermia occurs in cold environments.

**hypoxia**  diminished oxygen availability to body tissues.


I

**ideal culture**  the beliefs, values, practices, and feelings that people consider desirable, but which are not always practiced in reality.

**immunization**  the process of rendering a subject immune to a specific disease or agent, or of becoming immune.

**impaction, fecal**  hardened feces collected in the rectum.

**implementation**  the third stage of the nursing process; action-oriented nursing care.

**impotence**  a complete failure of sexual power or ability, especially in the male.

**incision**  a surgical cut into body tissue.

**incontinence**  inability to control elimination of feces or urine.

**indigenous**  originating in or characterizing a particular region or country.

**infection**  the presence of a pathogenic agent.

**ingestion**  taking in of nutrient material into the body's digestive tract.

**inspection**  visual examination to detect features perceptible to the eye.

**intentional wound**  wound produced for a specific purpose, e.g., surgical incision.

**internal respiration**  the gaseous exchanges between the body cells and their fluid medium.

**interstitial fluid**  fluid between the body cells: fluid outside the blood vessels.

**intracellular fluid**  that body water contained within the cells.

**intradermal**  tissue just under the surface of the skin (within the skin's substance).

**intramuscular**  within the muscle tissue.

**intrauterine device (IUD)**  small device placed in the uterus which interferes with the implantation of the fertilized ova; a mechanical form of contraception.

**intravenous**  within a vein.

**inversion**  a turning inward of a part.

**ion**  an element of an electolyte carrying an electric charge.

**IPPB**  Intermittent Positive Pressure Breathing device.

**ischemia**  decreased blood flow to a part.

**isolette**  a crib to which oxygen or air is supplied.

**isometric**  exercise in which muscles remain the same length but muscle tension is increased; body parts are not moved.

**insomnia**  sleeplessness: inability to fall asleep or remain asleep.

**isotonic**  exercise in which muscle is shortened and body parts are moved.


J

**jaundice**  yellowish hue of skin and sclera.

## K

**karaya**  a protective powder applied to the skin to prevent or heal decubitus ulcers.
**kosher**  food prepared as prescribed by Jewish law.
**Kussmaul respirations**  deep, rapid respirations: gasping for air.
**Kwashiorkor**  a protein deficiency disease of infants and young children.
**kyphosis**  a rounded thoracic convexity.

## L

**labia majora**  hairy skin folds on either side of the vulva.
**labia minora**  small inner skin folds on either side between the labia majora and vagina.
**laceration**  a wound in which body tissue is torn (not cut or incised).
**lactation**  secretion of milk from the breast; period of time during which a child is nursed.
**lacto-ovo-vegetarian**  one who avoids flesh foods but eats dairy products and eggs.
**larynx**  the structure that contains the vocal cords; located at the top of the trachea and below the base of the tongue.
**laxative**  a medication that loosens bowel contents and facilitates bowel emptying.
**legumes**  beans, peas, and lentils.
**leukocyte**  a colorless blood corpuscle capable of ameboid movement; protects body against disease-producing microorganisms.
**Levin tube**  a nasogastric catheter.
**licensing**  permission by an appropriate authority (e.g., the state) to offer to the public, in a selected jurisdiction, specific skills and knowledge.
**liniment**  a liquid drug preparation rubbed into the skin.
**listening**  an active process of hearing that involves full attention to the other person's communication.
**Lofstrand crutch**  a single aluminum tube topped with a metal cuff which fits around the forearm.
**lordosis**  an abnormal increase in the concavity of the lumbar spine.
**loss**  deprivation; being without something one has had or been used to having.
**lotion**  liquid used for external skin application.

## M

**maintenance functions of a group**  roles which aim to continue the group through such things as encouraging participation, providing support, resolving conflict.
**malignant hyperthermia**  unexplained fever occurring during use of certain anesthetic agents (e.g., halothane, succinylcholine).
**malnutrition**  poor nourishment resulting from improper diet or metabolic defect.
**mantra**  a word which is repeated during meditation to encourage relaxation.
**marasmus**  a disease of undernutrition in which there is an overall deficit in intake of both protein and calories.
**masturbation**  self-stimulation of the genitals through manipulation.
**maternal deprivation**  lack of a maternal relationship in infancy, possibly resulting in psychophysical symptoms. Mother may either be absent or unable to give emotional and physical care.
**meatus**  an opening; e.g., urinary meatus.

**meconium**   the dark green, mucilaginous material in the intestine of the newborn.

**medical asepsis**   keeping pathogens confined within a given area.

**medication**   a drug or remedy.

**medication compliance**   taking medication exactly as prescribed: what, when, how.

**meditation**   a relaxation technique in which one sits quietly for a set time period.

**megavitamins**   large doses of vitamins.

**melanin**   a dark pigment found normally in hair and skin.

**menarche**   the onset of menstruation.

**meniscus**   the crescent shape of the surface of liquid in a container.

**menopause**   the female climacteric, identified by cessation of menstruation.

**menstruation**   the discharge of blood and tissue from the uterus that occurs monthly from puberty to menopause except during pregnancy.

**mentor**   a wise and trusted counselor.

**metabolism**   the total of all physical and chemical activity occurring within the cells.

**midwife**   a person who assists women in childbirth. May be a nurse with special training or a layperson with training.

**milliequivalent (mEq)**   the number of grams of a solute contained in 1 ml of a normal solution.

**milligram**   one one-thousandth of a gram.

**minerals**   nonorganic substances necessary to cellular activity.

**micturition**   urination.

**mitered corner**   a sheet squared at the corner of a bed.

**motivation**   a need, problem, or inducement to action.

**mucus**   the secretion of a mucous membrane, composed of mucin, salts and body cells.

**mutuality**   characterized by give and take, sharing of responsibility, participation in another's destiny.

**myocardial infarction**   heart attack; formation of an infarct (localized necrosis) in heart muscle.

## N

**narcotic**   a drug that produces stupor or sleep. Can be legally obtained only with a prescription.

**naso-gastric tube**   tube inserted through nose into stomach for purpose of feeding or removing gastric contents.

**nausea**   the feeling that vomiting will occur.

**nebulizer**   a device that delivers a spray.

**necrosis**   cell death; usually resulting from injury or disease.

**nocturia**   excessive urination during the night.

**nosocomial infection**   infections contracted during hospitalization.

**NREM**   nonrapid eye movement sleep.

**nuclear family**   husband, wife and their children.

**nursing diagnosis**   the final product of the assessment step of the nursing process; collation of data so that a pattern of needs and problems can be identified.

**nursing process**   central to all nursing actions; an adaptable, organized and systematic structure allowing for necessary nursing actions through assessment, planning, implementation, and evaluation.

**nutrients**   necessary components of diet: water, protein, fats, carbohydrates, vitamins, minerals.

**nutrition**   the nourishment of the body by food.

**nutrition process**    the means by which the body uses food for energy, maintenance, and growth.

## O

**obesity**    weight greater than twenty percent more than ideal body weight.

**objectivity**    freedom from personal feelings or prejudice; correct perception of external reality.

**obstetrician**    a physician specializing in the care and treatment of women before, during, and after childbirth.

**official agency**    a tax-supported health care agency that assumes responsibility for the health of citizens within its jurisdiction and is governed by laws.

**ointment**    a semisolid preparation for external application.

**oliguria**    decreased urinary secretion to 100–400 ml per 24 hours.

**oral**    by mouth.

**orgasmic dysfunction**    an interruption of the female sexual response cycle caused by a biologic, psychologic, or social factor.

**orthopnea**    ability to breathe only when in the upright position.

**osmosis**    diffusion of water through a semipermeable membrane.

**osteoblast**    an immature bone-producing cell.

**osteoclasts**    large, multinuclear cells frequently associated with bone resorption.

**otitis**    inflammation of the ear.

**over-the-counter (OTC)**    medication available without a prescription.

**overnutrition**    obesity; specifically, increased caloric intake.

## P

**pain**    whatever the experiencing person says it is, existing whenever he says it does.

**pain reaction**    signs exhibited by person experiencing pain.

**pain threshold**    the lowest intensity of stimulus that will cause the sensation of pain when the stimulus is applied for a prolonged time period.

**pallor**    lightened skin color.

**palpation**    using fingers or hand to feel tissue and/or organ characteristics.

**palpatory estimate**    systolic blood pressure estimate; first pulsation felt in radial pulse as pressure is released.

**Papanicolaou (Pap) smear**    a simple, painless test used most commonly to detect cancer of the cervix: a sample of cervical secretions is examined for abnormal cells.

**paralytic ileus**    intestinal obstruction resulting from inhibition of bowel motility.

**parenteral**    in general practice, means given by injection.

**passive range of motion**    joint movement performed by another person.

**patent**    open (as in a patent airway).

**pathogen**    a disease-producing agent.

**pattern theory**    theory that perception of pain results from patterning of the nerve impulses generated by receptors.

**Pelvic Inflammatory Disease (PID)**    an infection in the female reproductive tract usually resulting from a sexually transmitted disease.

**perception**    the interpretation an individual makes of the sensory input from messages received.

**perceptual distortion**    an incorrect interpretation of sensory input.

**perceptual disturbance**    a problem in recognition and interpretation of stimuli.

**perineum**   the region between the vagina and anus (female) or scrotum and anus (male).

**periodontal disease**   gum disease; disease affecting the tissues surrounding a tooth.

**peripheral pulse**   pulsation felt at various sites on the body, e.g., carotid, brachial, temporal, femoral, popliteal, dorsalis pedis arteries.

**personification**   to embody a quality or idea in a real person or concrete object.

**perspiration, insensible**   virtually unnoticeable perspiration that evaporates immediately on reaching the skin surface.

**petechiae**   hemorrhages into the skin.

**petrissage**   a kneading motion used in back massage, involving taking large pinches of skin and muscle along sides of vertebral column and then the entire back.

**pH**   hydrogen ion concentration. Normal pH of arterial blood is 7.4.

**phagocytosis**   the envelopment of solid particles by living cells.

**pharynx**   the cavity (about 5″ long) behind the nasal cavities, mouth, and larynx, that communicates between them and the esophagus.

**phlebitis**   inflammation of a vein.

**physical assessment**   examination of the client for physical signs that may assist in clarifying his condition.

**physical fitness**   a state in which a person is able to complete all the required tasks of daily living without fatigue or exhaustion, and have energy left over for leisure activities.

**pill**   a globe-shaped solid form of a drug.

**pinocytosis**   a process by which substances of large molecular weight enter body cells by invagination of the cell membrane.

**placebo**   inactive substance resembling medication.

**placebo effect**   relief from discomfort obtained by psychological intervention.

**planning**   deliberate and systematic goal setting for client care; the second stage of the nursing process.

**plantar flexion**   bending the foot toward the sole of the foot.

**plaque**   see **dental plaque**.

**plasma**   fluid within the vascular system; noncellular portion of blood.

**pleura**   the serous membrane lining the thoracic cavity and covering the lungs.

**podiatrist**   a specialist who treats minor foot ailments.

**polyuria**   excessive excretion of urine.

**postural drainage**   a form of physical therapy in which the body is positioned so that secretions are removed from the lungs.

**posture**   the position of the body and the relationship of its parts to each other.

**potassium deficit (hypokalemia)**   a deficit of potassium in the extracellular fluid.

**potassium excess (hyperkalemia)**   an excess of potassium in the extracellular fluid.

**Povidone-iodine**   a skin cleansing solution made up of iodine and the polymer polyvinylpyrrolidone.

**precordial thump**   a blow delivered to the sternum during CPR.

**predisposing factors**   factors within a person such as knowledge, perceptions, values, and attitudes.

**premature ejaculation**   failure of the male to delay ejaculation long enough for the female to achieve orgasm in half of the couple's attempts at intercourse.

**preparatory depression**   a dying person's preparation for things that will be lost.

**prepuce**   cutaneous fold covering glans penis or glans clitoris.

**prescription**   a written direction, usually for compounding, dispensing and administering medication.

**problem-oriented medical records** a specific method for documenting patient care. An all-encompassing care plan.

**process** a systematic movement forward or toward a goal; a series of actions directed toward a specific end.

**projection** attributing one's own feelings or impulses to another.

**pronation** positioning the forearm so that the palm of the hand faces down.

**protein** a nutrient necessary for health, containing carbon, hydrogen, oxygen, nitrogen, and sulfur. Proteins break down into amino acids.

**proteinuria** protein in the urine.

**prothrombin** a blood clotting factor.

**psychosexual development** Freud's theory of maturational development in which the libido is the basic element.

**psychosocial assessment** assessment of the mental health and adjustment of the client considering the roles of family, religion, cultural diversity, and the community in the client's life.

**psychosocial development** theory of the interrelation of the individual ego and ever-present, ever-changing societal forces.

**psychotic** out of contact with reality.

**puberty** the attainment of sexual maturity, marked by menarche in females and production of spermatozoa in males.

**pubic area** genital area.

**pulmonary function tests** measures of ventilatory ability.

**pulse deficit** the difference between the apical beat and the radial pulse.

**pulse pressure** the difference between the systolic and diastolic pressures.

**puncture wound** a small opening in the skin made by a pointed object.

**purpura** bleeding under the skin.

**pyrogen** an agent that causes fever.

**pyuria** pus in the urine.

## R

**radiation** loss of body heat in the form of infrared heat rays.

**râles** bubbly breath sounds heard near the base of the lung on inspiration. Usually indicate presence of fluid in respiratory tract.

**range of motion** the normal extent of joint movement.

**rape** sexual intercourse forced on a person without consent. The most common sexual trauma.

**rationalization** justification for acts or decisions which are not necessarily rational or logical.

**RDA** Recommended Dietary Allowance.

**reaction formation** going to an opposite extreme to avoid carrying out an unacceptable impulse.

**reactive depression** an individual's response to past losses at the time of a present loss.

**rectus femoris** straight muscle of thigh that extends the leg and flexes the thigh.

**reference groups** groups to which an individual turns for reinforcement of values and a sense of identity.

**regularity** refers to bowel elimination on a patterned basis.

**reinforce** strengthen; e.g., dressings being added to already existing ones.

**reinforcing factors**   the supportive attitudes and behaviors of other persons; health professionals, peers, family members, and employers. Part of educational diagnosis.

**REM**   rapid eye movement sleep: the phase of sleep during which dreaming occurs.

**repression**   unconscious forgetting.

**reservoir**   the location in which a pathogenic agent lives and grows: human, animal, plant, rodent, insect or section of land.

**residential health care facility**   agency providing health care services on an inpatient basis, e.g., a hospital of either a general or specialized nature.

**residual urine**   urine remaining in the bladder after urination.

**respiration**   the exchange of oxygen and carbon dioxide in the body.

**respiratory center**   an area of the medulla oblongata that sends impulses down the spinal cord to the nerves that control diaphragm and intercostal muscles.

**retarded ejaculation**   inability of the male to ejaculate intravaginally. Also known as ejaculatory incompetence.

**retention (of urine)**   accumulation in the bladder of urine that cannot be eliminated.

**reticular activating system**   mechanism that controls central nervous system activity including wakefulness and sleep.

**reverse isolation**   barrier technique used in reverse to protect persons who are highly susceptible to infection.

**rheumatic fever**   a disease marked by fever and joint pains, believed to be a complication of an infection caused by streptococci.

**rhythm method of family planning**   biological method of contraception utilizing the natural rhythm of the female menstrual cycle, with abstinence during that part of the cycle when the woman is considered fertile.

**ritual**   a form or system of religious or other rite; customary, ingrained action.

## S

**sacrum**   triangular-shaped bone at base of spine.

**satiety**   a feeling of fullness (from food) and satisfaction.

**scoliosis**   lateral curvature of the spine.

**scrotum**   skin-covered pouch containing testes and accessory organs.

**sebaceous glands**   structures in the skin that secrete sebum, a lubricant.

**sedative**   medication that depresses the central nervous system and tends to reduce mental activity.

**self-actualization**   continuous striving of an individual to become or to reach his greatest potential.

**self-actualization group**   group aimed at providing an environment in which individual members can develop themselves in relation to others in a variety of ways.

**self-care**   the involvement of the individual in health matters: individual responsibility in managing common illnesses and injuries and increased awareness of wellness.

**self-concept**   the composite of a person's awareness of his own thoughts, feelings, hopes, strivings, fears, and fantasies.

**self-help groups**   coping groups formed to assist people who are attempting to adapt to changes which have occurred in their lives.

**sensory deprivation (deficit)**   reduction in amount and intensity of sensory input.

**sensory overload**   condition of highly intense, unpatterned stimulation.

**separation anxiety**   intense emotion of the toddler when left (e.g., in the hospital) without parents for even moments.

**sexuality** a deep and pervasive aspect of the total human personality that includes sexual feelings and behavior not only as a sexual being but also as a male or female.

**sexually transmitted disease (STD)** a disease transmitted through sexual contact.

**shearing force** a pushing force causing obstruction of subcutaneous blood flow because of the sliding of one tissue layer over another.

**shock** a circulatory disruption occurring when blood pressure is inadequate to force blood through tissues.

**single parent family** family consisting of one parent—father or mother—and children.

**sinusitis** inflammation of the sinuses.

**sitz bath** immersion in water of the hips and buttocks.

**sleep** a state of suspension of sensory and motor activity.

**Snellen eye chart** a device used for testing distance vision, consisting of block letters of decreasing size printed on a chart.

**sodium deficit** a condition in which the concentration of sodium in the extracellular fluid is below normal.

**sodium excess** an excess of sodium in the extracellular fluid.

**solutes** dissolved substances.

**sordes** accumulation of microorganisms, food, and epithelial tissue on lips and teeth.

**special care unit** hospital unit of concentrated care used for client who needs more than normal nursing, equipment, etc. (see **intensive care unit**).

**specificity theory** theory that specific pain receptors send pain signals by way of afferent pain fibers to spinal cord where some impulses are relayed to reflex arc and others to thalamus.

**sphincter** a circular muscle that contracts a passage or closes a natural orifice.

**sphygmomanometer** an instrument, either mercury or aneroid, that measures the level of blood pressure.

**spindles** quick bursts (14–16 cycles per second) on the EEG tracing.

**sterilization** 1. Procedure involving heat—autoclaving, boiling or dry heat—to kill all forms of bacteria, spores, fungi, and viruses. 2. Procedure whose purpose is to render an individual incapable of reproducing.

**stoicism** impassive behavior lacking in outward emotion, characterized by calm.

**stoma** an incised opening kept open usually for drainage, e.g., colostomy.

**stool** feces: fecal discharge from large intestine.

**streptococcal infection** infection caused by one of a variety of streptococcus groups. May be forerunner of rheumatic fever.

**stress** the usual wear-and-tear individuals experience in life; the condition caused by a stressor.

**stress incontinence** involuntary escape of urine caused by coughing or sneezing.

**stressors** causative agents of stress.

**stress-related illness** illness attributable to stressors.

**Stryker frame** an apparatus made of pipe and canvas designed so that one person can turn a client on it easily.

**stump** the distal end of a limb remaining after amputation.

**stupor** state in which the person appears unconscious but can be aroused sufficiently to respond to commands. Reflexes are usually present.

**subculture** a group of persons who have a distinct identity in some area of their lives, but are related to the larger culture in many ways.

**subcutaneous (sub-q)** the tissue layer under the skin; an injection into this tissue.

**subcutis**  the subcutaneous fatty layer of skin that lies beneath dermis.

**subjectivity**  personal, individual responses; opposite of objective.

**sublimation**  channeling the energy of an unacceptable drive or impulse into an adaptive, constructive pursuit.

**sublingual**  under the tongue.

**supination**  position of the forearm so that the palm of the hand faces up.

**suppository**  bullet-shaped solid mass of medication for introduction into a body cavity.

**surgical asepsis**  keeping an area free of microorganisms.

**susceptibility**  lacking defenses against a pathogen's attack.

**sutures**  stitches taken to secure edges of wound in proper position for healing.

**sympathy**  lack of objectivity in one's involvement in another person's problem.

**synthesis**  a process of reasoning which takes one from established or assumed principles to a proper conclusion.

**systolic pressure**  the first Korotkoff sound: a clear tapping sound heard when blood first flows through the compressed artery.


## T

**tablet**  a compressed, dry form of a drug. If scored, it may be carefully divided; also may be crushed.

**tachycardia**  abnormally rapid heart rate, usually over 100 beats per minute.

**tachypnea**  rapid rate of respiration.

**tapotement**  using edge of hand in a hacking (or tapping) motion over the back's surface in massage.

**task functions of a group**  the identified work of the group.

**teaching/learning group**  group formed for teaching needed knowledge and skills in a variety of areas.

**temperature**  the degree of sensible heat or cold.

**territoriality**  a tangible demarcation of boundaries.

**therapy group**  group that provides an environment for personal development and improved functioning.

**thermometer**  an instrument for determining temperature.

**third-party payment**  payment of fees for medical or other services not by the recipient of the services but by another party, e.g., an insurance company.

**tidal volume**  amount of air used with each respiration.

**topical**  applied to skin or another body surface. Usually intended for direct action at site where applied.

**trachea**  the air passage extending from larynx to the bronchi; windpipe.

**tracheostomy**  an opening through the neck into the trachea for insertion of a tube to facilitate air passage or removal of secretions.

**tracking**  presence of medication in tissues above depth where it was injected.

**tranquilizer**  medication that calms an anxious person but does not cause drowsiness.

**transportation**  the delivery of nutrients to body cells.

**traumatic wound**  a wound that occurs by accident.

**trigeminal neuralgia**  pain arising from irritation of fifth cranial nerve.

**triglyceride**  a neutral fat that is the usual storage form of lipids. Normal blood triglyceride: below 160 mg/100 ml.

**trocanter roll**  a blanket or sheet rolled and placed along the femur to keep the leg in proper alignment.

**tubal ligation**   sterilizing the female by severing the fallopian tubes, thus preventing ova from traveling to the uterus. A surgical contraception.

**turgor**   elasticity present in tissues with normal fluid fullness.

## U

**ulcer**   a defect of skin or mucous membrane produced by sloughing of tissue.

**undernutrition**   another term for malnutrition: specifically, decreased caloric intake.

**unit dose system**   organized plan for medication administration in which the drug is premeasured and individually packaged and labelled.

**urgency**   a great desire to void.

**urinal**   a container used to receive urine.

**urinary meatus**   opening of urethra on body surface through which urine is expelled.

**USDA**   United States Department of Agriculture.

## V

**vaginal orifice**   entrance or opening to vagina.

**vaginismus**   involuntary contraction of the outer one third of the vagina that prevents insertion of the penis.

**validation phase**   subjective and objective feedback from client, records, peers on effects of nursing assessment and nursing actions.

**vasectomy**   surgical sterilization of the male. Severing of the vas deferens or sperm duct.

**vastus lateralis**   muscle that originates on lateral aspect of femur and extends the leg.

**vegan**   a strict vegetarian: one who avoids all foods of animal origin.

**vegetarian**   one who avoids red meat and eats only fish and poultry in addition to vegetable foods.

**venereal disease (VD)**   diseases communicated through sexual contact, such as syphilis and gonorrhea.

**venipuncture**   puncture of a vein for taking blood or administering medication or fluids.

**ventrogluteal (muscle)**   a site for intramuscular injections: gluteus medius and minimus. See **Hochstetter's site.**

**venules**   small veins.

**vial**   a small medication bottle with a rubber stopper. A closed system.

**visceral**   pertaining to any large internal organ.

**viscosity**   a physical property of a substance that depends on the friction of its molecules as they slide by one another: fluidity.

**vitamins**   organic substances present in minute quantities in foods and necessary for metabolism.

**voiding**   micturition; to empty of waste matter, e.g., urine.

**voluntary agency**   health care agency supported by funds and donations, usually focusing on a particular health problem, governed by a group of private citizens with a paid support staff.

**vomiting**   the ejection of stomach contents through the mouth.

## W

**wheeze**   musical, high-pitched sound heard on expiration as air passes through a narrowed lumen.

**Workman's Compensation** state-regulated requirement that employers assume financial responsibility for injuries incurred by an employee while on the job.

**wound** an interruption in the continuity of any surface caused by physical trauma. See also clean, contaminated, intentional, puncture, traumatic wounds.

## X

**xiphoid** the sword-shaped cartilage connected to the lower end of the sternum.

## Y

**Yoga** therapeutic postures, breathing, relaxation, concentration and meditation exercises adapted from the Eastern way of life.

## Z

**z-track injection** a method of tissue displacement that permits the intramuscular needle to be placed deep in the muscle and which prevents "tracking."

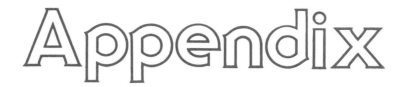

# Appendix

# Nursing History Guide
# and
# Nursing Care Plan

by Charlet Grooms, R.N., M.S.N.
Curriculum Coordinator, North Technical Community College

Patient's Name __Carla Smith_____ Diagnosis __CVA - Lt sided weakness__

Age __69__ Sex __Fe__ Occupation __Housewife_____

Information obtained from ____self_____Relationship_____

A. Safety and Security

1. Do you need help with your bath while in the hospital? Yes __X__ No____
   If yes, describe:
   Can wash self except for rt. arm and back.
   Likes tub. bath.

2. When do you prefer to bathe? Morning____Afternoon____Evening_____

   No preference __X____

3. Is your skin usually: Dry __X__ Normal _____ Oily_____
   What, if anything, do you normally use on your skin?
   Vaseline Intensive Care

4. Do you need help brushing your teeth? Yes __X__ No _____
   If yes, describe:
   Cannot brush them due to Lt sided weakness
   Cleans teeth in morning and at bed time
   Uses Efferdent to soak dentures
   Uses Cepacol mouth wash

5. What is the condition of your teeth? Dentures __X__Good____Poor_____

6. What is the condition of your mouth? Dry____ Sores____Good __X____

7. Does the condition of your teeth or mouth limit your ability to
   eat? Yes____ No __X__    If yes, describe:

8. Do you have difficulty seeing? Yes __X__No_____
   If yes, describe:
   Cataract lt. eye

9. Do you wear glasses? __X__Contacts?_____
   If yes to either, do you wear them all the time? __X__Part of the
   time?_____

10.  Do you have difficulty hearing?  Yes_____No__X__
     If yes, describe:

11.  Do you wear a hearing aide?  Yes_____ No__X__

12.  Do you wear any prosthesis?  Wigs____Arm____Leg_____ Eye_____

                                  Pacemaker_____   Breast_____

13.  Are you allergic to any medications?  Yes__X__ No_____
     If yes, list:  Codiene
                    Aspirin

     a.  Are you presently taking any medications?
         If yes, list:

14.  Level of sensorium.
     Alert, oriented to time, place, and person

15.  Other observations or information related to personal safety and
     security; i.e. condition of skin, deformities, bruises, loss of
     tactile sensation, etc.
     Left sided weakness of arm and leg,
     Reddened area on coccyx and lt. hip.

B.  Activity and Rest

    1.  Have you had any pain or discomfort since admission __NO__Before
        admission_____What did you do to relieve the discomfort?

        a.  Describe the pain or discomfort.

    2.  Do you have trouble going to sleep?  Yes__X__ No_____
        Usual bedtime__11 p.m.   Need radio with soothing music

        Number of hours of sleep__7__

        Do you have trouble staying asleep?  Yes_____No__X__

        Do you get up at night?  Yes__X__No_____
        If yes, describe:
                       Gets up x1 to use bathroom

        What have you done in the past to help you get enough rest or
        sleep?

3.  Do you have any difficulty moving or walking?  Yes__X__ No_____
    If yes, describe:
      Lt sided weakness - has difficulty turning to rt. side.

4.  Do you need assistance in moving about?  (i.e. wheelchair, cane,
    etc.)
      Uses wheelchair - goes to P.T. x 2 per day -
         learning to use walker

5.  Do you maintain an exercise schedule?
      Active R.O.M. to rt. side x 4 /day
      Active and passive R.O.M to left side x 4 /day

6.  Do you wear any braces (i.e. back, neck, etc.)?

7.  Other observations or information related to activity and rest;
    i.e. contractures, deformities, etc.

C.  Nutrition and Elimination

1.  Usual eating habits:

| | Time | Usual Foods |
|---|---|---|
| Breakfast | 7 a.m. | cereal, juice, coffee |
| Lunch | 12 noon | soup, sandwich, coffee |
| Dinner | 6 pm. | meat, potatoes, vegetable, fruit coffee |
| Snacks | | |

2.  Have you been on a special diet?  Yes__X__ No_____
    If yes, describe:
      lo cholesterol

3.  What foods do you dislike?
      none

4.  Do you have any food allergies?  (If yes, please list.)
      no

5.  What are your fluid preferences: _____.

           dislikes: _____.

6. Do you have nausea or vomiting?  No
   If yes, describe:

7. Bowels

   a. Usual bowel habits:  Frequency _Q.O.D._ Usual Time after break.
      Color _brown_

   b. Do you have any bowel irregularities?  Diarrhea _____
                                             Constipation _X_

   c. What do you do to relieve your irregularity?
      Metamucil Q.O.D.

8. Bladder

   a. Do you have trouble passing your urine (water)?  Yes ____ No _X_
      If yes, describe:

   b. Do you have Ureterostomy ____ Colostomy ____ Ileostomy ____?

   c. Do you get up at night for B.R.?
      If yes, describe:       x ī to urinate

9. Other observations or information related to nutrition and
   elimination (i.e. weight and height).  wt. 146 lbs

D. Oxygenation

   1. Vital signs:  T 98.8 P 76 R 16 BP 133/70

   2. Do you have a cough?  Yes ____ No _X_
      Is it productive?

      a. How long have you had a cough?

      b. Describe the material you cough up.

   3. Do you smoke?  Yes ____ No _X_
      If yes, describe how long and how many packs per day.

E.   Sexual Role Satisfaction

   1.   Marital Status:  (M)   W   S   D   Sep.

   2.   Menstrual history and pattern.
       menses ceased at age 56

   3.   Date and result of last pap test. negative  12/18

   4.   When was the last time you did a breast examination?  Would you
      like more information on doing a self-breast examination?
      Has never done BSE, not interested in learning now.

   5.   When was the last time you did a testicular examination?  Would you
      like more information on doing testicular self-examination?

   6.   Do you have any discharge?  Yes_____No X

      Burning?  Yes_____No_____

      Itching?  Yes_____No_____

      If yes to any of these, describe.

   7.   Has your illness affected your sexual functioning?  Yes X No_____
      If yes, would you like to talk about it?  yes

   8.   Do you expect a change in your sexual functioning when you go home?

      Yes X No_____    If yes, would you like to talk about it?  yes

   9.   What effect has your coming to the hospital had on your family (i.e.
      how they feel about it, changes they had to make.)
      husband visits x2/day       daughter provides meals and
      husband calls in a.m,              transport for father
      daughter and son visit qd.

  10.   What changes have you had to make prior to admission (i.e. job
      appointments, family responsibilities, financial responsibilities).
      Did not have time to make any preparation
      Daughter is caring for father; "That's the only arrangement
        that needed to be made."

11. Other observations or information related to sexual role adjustments. (i.e. number of children)
    2 children - married and living away from home. Husband has heart disease. Unable to do any work, at times needs assistance dressing.

F. Mental Health and Behavioral Adjustments

1. What is your religion? Jewish_____ Catholic_____ Protestant_X_____

   Other_____

2. Are there any restrictions placed on you by your religion that will interfere with your treatment and care in the hospital? Yes_____ No_X_____ If yes, describe:

3. How do you feel about your illness?
   "I have to get strong again. My husband cannot get along without me."

4. Have you ever been in a hospital before? Yes_____ No_X_____

   a. Any special memories about your previous hospitalization?

5. Why do you think you were admitted to the hospital?
   "Because of my stroke and high blood pressure."

   a. How long do you expect to be in the hospital?
   "Not too long."

   b. What has the doctor told you about your illness?
   "That my pressure caused it."

6. What do you enjoy doing for recreation or as a pastime (i.e. reading sewing, etc.)?
   crochet and knit

7. Other observations or information related to mental health or behavioral adjustments (i.e. non-verbal communications, tone of voice, patterns of behavior, cultural implications, language or speech barrier, etc.)
   Readily cries when talking about inability to move and use lt. side.
   Very determined to regain total use of lt. side.
   Works on exercising lt. side to the point of exhaustion

G. Discharge Planning

1. Do you expect to go to your own home when discharged? Yes __X__ No____
   If no, what arrangements have been or are being made?

2. Is there someone living with you at home who will be able to assist you if necessary?

   "My husband, but he cannot help me."

3. What instructions has the doctor given you concerning your care at home?

4. Other observations or information related to discharge planning.

   Lives in own home. One floor plan. Has basement.

Statement of Problem (Assessment)

Validation of Stated Problem

| Assessment | NSG Diagnosis | Plan | Evaluation |
|---|---|---|---|
| Lt. sided weakness likes tub bath unable to wash Rt. side and back. | needs assistance c̄ bath | ① Take to B.R. in wheelchair ② Assist into tub, (a) place wheelchair c̄ pt. rt. side next to tub. (b) Have her stand and get balance. (c) Instruct her to use rt. side to get into tub. (d) You support left side. ③ Wash her rt. arm and back ④ Allow her to finish rest of bath. | Enjoys tub bath and the accomplishment of performing personal hygiene herself. This method of getting her into the tub works very well. |
| skin dry uses Vaseline Intensive Care lotion | dry skin | ① provide Vaseline Intensive Care lotion. ② Apply to those areas of skin that she cannot reach. ③ lotion to be applied T.I.D. | T.I.D. application of lotion has controlled dry skin. |
| Lt. sided weakness cannot hold dentures to brush them. | Needs assistance c̄ denture care. | ① Provide denture cup, water, and efferdent for teeth. ② Provide cepacol mouth wash. ③ Investigate obtaining tooth brush c̄ suction bottom. ④ Brush dentures until above brush is obtained. ⑤ Provide oral care in morning (before breakfast) and at bedtime. | This plan for oral care is effective in maintaining oral hygiene. Toothbrush c̄ suction bottom has been ordered. |

510

Statement of Problem (Assessment)

Validation of Stated Problems

| Assessment | NSG Diagnosis | Plan | Evaluation |
|---|---|---|---|
| Cataract Lt. eye wears glasses at all times while awake. | Limited vision | ① Approach from rt. side ② Place bedside stand on rt. side of bed. ③ Have glasses readily available for her to put on. | Is able to see people when they enter the room and able to get things she needs from the night stand. Puts on own glasses when awakening in AM. |
| Allergic to Codiene and Asprin. → | | ① Check medication for presence of codiene or asprin. ② place alergy sticker on chart. | at present no medications contain these substances done |
| Lt sided weakness reddened area on coccyx and Lt. hip. Has difficulty turning to right side. | skin breakdown | ① massage all bony prominences T.I.D. ② Place on alternating pressure mattress. ③ Turning schedule. a. 8 am - Supine b. 10 am - rt side c. 12 noon - Lt. side d. 2 pm - supine etc. ④ Instruct her on turning schedule. Allow her to maintain schedule. ⑤ Assist her in turning to rt. side at scheduled time. | Reddened areas are subsiding. She is maintaining own turning schedule. Calls when it is time to be placed on rt. side. |

511

Statement of Problems (Assessment) | | Validation of Stated Problems | 

| Assessment | NSG Diagnosis | Plan | Evaluation |
|---|---|---|---|
| Lt. sided weakness learning to use walker in P.T.<br><br>Uses wheelchair for mobility. | Limited mobility | ① Cough and deep breathe 2 hrs.<br>② ⓐ Active R.O.M. to Rt. side<br>Q.I.D.<br>ⓑ Active and passive R.O.M to Lt. side Q.I.D.<br>③ elastic hose<br>④ I+O - maintain positive fluid balance. (600 cc. over output per 24 hrs.)<br>⑤ place in wheel chair when turning schedule indicates supine position.<br>⑥ Place Stryker floatation pad on wheelchair. | Lung sounds clear.<br><br>Maintaining schedule. No stiffness or contractures developing<br><br>Intake ranges from 1000 to 700 cc. over output. Urine clear amber in color.<br><br>Enjoys being in wheelchair and sitting in lounge. |
| Needs radio to go to sleep →<br>Gets up x1 during the night to void. → | | ① ask husband to bring in clock radio.<br>① Determine approximate time when she has to void during the night.<br>② Provide assistance to B.R. | done. She now has no difficulty going to sleep<br><br>Gets up about 4 AM to void. Able to go back to sleep. |
| Lo Chol. diet.<br>Chol. lab test?<br>wt. 146 lbs. | ↑ Chol. Bld. level | ① check tray for lo chol. foods<br>② Determine her knowledge of lo. Chol. diet.<br>③ Develop teaching plan for ↓ chol. diet. | This is 1st experience c̄ ↓ Chol. diet. Dietician notified to begin diet instructions |

Validation of Stated Problems

Statement of Problems (Assessment)                                    Validation of Stated Problems

| Assessment | NSG Diagnosis | Plan | Evaluation |
| --- | --- | --- | --- |
| Has difficulty c̄ constipation. Bowels move q.O.D. Uses Metamucil q.O.D. | Constipation | ① Maintain record of B.M.'s ② Adm. Metamucil q.O.D. ③ Assist to B.R. after breakfast for B.M. | Bowels move q.O.D. must get to bathroom as soon as breakfast tray removed. |
| Admission B.P. 194/100 on Aldomet | Control of hypertension | ① Adm. Aldomet ② Check B.P. q.I.D ③ Report B.P.↓ 150 Systolic or 80 diastolic ④ Determine knowledge level of hypertension. ⑤ Develop teaching plan for hypertension. | B.P. ranging 130/70 - 146/78 Has been on B.P. pills for 2 years. Understands hypertension. Needs instruction on Aldomet, and taking of B.P. |
| Husband has ht. disease. Unable to do any work around house. At times needs assistance dsg. Pt. has cared for husband, is manager of the home. States "I have to get strong again - my husband cannot get along without me." | Needs assistance in the home when pt. is discharged. | ① Talk c̄ family about availability of someone to live in the home to assist pt. + husband in ADL and managing home. | Family does not have anyone who could stay c̄ parents all the time. Referral sent to soc. service. |
| Readily crys when talking about her condition. States "I have to get strong my husband cannot get along s̄ me." | Needs asst in the grieving process. | ① Allow her the opportunity to ventilate her feelings. ② Encourage her to talk about her condition by using therapeutic communication skills. | Continues in the anger stage but is improving. |

513

Statement of Problems (Assessment)

Validation of Stated Problems

| Assessment | NSG Diagnosis | Plan | Evaluation |
|---|---|---|---|
| Works on exercising. Lt. side to point of exhaustion. | | ③ Assist her in establishing short range realistic goals.<br>④ Praise her as she accomplishes tasks. | |

514

# Index

Abduction, 381
ABG (arterial blood gases), 253
Abortion
  induced as birth control method, 57–58
  spontaneous, 57
Abrasion, 223
Absorption, step in nutritional process, 284
Acceptance, stage of dying process, 74–75
Accessory muscles of inspiration, 243
Acid-base balance, 327–328
Acidosis, 327–328
Active range of motion, 382
Active transport, 326
Activity and rest, need for balance of, 393
Acupuncture, effectiveness with pain, 437
Acute (episodic) care, 471–472
Adaptation
  to stress, 180–181
  to loss, 66
Adduction, 381
Adenosine triphosphate, 326
Adipocytes, 285
Adolescents
  defined, 31
  developmental tasks of, 32
  need for calcium of, 278
  need for carbohydrates of, 277
  need for protein of, 277
  and nurse-client relationship, 161
  and peer group influence on hygiene, 204
  responses in caring relationship of, 10
  sexual development of, 43–44
  sleep requirements of, 396
  and touch, 10
Adults
  changes in dietary requirements of, 279
  defined, 44
  sexual development of, 44–46
  sleep requirements of, 399
  See also Late adulthood; Middle adult; Young adult
Afro-American culture

effects of skin color, 125, 126
family importance for, 127
religious beliefs of, 127
special medical problems of, 126
time orientation of, 127
Age
  change in nutritional requirements, 276
  effect on body temperature of, 405
  effect on healing of, 225
  effect on skin of, 222
  effect on sleep of, 397
  as related to pain, 441
Agency. See Health agency
Aging process, 64–65
Air pollutants, 135
Airway
  artificial, insertion of, 267
  correction of obstruction, 267
  patent, 267
Alcohol, and medications, 348
Alcohol, Drug Abuse and Mental Health Administration, 473
Alcoholics Anonymous, 100
Alertness. See Consciousness
Alkalosis 327–328
Allergy, 346
Alopecia, 222
Alpha rhythm, 396
Alveoli, 237
Ambulatory care, 108, 472
American Association of Industrial Nurses (AAIN), 456
American Association of Sex Educators, Counsellors and Therapists (AASECT), 47–48
American Civil War, effect on nursing, 454
American culture
  Kinsey reports on sexuality of, 46–47
  and sexuality, 41
  See also Afro-American culture; American Indian culture; American middle-class culture; Asian American culture; Spanish American culture

Bronchoscopy, 253
Browen, Phyllis and Dorothy Hicks, and immobilized muscles, 391
Brown, Esther Lucille, study of nursing (1948), 458
Bryar, Rosamund, on self-care, 344
Buccal, 369
Burgess, Ann Wolbert, sleep, 395

Cady, Jane, distraction from pain, 443
Calcium, nutritional needs for, 278
 *See also* Nutrition
Calisthenic, 378
Calorie, defined, 276
Cancer
 effect on healing of, 225
 importance in fiber in, 282
 preventive measures, 477
 reproductive organs and, 48
 smoking and, 136
Cancer Institute, 116
Cancer Society, 474
Cannula, 264
Canthus, 207
Carbohydrates, nutritional need for, 277
 *See also* Nutrition
Carbon dioxide, 237
Carcinogens, 282
Cardiac arrest, 254–257
 *See also* Cardiopulmonary resuscitation
Cardiac catheterization, 254
Cardiopulmonary resuscitation (CPR), procedure, 254–257
 for adults, 257
 for infants, 257
Cardiovascular disease
 and cholesterol, 282, 283
 obesity as cause of, 285
 *See also* Heart
Caring, concept of
 and nursing, 6–10
 definition, 6
 process, major ingredients of, 6–7
 relationship, 7–8
Carotid sinuses, 239
Carrier, of pathogenic agents, 138
Carty, Rita, and deaf clients, 429
Cathartics
 and body fluid imbalance, 329
 defined, 302
Catheterization
 bladder irrigation, 319
 description of, 316
 indwelling, procedure for removal, 316–317
 procedure, 317
 removal of, 320
 straight, procedure, 316–317
Cations, 325
Celibacy
 as birth control method, 44–45

as sexual lifestyle choice, 56
Center for Disease Control in Atlanta, 142
Centigrade (Celsius), conversion formula to Fahrenheit, 408
Certification, of nurses, 463–464
Change groups, 100
Charting. *See* Recording; Nurse's notes
Chemoreceptors, 239
Chest percussion and vibration, 263
Chest X ray (fluoroscopy), 252
Cheyne-Stokes respirations, 243
Childbearing centers, 54
Child-rearing, in American Indian culture, 124
Children
 development of, 27–30
 fecal incontinence in, 307
 medications for, 369–371
 need for protein of, 277
 and nurse/client communication, 161
 obesity in, 285
 resuscitation of, 257
 sensory screening of, 428
 sexual development of, 42–43
 sleep requirements of, 396
 stages of understanding death in, 72
 and touch, 9–10
Children's Bureau, 473
Chinese, and religious beliefs, 121
 *See also* Asian-American culture
Cholesterol, 282–283
 low, diet, 290
Christianity, and high regard for care of sick, 454
 *See also* Religious and spiritual beliefs
Christakis, on hypertension, 283
Chronic bronchitis, and smoking, 136
Chronic disease
 and caring relationship, 10
 Commission on, 475
 coping with, 476
 defined, 475
 similar stages of, and death and dying, 75
 stress and, 476
Church. *See* Christianity; Religious and spiritual beliefs
Circadian rhythms, 397–398
Circ-o-lectric bed, 386
Circulation
 assessment of, 242–254
 blood pressure and, 245–249
 description of, 239–240
 diagnostic tests, 252–254
 overload, with use of IV, 336
 pulse and, 244
 *See also* Respiration/circulation
Cleanliness
 in avoiding colds, 241
 dominant value of middle-class culture, 115
 effect of, on growth and development, 15
 of equipment, 138

# COMMON ABBREVIATIONS

| | | | |
|---|---|---|---|
| a̅a̅ | of each | E.R. | emergency room |
| ABG | arterial blood gases | et | and |
| a.c. | before meals | fl. | fluid |
| A.S.A. | acetylsalicylic acid (aspirin) | F. | Fahrenheit |
| | | G.I. | gastrointestinal |
| B.M. | bowel movement | G.U. | genitourinary |
| b.i.d. | twice a day | Gm., gm. | gram |
| B.P. | blood pressure | Gr., gr. | grain |
| B.R.P. | bathroom privileges | Gr. X̄ | 10 grains |
| | | Gr. ī̄s̄s̄ | 1½ grains |
| c̄ | with | $H_2O$ | water |
| C. | Celsius | h.s. | bedtime |
| ca | cancer | IM | intramuscular |
| cc | cubic centimeter | I and O | intake and output |
| CBC | complete blood count | IV | intravenous |
| | | Kg. | kilogram |
| CHF | congestive heart failure | Lab. | laboratory |
| | | l. | liter |
| CNS | central nervous system | m. | minim |
| | | mEq. | milliequivalent |
| c/o | complains of | NPO | nothing by mouth |
| COLD | chronic obstructive lung disease | $O_2$ | oxygen |
| | | O.D. | right eye |
| COPD | chronic obstructive pulmonary disease | O.B. | obstetrics |
| | | O.O.B. | out of bed |
| | | O.R. | operating room |
| $CO_2$ | carbon dioxide | O.S. | left eye |
| CVA | cardiovascular accident | O.U. | each eye |
| | | p.c. | after meals |
| D/C | discontinue | per | by |
| $D_5W$ | 5% dextrose in water | p.o. | by mouth |
| | | postop. | postoperative |
| dil. | dilute | p.r.n. | when necessary |
| ECG *or* EKG | electrocardiogram | pt. | patient |
| EEG | electroencephalogram | P.T. | physical therapist |
| | | q. | every |